CONTINUITY
AND
CHANGE
IN
ART

The Development of Modes
of Representation

CONTINUITY
AND
CHANGE
IN
ART

The Development of Modes
of Representation

Sidney J. Blatt
in collaboration with
Ethel S. Blatt

LEA LAWRENCE ERLBAUM ASSOCIATES, PUBLISHERS
1984 Hillsdale, New Jersey   London

Lawrence Erlbaum Associates, Inc., Publishers
365 Broadway
Hillsdale, New Jersey 07642

Library of Congress Cataloging in Publication Data

Blatt, Sidney J. (Sidney Jules)
    Continuity and change in art.

    Bibliography: p.
    Includes index.
    1. Visual perception.   2. Art and society.   3. Art—
Psychology.   4. Painting—Psychological aspects.
I. Blatt, Ethel S.   II. Title.
N7430.5.B55   1984   750'.1'9   84-4201
ISBN 0-89859-342-5

Printed in the United States of America
10 9 8 7 6 5 4 3 2 1

To our family —
    past, present, and future.

Contents

List of Illustrations

Preface

Jean Piaget's extensive studies of individual cognitive development were based on a fundamental assumption—that his observations define a genetic epistemology, a theory about the natural evolution of knowledge that occurs in multiple contexts. Piaget assumed that his observations about the structural development of thought in the individual were applicable to the study of culture as well; he assumed that there is a fundamental parallel in cognitive development in individuals and in culture. Although there has been considerable investigation of individual psychological development based on Piaget's formulations, relatively few studies have examined Piaget's hypothesis that his observations are equally applicable to cultural development. This book is an attempt to test this hypothesis—to examine the extent to which a theory of cognitive development gained primarily from the study of individuals can provide understanding of sequences in cultural development.

This book considers the development of the concept of the form of objects and of space in the history of art and science in Western Civilization and examines the extent to which this process follows the basic developmental principles articulated in Piaget's genetic epistemology. The model of cognitive development, presented in Chapter 2, derives primarily from the work of Jean Piaget and Heinz Werner, and as extended by investigators in developmental psychology including Larendeau and Pinard, Olson, Feffer, Gardner,

Kaplan, and Dolle. These observations and formulations of developmental psychology are supplemented by concepts from developmental psychoanalysis, particularly the important issue of the development of the subjective vantage point and its essential role in the development of the capacity to represent the three-dimensional form of objects and of space, and to use affects as a source of information about the personal meaning of experience.

This developmental psychological model is applied to an examination of the development of the capacity to represent the form of objects and of space in three major epochs in the history of Western Civilization: from Ancient to Medieval, from the Renaissance to the Baroque, and from Impressionism to contemporary time. Chapters 3, 4, and 5 consider the hypothesis that the modes of representing the form of objects and of space in painting follow a basic progression toward increased differentiation, articulation, integration, and complexity. While cultural development, like individual development, does not follow a fixed, monotonic, linear sequence without variation, reversions, or sudden surges of progress, it does proceed systematically toward developmentally more advanced levels of representation. This is not a progression toward a fixed, predetermined, ideal goal or telos, but a natural, unending, developmental unfolding. Such a developmental progression does not lead to any conclusion about the importance or worth of earlier or later modes of representation. Instead, it simply assumes that different modes of representation occur in different phases of the developmental sequence and that later modes are built on earlier accomplishments and achievements. Such a developmental progression also does not imply a commitment to a conceptualization of a "recapitulation" across contexts or of ontogony and phylogony. Rather, it is based only on the assumption of a "formal parallelism" (Brunswik, 1959) in the development of all cognitive endeavors whether they occur in the culture or in individual psychological development.

Individual and cultural development of modes of representation unfold from an initial mode based primarily on the extension of action sequences (a sensorimotor mode), to an intuitive coordination of a few dimensions (a preoperational-intuitive mode), to a systematic coordination and integration of different dimensions of the manifest, external form of objects (a concrete operational mode), to the coordination and integration of more abstract, internal form and structure (a formal operational mode). This developmental sequence also involves a progression from an initial emphasis on the surfaces and boundaries of objects in isolation (topological concepts of space), to an emphasis on the relationships among different parts of a single object or among different objects in space that are initially specified intuitively and later in increasingly precise mathematical terms (projective-Euclidean concepts of space), to an emphasis on space, not as an absolute, but as defined in reference to the particular location and movement of a participant-observer (Riemannian concepts of space). This progression essentially involves the development of increasingly complex mathematical concepts and scales (Stevens, 1951) proceeding from a nominal scale in which observations are placed in discrete, mutually exclusive categories; to an ordinal scale in which observations are placed in a simple qualitative, comparative order based on comparison and contrast; to an interval scale in which the relationships among observations are defined by a common, but arbitrary, quantitative metric system; to a ratio scale in which observations about the relationships among objects are defined by a precisely defined metric system based on an experientially relevant reference point and scale values. Although there are periods of cultural development that contain ambiguous and at times inconsistent data, such as the occasional foreshortening and the sense of action in the animal forms of Paleolithic art or the undulation in modes of representation in art during the complex and controversial Middle Ages, there is a major progressive linear trend in the cultural development of modes of representing the forms of objects and of space on a two-dimensional surface.

Art is an integral part of the culture's predominant mode of conceptual or symbolic construction. Thus, the different phases in the development of modes of representation do not occur in painting alone. Painting is only one expression of a basic *Weltanschauung* that appears in the interests and preoccupations of a culture and in its multiple cognitive endeavors. The natural sequence in the development of modes of representation may be particularly apparent in painting, but it can also be observed in the concepts of natural science. Thus, at the conclusion of Chapters 3, 4, and 5, the parallels between the forms of objects and of space in painting and in science are explored. Also, in each chapter some consideration is given to relationships between the concepts of the form of objects and of space and the general world view of the period, especially the development of concepts of perspective and infinity and their relationship to cultural humanism and the emphasis on the individual during the Greco-Roman period and in the Renaissance.

There are, however, inherent limitations to this analysis of the development of modes of representation, because psychological processes and cultural phenomena are at different levels of discourse and utilize different concepts and notational systems not easily transferred from one area to another. The term representation, for example, has different meanings in different areas—in painting it refers to technical procedures for recreating a segment of nature on a two-dimensional surface, in psychological theory the term refers to a construction of a sense, image, or conception of a segment of nature in one's mind, and in science the term refers to a model of a physical structure. Yet, in all these realms, representation refers to a process of symbol construction and in this sense they are equivalent terms despite differences in the media in which the symbol construction occurs. Another limitation in this study of changes in the representation of the form of objects and of space in painting is that a host of other dimensions important to painting are ignored, as are other artistic forms, such as sculpture, architecture, literature, music, and dance. Also, the investigation of a long-term developmental sequence tends to omit fine-grain analyses of particular periods and by necessity some important artists and important periods. And a consideration of a long-term developmental sequence does not preclude the possibility that some subcycle sequences occur within shorter time periods. Further, the use of a psychological analysis based on the development of concepts of the form of objects and of space ignores other psychological processes such as the development of concepts of time, causality, and affects.

Despite these limitations, cultural continuity and change as seen in the modes of representation of the form of objects and of space in painting and in science follows a basic developmental progression. In subsequent research, it would be valuable to consider the application of developmental psychological principles to a more detailed analysis of particular periods, to the study of other art forms such as sculpture and architecture, or to the long-term development of psychological dimensions other than the form of objects and of space, such as concepts of time and their developmental unfolding in literature, poetry, and music.

From the inception of this book in 1975, I have been keenly aware that this has been an ambitious undertaking. It has been a labor of love that has given me moments of great exhilaration that came with insight and discovery, and moments of despair. I have been tempted several times since beginning this effort to abandon the project because I felt overwhelmed by the range of material I was seeking to understand and integrate. Support of friends and colleagues, as well as the excitement of interdisciplinary synthesis, however, provided the impetus to continue. I present this material to colleagues in my field, not as an art historian, but as a psychologist and psychoanalyst interested in cognitive processes, with the hope of encouraging further exploration of cultural phenomena and the use of psychological theory in interdisciplinary investigation.

Over the years, much of my research as a psychologist and psychoanalyst has been in the area of cognitive processes and especially the development and impairment of mental representation in different forms of psychopathology. Thus, this work on the development of cultural modes of representation is an extension of my prior work. My interest in the application of individual psychological concepts to cultural phenomena has been stimulated in part by the interdisciplinary emphasis that has developed at Yale and in the New Haven community in the past decade. Of particular relevance has been the Kanzer Faculty Seminar in Psychoanalysis and the Humanities, as well as the work of several colleagues at the Western New England Institute for Psychoanalysis, especially Drs. Hans Loewald, Theodore Lidz, and Stanley Leavy. Dr. Leavy's seminar on structuralism, offered in collaboration with Professor Edward Casey of the Philosophy Department at Yale, was of special importance to me.

This study of cultural development would not have been possible without the collaboration and advice of numerous friends and colleagues. I am grateful first and foremost to Ethel, my wife and collaborator, who introduced me to the excitement of art history and guided my studies in this area. These experiences have enriched my life and provided the basis for this work. My interests in concepts of form and of space derive partly from my earlier collaboration with Dr. David Roth in which we investigated concepts of space in different types of psychopathology.

A primary factor facilitating my work on this book was the opportunity I had to spend an academic leave in 1977 at the Warburg Insti-

tute for Renaissance Studies. I am grateful to Professor Joseph
Trapp, Director of the Warburg, for his generous assistance and for
providing me access to the resources and facilities of the Institute. Sir
Ernst Gombrich was generous of his time and comments. Although
impatient with a developmental psychological analysis of cultural
phenomena, Professor Gombrich's incisive comments and criticisms
forced me to clarify further many of my concepts and assumptions.
Dr. Kim Veltman, a former student and colleague of Sir Ernst, enriched my stay at the Warburg both personally and professionally. His
comments and criticisms of an earlier draft of this manuscript contributed substantially to my understanding of aspects of the history of
art and science. Likewise, Professor Michael Gross of Hampshire College provided consultation in the history of science and he patiently
reviewed several drafts of the manuscript. His advice, consultation,
and encouragement were important at critical moments. Professor
Stanley Weintraub of The Pennsylvania State University read an early
draft and provided constructive criticism. Professor Michael Kubovy,
of Rutgers University, also reviewed the entire manuscript; Professors Jean Schimek of New York University, Gerald Gratch of the
University of Houston, and Stanley Rosenberg of Dartmouth College
reviewed the introductory theoretical chapter and Chapter 2, the developmental psychological model, and I am grateful to them for their
advice. Numerous friends and colleagues at Yale shared observations
and thoughts during the course of this work including Professors Joel
Allison, Marshall Edelson, Jack Greenberg, Harry Frankfurt, Anne
Hanson, Geoffrey Hartman, Jay Hirschfield, Irving Janis, Walter
Kahn, Hillel Levine, Theodore Lidz, Lottie Newman, and Jerome
Singer. Portions of this manuscript were presented at the Kanzer
Faculty Seminar in Psychoanalysis and the Humanities at Yale on
March 27, 1980, and I am grateful for the comments of the participants of that meeting, especially Professor Anne Hanson. I am also
grateful to the participants of an undergraduate senior-graduate
seminar I offered at Yale on this topic in the spring of 1979, and
especially to Professor Jean Henry of the University of New Haven
who participated in that seminar and later also reviewed the entire
manuscript. Editorial advice and consultation were provided by Professor Adrianne Munich, Rosemarie Wellner, and Henry and Susan
Schwab. Several research assistants and secretaries contributed to this
work over the years, including Dr. Mary-Rose Coiner, Barbara Mac-
Kinnon, Meg Turner, Janet Stein, Janet Powell, Toni Suarez, John
and Judith Casey, and Suzanne Whang.

I am also indebted to Helen Chillman, Librarian of the Slides and Photographs Collection at Yale, and to her assistant Ann Gaspari, for their assistance in locating the illustrations for this book. Illustrative material was obtained from the following sources and I am grateful for their assistance: Alte Pinakothek; Alinari (E.P.A.); Archives Photographiques; Art Gallery of Ontario; Art Institute of Chicago; Bayerische Staatsbibliothek; Bibliothèque Nationale; Brera Gallery; British Library; British Museum; Cairo Museum; Courtauld Institute Gallery; Carlo Gandini; Photographie Giraudon; Professor P. Graziosi; Hirmer Verlag; Hirshhorn Museum and Sculpture Garden of the Smithsonian Institute; Houston Museum of Fine Art; Kunsthistorisches Museum; Larousse; Louvre; Martinus Nijhoff; Mauritshuis at the Hague; Metropolitan Museum of Art of New York; Michigan-Princeton-Alexandria Expedition to Mount Sinai and Professor Kurt Weitzmann; Museum of Modern Art; National Gallery, London; National Gallery, Washington; National Museum, Athens; National Museum, Naples; Philadelphia Museum of Art; Prado; Princeton University Press; Rijksmuseum; St. George's Gallery; Studelsches Kunstinstitut; Tate Gallery; Uffizi Gallery; University of Chicago Press; The Vatican; Villa Giula Museum; Wallace Collection; Mrs. John Hay Whitney; Professor Neil Welliver; Yale Center for British Art; and Yale University Art Gallery.

I want to express my appreciation to Lawrence Erlbaum and his associates, Jack Burton and Philip Young. They have been more than just publishers in their interest in and commitment to this book.

Finally, I want to express my gratitude to the A. Whitney Griswold Fund of Yale University for its support of this endeavor.

Sidney J. Blatt

February 1, 1984
Woodbridge, Connecticut

1
The Form of Objects and of Space in the History of Art

INTRODUCTION

In a provocative and controversial statement, Erwin Panofsky (1924/25) discussed the representation of space in art as a symbolic form that reflects the *Weltanschauung* of its period—the culture's conception of nature expressed in the form of objects and of space. Panofsky was particularly interested in the development of linear perspective as the symbolic form of the Italian Renaissance and how it reflected the culture's view of space as infinite, homogeneous, and isotropic. But he stressed that while linear perspective was a unique and most realistic representational construction, it was only one phase in the development of symbolic form, or modes of representation, in the history of art. The goal of this book is to explore the sequences through which the modes of representing the form of objects and of space have developed in the history of painting and to consider these modes of representation as expressions of the symbolic form and the predominant world view of major epochs in the history of Western Civilization.

The form of objects and of space is a basic aspect of human consciousness, a basic dimension for experiencing and understanding nature. Form defines the intimate relationships between individuals within a culture and the relationship of the culture to nature (Focillon, 1934/1948). Concepts of form and of space are evolving conceptual structures, inherent and basic to the multiple cognitive endeavors of a society—its art, literature, philosophy, and science (Jammer, 1954/1969). Form is the very essence and substance of art and the tendency to create "new families of form" is a primary characteristic that defines particular periods of art (Focillon, 1934/1948). A fundamental hypothesis of this book is that the creation of these families of form and concepts of space follow a basic, natural, developmental progression toward increasing differentiation, articulation, integration, abstraction, and complexity.

Throughout history, from Paleolithic to contemporary time, there have been consistent and systematic changes in the mode of representing a segment of nature on a two-dimensional surface. The development of a new mode of representation in painting involves a cognitive-perceptual reorganization and the construction of new cognitive schemata (Olson, 1970). These new cognitive schemata are the consequence of artists' attempts to revise and extend modes of representation already available in the culture. Changes in the modes of representation in the history of art have followed a fundamental developmental progression that is characteristic of all cognitive, intellectual endeavors. This progression occurs in cultural development, in art, literature, and science, as well as in the psychological development of the individual. There is a "formal parallelism" (Brunswik, 1959; Kaplan, 1966; Piaget, 1971; Werner, 1948, 1957; Werner & Kaplan, 1956, 1963) in all cognitive development. Understanding the structures of cognitive development in one domain provides guidelines for understanding development in other domains. Thus, the extensive understanding that has been achieved about the developmental unfolding of cognitive processes within the individual (e.g., by Piaget and Werner) provides a model for the study of cultural development and particularly changes in modes of representation in the history of painting. It was for these reasons that Piaget thought of his discoveries in developmental psychology as defining a genetic epistemology.

To use a psychological model of the individual's development of cognitive processes for the study of cultural phenomena does not imply that earlier levels of cultural development are either childlike or primitive. Because they are earlier in development they are less differentiated, articulated, and integrated, but they are neither childlike nor primitive. Earlier levels are, in fact, vital steps that capture

and highlight certain experiences or dimensions that may be lost in subsequent elaboration and complexity. A model of cognitive development, equally applicable to individual and cultural development, assumes only a formal parallelism among developmental sequences in a variety of endeavors. This developmental sequence is "an ideal or natural order" (Toulmin, 1953, 1972) that can be studied in diverse contexts without any assumption of priorities among the various developmental sequences. There is no commitment to a "recapitulation" across contexts or of ontogeny and phylogeny, only an assumption of parallel sequences in various contexts. Earlier developmental phases are essential steps that are integrated hierarchically in more differentiated, articulated and integrated constructions (Werner, 1948; Werner & Kaplan, 1963).

While there are many dimensions that must be considered in a full analysis of cultural development, the representation of the form of objects and of space is central. The structural organization inherent in the representation of form and space expresses the general conceptual schemata of the society, what Foucault (1970) calls its cultural episteme. Changes in this structural organization reflect transformations in the culture's interpretation of the universe (e.g., Frankl, 1960; Malraux, 1954; Panofsky, 1924/25; Riegl, 1901/1927; Weitz, 1970; Wölfflin, 1915/1932). Changes in the representation of the form of objects and of space are structural changes that are expressed in the multiple cognitive endeavors within the cultural period. Each cultural epoch is a complete and articulated whole (Burckhardt, 1860/1950), with a particular cognitive organization that is expressed in its art, religion, science, and social order. At the height of each culture there is a structural unity of the elements of the culture (e.g., Burckhardt, 1860/1950; Dilthey, 1927/1957; Dvořák, 1918/1967; Gombrich, 1969a; Hauser, 1951/1960, 1965; Lovejoy, 1936/1964; Panofsky, 1960/1972). This structural unity, derived from the social structure, values, meanings, and *Weltanschauung* of the culture, is expressed in the configurations of art, literature, music, poetry, philosophy, theology, and science. An analysis of the predominant mode of representing the form of objects and of space in art can aid in the identification of the conceptual structure and unity inherent in the multiple cognitive endeavors of the major epochs in the history of Western Civilization.

Numerous art historians, beginning with Johann Winckelmann, Jacob Burckhardt, Alois Riegl, Max Dvořák, and Johan Huizinga,

considered art history within the broad context of cultural and intellectual history. They believe art reflects the *Weltanschauung* and provides insight into the thought, will, and feeling of the historical
period. Art is an expression of the period and it reflects the attitudes
and institutions of its time, but it is only one of many expressions of
the basic cognitive structure that underlies all intellectual endeavors
of the society. Art is "part of the history of ideas, of the development
of the human spirit" (Dvořák, cited by Antal, 1949a, p.49); it is a
historical document of the individual artist and the prevailing *Weltanschauung* and style of the particular period (Kleinbauer, 1971).
But as stressed by Benjamin (1977), the meaning of the style and the
period can be fully realized only subsequently as the relationship
between the style and its period become clarified. Art is an expression
of its time, but its full meaning can only emerge with time. Art can
only be understood in a historical context; the potential importance of
a contribution is discernable only with the passage of time, in relation
to its prehistory as well as its post-history (Benjamin, 1977). "To explain a style can mean nothing more than to place it in its general
historical context and to verify that is speaks in harmony with other
organs of its age" (Wölfflin, 1898, p.79; see also Schapiro, 1953). Art,
as an aesthetic and cognitive expression of the intellectual conceptions
and experiential forms of a society, has its origins in the historical
process (Pepper, 1942). While it is logically impossible to predict the
future course of history (Popper, 1957), it is possible subsequently to
discern and specify the systematic principles involved in revisions of
artistic style and in the reorganization of the cognitive structures that
are basic to the various epochs in Western Civilization.

In this book we seek to articulate a theoretical model of the development of the capacity to represent the form of objects and of
space and to apply this model to the study of changes in modes of
representation in the history of painting. This attempt to identify the
conceptual structure inherent in major epochs in the history of art is
congruent with the persistent call of many art historians for the establishment of a "vocabulary of form," a "system of schemata" (e.g.,
Gombrich, 1960), or a "semantics of the visual arts" (Janson, 1961)
that can provide a consistent theoretical matrix for art historical
analysis. We also seek to demonstrate that the modes of representing
the form of objects and of space in art express important dimensions
of the culture's fundamental cognitive structure that is inherent in its
multiple cognitive endeavors, especially in its conception of the uni-

verse. This cognitive analysis of cultural development is consistent with the contemporary emphasis upon structuralism as a theoretical orientation and as a method of inquiry.[1]

This introductory chapter considers some of the basic theoretical assumptions involved in evaluating patterns of cultural change through a structuralist analysis of the modes of representing the form of objects and of space in the history of painting. The second chapter presents a model of individual development of the capacity to represent the form of objects and of space. This model is based on an integration of cognitive developmental and psychoanalytic theory and research. Chapters 3, 4, and 5 apply this psychological developmental model to an analysis of the changes in the representation of the form of objects and space in art in the major epochs of Western Civilization. The concluding sections of Chapters 3, 4 and 5 consider the parallel

---

[1] In addition to the study of the development of cognitive structures through history (a diachronic analysis) and their simultaneous expression in the multiple cognitive endeavors of a culture (a synchronic analysis), one can also investigate the relationships of the development of these cognitive structures to major changes in social organization—the influence of economic, political, and social forces on the intellectual endeavors of a society (a dynamic-causative analysis). The search for causal explanations for the appearance of cultural phenomena assumes a complex transaction between art and the embedding culture, in which the culture stimulates the art, and the art, in turn, has important functions within the culture. A dynamic-causal analysis integrates cultural and intellectual history with social history in order to understand the social, political, economic, religious, and psychological factors as the context from which fundamental ideas of the culture emerge (e.g., Antal, 1953b; Hauser, 1951/1960; Schapiro, 1953). Hauser (1951/1960), "in the most ambitious and most adversely criticized social history of art" (Kleinbauer, 1971, p. 77), examined the role of economic and social forces in creating changes in artistic style. He viewed, for example, the 16th century Mannerist style "as an expression of the unrest, anxiety, and bewilderment generated by the process of alienation of the individual from society and the reification of the whole cultural process" that was part of the social crisis of the 16th century (Hauser, 1965, p. 111). Likewise, Antal (1953) discussed the neoclassicism and romanticism of the 18th century as a characteristic bourgeois outlook on the eve of revolution (Kleinbauer, 1971). Though there is considerable controversy about the more neo-Marxist views (e.g., Antal, 1953; Hauser, 1951/1960) that social, political, and economic conflicts and upheaval are the activating force that creates cultural change, most art historians generally agree that the structure and content of art express the historical, social, political, scientific, religious, and economic tendencies of the period.

between the development of modes of representing space in art and the development of concepts of space in science and cosmology. This analysis is based on Panofsky's (1924/25) hypothesis that aesthetic and scientific concepts of space develop in an interdependent fashion. Art and science are two major conceptual schemes for representing nature. Though the concepts of space are expressed in somewhat different terms in the two disciplines, they evolve from the same cultural matrix (Gabo, 1937). Thus, the development of modes of representation of space in the history of art should be paralleled by similar changes in the development of the concept of space in science.

In these latter chapters we also seek to demonstrate that changes in conceptual schemata involve revisions in the fundamental metric and mathematical structure utilized by the culture. These changes in basic mathematical structure range from an initial emphasis upon simple nominal designation, to ordinal sequences based primarily on qualitative comparisons, to more complex, quantitative, interval metrics established in terms of arbitrarily defined reference and scale points, and later, to an emphasis on quantitative ratio scaling defined in terms of stable, consistent, numerically and experientially relevant, reference and scale points (Stevens, 1951).

PATTERNS OF CHANGE

The representation and conceptualization of space in art and science characterize the *Weltanschauung* of a culture. Changes in social conditions and increases in knowledge create a social climate in which innovative individuals within the culture can develop a new mode of representation that resolves ambiguities, inconsistencies, and contradictions that have become increasingly apparent about current as well as previous modes. The history of art and the history of science are both part of a basic cultural developmental progression toward increasing levels of differentiation and integration. The transitions between stages of this developmental progression are the result of attempts to resolve dilemmas, inconsistencies, and contradictions that become apparent with sufficient mastery of the then-traditional modes of conception and representation. As Schäfer (1919/1974, p. 149) noted, "one generation takes up the representational types of another and hands them on because that's 'how it is done'. *The great force of tradition is at work.*" (Schäfer's Italics). But the new is not simply a continuation of the old; it involves a transformation of structure, meaning, and function in the creation of a new style that integrates and extends previous styles (Hauser, 1953/1959).

The representations of space in art and science are essential parts of a continuous transformation of society's understanding of nature. Major changes in the conception of space mark particular nodal points in the history of civilization. While there are interruptions and discontinuities as well as long periods of stability in cultural development, there is also a basic continuity in the major transformations of the conception of space. Concepts of space are constructions of human thought that express the society's attempt to develop conceptual schemes for understanding nature. Major transformations of these schemes usually evolve through a long and continuous process and they eventually pervade the entire society.

Transformations of the modes of representation and conceptualization of space in art and science are built upon prior stages. Developments in the modes of representation progress, although sometimes somewhat erratically, toward greater complexity and diversity. Individuals and cultures weave diverse elements into coherent wholes within their own age or epoch. Successive waves of intellectual and conceptual revolution are dynamic transformations of structures that result, at least for a time, in an era of relative intellectual calm and stability (Kuhn, 1962/1970). As Kuhn has articulated, the everyday activity of "normal science" (and art) is guided by existing "paradigms"; but this eventually leads to contradictions and an awareness of inadequacies and inconsistencies in the paradigm. Eventually, these anomalies inspire pioneers to seek a new and possibly discontinuous (and, at times, initially disconcerting) innovative paradigm that provides a resolution and integration for the anomalies. Innovations usually occur at a time of social freedom and stability and are part of a much broader social transformation. New conceptual structures often appear as a "conversion experience" (Berger & Luckmann, 1966; Kuhn, 1962/1970). Innovation in science and art is often produced by a comparative outsider to an ongoing tradition, but nonetheless one with a competent grasp and mastery of the existing paradigm, but only after a relatively brief period of exposure—brief enough to have avoided developing a full and intense commitment to it. Innovation is achieved by individuals who possess both a competence and a comprehension of the current world view as well as some psychological distance, distress, confusion, and unrest.

An emerging new conceptual matrix, often embodied by a new social group, and an individual sense of personal crisis as well as competence, lead some people of remarkable talent to articulate a new conceptual structure that resolves the anomalies and inconsistencies for the new social movement as well as for themselves (Berger & Luckmann, 1966; Kuhn, 1962/1970).

Moore (1963/1974) discussed a number of basic patterns of cultural change. Change can be "gradual or rapid, peaceful or violent, continuous or spasmodic, orderly or erratic." Change can occur in a repetitive, "trendless cycle" (p. 44) in which themes of rise and decline occur in successive reoccurring sequences. Change can also occur as an evolving long-term developmental process that follows a simple, gradual, continuous, monotonic, linear function. There can be various discontinuities, stages, minor undulations, uneven rates, or subtle short-term cycles within a long-term developmental process. In long-term change there can also be temporary retrogression followed by a sudden, rapid, extensive developmental surge. One alternative to a long-term linear developmental progression is a pattern of change that combines both a unity and a diversity of change within a single conception of a "branching evolution" (p. 39). This allows for the specification of a single developmental line as well as branching processes that proceed at different rates and in somewhat different directions. There are also processes of change that can be described as asymptotic or exponential in which there are markedly different rates of development either early or late in the process. Moore points out, however, that the pattern of change can depend upon the time periods and the observational units used, the details demanded, and whether the data are essentially qualitative or quantitative. Quantitative data allow for much greater diversity and precision in the description of the patterns of change. Moore cautions that value judgments can influence a formulation of change associated with progress and maturity or with a retrogressive return to a prior "happy" or "Golden Age." But, as will be stressed throughout this book, distortion in evaluating change in the history of art can be limited and contained by specifying variables and dimensions in a theoretical system established and defined independent of the phenomena to be evaluated. A theoretical model of the psychological development of concepts of space provides a model that has validity external to the development of modes of representation in art. Therefore it can limit the intrusion of value judgments in the investigation of changes in modes of representation in the history of art.

Different types of patterns of change of style have been discussed in the history of art, including cyclical, polar, and progressive developmental theories, and various combinations of these (Kleinbauer, 1971; Schapiro, 1953; Weitz, 1970). In a cyclical theory, each stage has a characteristic style and the stages follow an irrestible course, often based on a biological analogy of the natural life cycle from birth, infancy, maturity, senility to death. There is an implication within each style of a rise, growth, and eventual decline and decay. Schapiro (1953) notes that there can be short-term cycles within one or more periods, such as the rise and fall of a Greco-Roman or a Gothic style, or there can be long-term cycles. Schapiro (1953), however, finds these cyclical theories unconvincing because new styles are often created without the complete decline of a preceding style. Winckelmann (1764) was the first art historian to articulate a normative historical course marked by repeated phases of growth, decline, and decay. In the mid-18th century, he discussed Greek sculpture as proceeding from origins, to mature perfection, to a decline and fall and applied this biological analogy to the various periods, especially the history of ancient art. Actually, Vasari (1550/1965) had developed a similar scheme in his analysis of the lives of Renaissance artists when he discussed the infancy, adolescence, and maturity of the Renaissance (Kleinbauer, 1971).

Cyclic conceptions of changes in style are often based on a definition of a set of polarities, and changes are described as recurrent movement between two poles either within, or across, periods of style. Alois Riegl (1858–1905) was among the first art historians to offer an alternative to the conception of Winckelmann by regarding the progression from archaic to classical art as a single developmental process across two antithetical categories or poles of perception that he termed "haptic" (tactile) and "optic" (visual). He considered this process a basic universal principle that determined change in style both within particular eras as well as over much longer time spans in the history of Western Civilization.

One of the most influential polar conceptions in art history was Wölfflin's (1915/1932) formulation of five polarities that he used to contrast the art of the Renaissance with that of the Baroque. Wölfflin's polarities include linear and painterly, planar or parallel surface form and diagonal-recessional depth, closed (tectonic) and open (atectonic) form, composite and diffuse composition, and clear and unclear form. These five polarities defined two major modes of vision, the "linear" and the "painterly." According to Wölfflin, there is an immanent, inevitable development that has an internal logic, which can proceed in only one direction—from linear to painterly. For Wölfflin (1915/1932, p. 18), the painterly mode "is not truly intelligible without the earlier" linear mode. Wölfflin's morphological analysis of visual modes and his emphasis on visual forms were particularly effective in the study of the art of the Renaissance and the Baroque. Wölfflin believed that these polarities were applicable to the entire history of art as well as to development in literature and science.

There is considerable controversy about Wölfflin's formulations. Schapiro (1953) and Hauser (1953/1959), for example, note that throughout the history of art there have been various combinations of these polarities, and the second pole does not necessarily follow from the first one since other options exist. Paul Frankl (1960) integrated Wölfflin's polarities with a cyclical conception of preclassic, classic, and post-classic periods of being and becoming that occur in the repetitive movement through these polarities in the development of elementary forms (Kleinbauer, 1971; Schapiro, 1953). In addition to Wölfflin's five antithetical polarities and Riegl's (1901) haptic and optic modes of perception, there have been other polarities used in the history of art such as idealism and naturalism (e.g., Dvořák, 1918/1924), geometric or abstract and organic or naturalistic (e.g., Worringer, 1907/1953).

Some art historians discuss the development of artistic forms and styles as revisions and alterations of a prior mode, while others discuss a long developmental sequence throughout the history of civilization. Art historians discuss a variety of developmental sequences ranging from a short-term repetitive cycle to a long-term developmental process, but there is general agreement that the development of artistic forms and styles does not proceed toward a fixed or predetermined ideal style. Even within a long-term developmental process, progress in the development of artistic form is seen as based on revisions and extensions of prior forms and styles.

One of the primary models of change of style in the history of art is the conception of change as a continuous, long-term, developmental process. This linear conception of development is essentially Aristotelian (Kleinbauer, 1971) in its assumption of a serial developmental order from simple to complex forms. But such a model need not be a teleological conception of development as proceeding toward a predetermined, fixed, ideal goal (Kuhn, 1962/1970). Progress in art is viewed as developing out of a dialectic between currently available cognitive structures and the impulse to seek new understanding of nature and new symbolic forms. Revisions in style occur as the result of constant attempts to achieve and establish a more comprehensive understanding of nature through a repetitive process of thesis–antithesis–synthesis. Revisions of inconsistencies and contradictions in current modes of understanding and representing nature facilitate the development of more comprehensive cognitive structures. The rate of cultural change can be influenced by significant changes in the social context. Increases in knowledge and/or major revisions in social, political, and economic conditions facilitiate cultural development. New structures of artistic form are influenced primarily by the structure of prior accomplishments, but the rate at which structures are revised and transformed into new structures is determined primarily by social conditions. The concerns, interests, and preoccupations of a culture are reflected primarily in the content and themes of its art. Revisions and transformations of structures are determined primarily by the form and organization of the prior cognitive structures and the freedom within a culture to seek new understanding of nature.

A linear model of development is also Darwinian in that changes in the modes of representation are viewed as becoming increasingly comprehensive and complex through gradual modification as well as dramatic shifts (Kleinbauer, 1971). But it is important to stress that this progression is never exact and perfect. Given the broad sweep of any developmental sequence, there are occasional discontinuities and even temporary regressions or sudden progressions. As seen in the Middle Ages, or as Meiss (1951) so carefully documented in his study of the impact of the Black Death on painting in Florence and Siena from 1350 to 1375, major social upheaval can interfere and even cause short- or long-term temporary setbacks in the development of cognitive structures (Peckham, 1965). Thus, the delineation of a linear progression in cultural development need not be dependent upon the identification of a fixed, monotonic, linear sequence, but rather on the specification of a "curve of best fit" which, while not accounting for every observation, still accounts for a major portion of the observations in a more precise form than alternative descriptions. Cultural development, like all developmental sequences, can have temporary reversions or proceed at variable rates at different times in the sequence, but a broad overview of the process indicates a clear developmental progression. Hauser (1953/1959, p. 224) stresses that continuous developmental progression is not simply a straight linear process; progress can be irregular and marked by disruptions, disturbances, and interruptions.

Kubler (1962) discusses continuous, long-term changes in the fundamental morphology of art. Kubler, in a historical, rather than a biological conception of time and change, describes the formal sequence of "linked solutions" of successive problems in art. Kubler examined the continuous change in the solution of artistic problems; these solutions are interrelated and open to revision and elaboration by new solutions. He sought to identify and describe the series of changes that occur in significant, minute, and, at times, dramatic variations and solutions. Early solutions (promorphic) are technically simple, energetically inexpensive, and expressively clear. Late solutions (neomorphic) are costly, difficult, intricate, recondite, and animate. Kubler used the terms promorphic and neomorphic to avoid more value-laden terms such as "primitive," "decadent," "archaic." Promorphic and neomorphic are determinants that are only relative to a "pertinent form-class . . . , (and) a defined starting point" (Kubler, 1962, p. 56). Inventions in art, according to Kubler, "are not isolated events, but linked positions" in a formal sequence. There is "a structural order in the sequence of inventions which exists independently of other conditions. . . . Under certain circumstances an inherent structural order in the sequence of new forms is readily apparent . . . where linked runs of related solutions follow one another in a recognizable order as if following out the conditions of a prior program common to these various evolutions" (Kubler, 1962, pp. 85–86).

Schapiro (1953, p. 303) also proposes a long-term developmental model in his discussion of progress from ancient Greek to medieval and modern western Europe as a sequence from "archaic linear" to "pictorial" representation and naturalistic art. Schematized representations of isolated objects are replaced by perspective representations in which there are "continuities of space, movement, light, shadow and atmosphere." Schapiro (1953), as Hauser (1953/1959), finds concepts of a continuous process in the history of art more accurate and convincing than the doctrine of inevitable cyclical recurrences. Schapiro believes that many of the cyclical theories of the history of art are essentially descriptions of shorter phases in the progressive development of representations, and he stresses the need to investigate the formal properties of the long-term developmental progression of various modes of representation.

The formulations of the history of art as a continuous developmental progression are often derived from the application of concepts of psychological theory to the history of art. Emanuel Loewy (1900/1907), for example, discussed the representation of natural forms as progressing from concrete representations based on a memory image of the actual object, to perspective representations based on a specific perception of the object. Loewy provided an articulation of the forms of archaic representation and their development through various stages to naturalistic art.

Riegl was among the earliest to conceptualize artistic development as a single, continuous process with transitions at world-historical epochs. His conception of progress was based on a move from the haptic (tactile) to the optic (visual) mode of perception, a long developmental process that extends across the entire culture. According to Schapiro (1953):

> The history of art is, for Riegl, an endless necessary movement from representation based on vision of the object and its parts as proximate, tangible, discrete, and self-sufficient, to the representation of the whole perceptual field as a directly given, but more distant, continuum with merging parts, with an increasing role of the spatial voids, and with a more evident reference to the knowing subject as a constituting factor in perception. (p. 302)

Riegl stressed the change from an objective to a subjective relation to the world. The object in the haptic mode is a concrete, tangible, self-contained, isolated entity. In the optical mode, the perceptual field is a totality in which objects and parts of objects are integrated with the surrounding space. The viewer has a conscious, self-reflective role in the representation of the perceptual field. The shift from a tactile to an optical mode of apprehending the world initially occurred with objects in isolation and later once again in the relation of objects to their spatial context. Though Riegl did not have available a sophisticated psychological or sociological theory, he developed a broad view based on a sensitive appreciation of psychological processes. He emphasized dimensions such as "will, feeling and thought" as changing people from having "a predominantly objective to a sub-jective" relationship to the world. Riegl did not consider this shift from the objective to the subjective as simply "a development of natu-ralism from an archaic to an impressionistic stage," but as a conse-quence of fundamental changes in "the intimate structure of styles, the principles of composition, and the relations of figure to ground" (Schapiro, 1953, p. 302). For Riegl, the history of art is an autono-mous dialectical process that expresses the development of successive world views.

There is considerable controversy and debate (e.g., Gombrich, 1960), however, about whether there is a long-term developmental sequence in the modes of representing the form of objects and of space in the history of art. These criticisms provide appropriate cau-tions about some of the limitations of such a hypothesis. Some art critics and historians (e.g., Ackerman, 1960; Croce, 1953; Venturi, 1936), for example, maintain that each work of art must be ap-preciated and understood in its own right as a complete, integrated expression of an individual artist within a particular cultural context. They believe that concepts of style or historical development cannot explain the creative endeavors of individual artists. Works of art can be understood only through an analysis of the artistic sensibility of the artist and the attitudes that prevailed at the time the work of art was produced (Kleinbauer, 1971). Ackerman (1962) maintains that an excessive concern with historical, developmental trends tends to di-minish the appreciation of the artist and the work of art. He believes that art must be free of arbitrary classifications and should be ap-preciated and understood in terms of its own intrinsic qualities and cultural context. Art can best be understood by studying the creative activity of the artist, and not by formulating abstract constructs such as a myth of a developmental process. While Ackerman acknowledges that the artist does not work in a historical vacuum and has contact with a cultural context, he believes that art history needs to be particu-larly concerned with the autonomy of the individual work of art and the experiences of the artist who produces it. Ackerman stresses the need to appreciate art and the artist in terms of the historical, polit-ical, economic, social, and cultural context, and not as a point or place in a hypothetical developmental process. Despite Ackerman's concerns, it is possible that an understanding of a particular style within the context of a long-term developmental process may facilitate a fuller appreciation of the emergence of that style in the work of an individual artist during a particular historical period.

Several art historians (e.g., Ackerman, Gombrich, Hauser, Schapiro) are concerned that the history of art not be fashioned like "another version of the materialist success story," (Ackerman, 1962/ 1967, p. 231), or Hegelian "romantic mythologies" of the "great drama of mankind's evolution from childhood to maturity" (Gombrich, 1960, p. 19). They are concerned that the primary judgment of the value of art would be based on an evaluation of the work's contribution to subsequent phases of the developmental sequence. In addition, Gombrich (1969a) rejects a Hegelian conception in which each cultural epoch is seen as a necessary stage in the progressive ascent toward a higher plane of articulation primarily because he rejects Hegel's underlying theological assumption that this process is an unfolding based on divine reasoning leading toward a preordained destiny or goal, that it is a search for the Absolute Spirit. Gombrich also rejects the conception of a progression in the development of artistic style because of Hegel's assumption that such a progression indicates that individuals, in the course of history, have undergone profound biological and psychological change. Because of these underlying theological assumptions, Hegel was unable to allow for the possibility that there could be temporary setbacks and declines in the attempt to achieve the Absolute Spirit. But one can consider the possibility of a long-term developmental progression independent of theological assumptions. Developmental sequences can emerge as revisions of prior stages without proceeding to a preordained goal, without judgments of intellectual, biological, or aesthetic superiority or inferiority, and with the possibility that temporary reversions can occur within the long-term developmental process (see also Gablik, 1976).

Many art historians object to suggestions that art history parallels individual psychological development. These suggestions raise anew the controversy, most prominent in biology, of ontogeny recapitulating phylogeny (see Gould, 1977). But a parallel in the development of art and individual psychological development need not be based on an assumption of recapitulation, but rather of assuming only a formal parallelism between developmental sequences (Brunswik, 1959; Piaget, 1971; Werner & Kaplan, 1963). Gombrich (1960) takes exception to the comparison of art history to individual development because he believes it is based on an implicit assumption that earlier societies were as unskilled as children because they had the mentality of children or because they lacked the motivation to seek more complex modes of representation. Gombrich is concerned by the implications that modes of representation in earlier stages in the history of art be considered primitive and that early artists (or artists of any period for that matter) be considered biologically, psychologically, and intellectually inferior or childish. A developmental progression in the history of art, however, can be viewed as similar to developmental progression in the history of science. While Aristotle's concept of the universe, for example, may be simple and primitive in comparison to contemporary conceptions of the universe, one would not consider Aristotle biologically, intellectually, or psychologically inferior. Likewise, in the history of art, earlier modes of representation in art, although simple and primitive compared to later ones, are not the product of simple people or primitive minds. Gombrich (1977) himself, in fact, points out that art serves different functions in different societies (magical, religious, ceremonial, functional, and narrative) and different modes of representation are more effective for different functions.

Gombrich's objections to the formulation of a long-term developmental sequence in the history of art may be due, in part, to his reliance on a model based on perceptual theory and research. Perceptual processes are basically innate and essentially the same in form and structure in every culture. As Gombrich (1954) has commented, art has a history, perception does not. Thus, an analysis of art history based on a theory of perception could be interpreted as implying either cultural or biological inferiority. But throughout the history of civilization there has been a clear progressive development in modes of representation in art, literature, and science. An analysis of art history based on a theory of representation can acknowledge the important progressive contribution of prior cultures and societies without assuming aesthetic, cultural, or biological inferiority.

Cognitive structures develop over the epochs of civilization or the brief time span of the individual life cycle, in a basic progression toward increasingly complex, articulated, differentiated, and integrated forms. Prior phases provide the essential basis and matrix for subsequent development. The developmental progression of symbolic forms and of cognitive structures in individual and cultural development unfolds according to a basic structural pattern that occurs relatively independent of content. The basic dimensions of this natural developmental process can be observed and defined in a number of different areas of discourse. Probably because children provide an immediate availability of primary data and an endless opportunity for the direct observation of the various stages in the unfolding of this basic developmental sequence, the basic process of the development of cognitive structures and symbolic forms has been most fully described within the human life cycle. The development of cognitive structures in the child does not imply any judgment that earlier stages are inferior, primitive, or less valuable. Earlier stages in any developmental progression are less differentiated and less integrated than later stages, but each stage has its unique qualities and is an essential contribution to the basic developmental process. Understanding individual development may provide a model for differentiating and understanding parallel sequences in a variety of endeavors, including the history of art and the history of science. Such a developmental model can provide the concepts necessary for defining a "vocabulary of form" or a "system of schemata" that could be applied to the study of development of modes of representation and of symbolic forms in a variety of intellectual endeavors.

While in most developmental theories there is implicit admiration for higher levels of development and for the most advanced contributions, one cannot simply take for granted the impressive achievements of earlier stages of the developmental process. Earlier stages are major accomplishments and are essential for later development. Aspects from the contributions of each stage are retained in subsequent extensions, revisions, and transformations. In child development, the representations of early stages are often the modes for experiencing more direct, affect-laden experiences, particularly in bodily terms. Later stages of development contribute to more abstract and conceptual representations that allow for greater generality, but they may be somewhat removed from immediate, affective experience (Blatt, 1974). Concepts in art and science have evolved from being relatively simple and direct to being more complex and abstract, and this development can be described independently of any judgment about the value of the contribution or the mentality of the culture. There is little indication that basic perceptual processes or mental capacities have changed significantly since Paleolithic man. There is no doubt, for example, that individuals in early civilization perceived depth and had some conception of perspective. But it required time to conceptualize these experiences and to develop the cognitive schemata and the techniques for representing three-dimensional experiences on a two-dimensional surface. Later epochs, building on earlier contributions, invented increasingly precise techniques for highly realistic representations of these three-dimensional perceptual experiences.

Gombrich, Ackerman, and Schapiro caution that there is a temptation to define any conceptualization of a process as a natural sequence because historical evidence highlights cause-and-effect sequences within the process. Ackerman (1962/1967, p. 231), for example, stresses that artists are not aware of what will succeed their work; they only know the past and the present, and they attempt to take "a step—sometimes a leap—away from the past." Ackerman, like Schapiro (1953), rejects a deterministic theory of a preordained pattern in the development of style in the history of art. They believe that in order to appreciate and interpret a work of art, we need to understand its context rather than its effect. Ackerman (1962/1967, p. 232) argues that the development of art should not be described as the succession of steps toward the solution of a problem, but instead as a "succession of steps away from one or more original statements of a problem." He argues that patterns can be detected because succeeding works both retain and reject aspects of prior statements. He points out that a pattern or configuration of change may appear purposeful or predestined only because each work retains aspects of its predecessor. Thus, unique contributions and innovations in style can often be coherently related to earlier works without necessarily defining an overall long-term developmental sequence or pattern. For Ackerman, changes result from probing the unknown, rather than from a sequence of steps toward a predetermined solution.

Ackerman takes the position that overemphasizing chronological succession should be avoided because it is based on the questionable assumption that each work of art is necessarily more closely related to its immediate predecessors than to works of an earlier stage or style. He considers works of art as occurring in an open system, as "a repository of experiences entering from every direction in the artist's surroundings" (1962/1967, p. 233), from distant as well as from recent past and from factors both within as well as external to the style itself. But Ackerman is also impressed with the similarity of sequences and patterns of change that have occurred in very different cultures. He notes a cyclical similarity, for example, in Greek, Gothic, and Renaissance art, in which a phase of equilibrium (usually described as classic) is preceded by a more formal phase and followed by a freer period. These recurring cycles transcend historical forces and reflect the artists' attempts to refine the solutions of their predecessors. Changes are a product of the tensions in the society experienced by the artist—the tensions between the stability and security of established schemes and the desire to create something unique and different. There is a tension between "the reproduction of existing forms and the invention of new ones, by necessity, not by choice" (1962/1967, p. 228). The unique balance of the forces for stability and for change in each culture results in differential rates of change. Despite the reservations expressed by Ackerman, Gombrich, Schapiro, and others, it is still possible that there could be a logical and natural progression in cultural development in which the pattern of change of style is not determined by any preordained destiny, nor by a common goal, but by a hierarchical succession of complex decisions, each made in response to prior solutions and statements.

Kleinbauer (1971, p. 33) expresses some concern that attempts to relate the visual arts to theories of development and progress are attempts "to make art history a science, to create an objective and systematic investigation of the arts." Kleinbauer is critical of Hans Sedlymayr's configurational analysis of the 1930s as an attempt to discuss art history in terms of the methods of science, such as the creation of a qualitative and historical taxonomy, and the analysis of the principles of structural composition. Some art historians consider structural principles and the methods of natural science as inapplicable to art historical inquiry because they empty art of its aesthetic significance and integrity. But the definition of principles of structural organization is necessary if art historians are to verify formal relations among underlying principles in works of art. Despite his reservations, Kleinbauer (1971) believes that there may be some value in the application of the methods of natural science to the identification and explanation of major structural characteristics and underlying compositional principles in works of art.

Though a number of art historians express concern that a search for a developmental progression of structural principles over large epochs detracts from the appreciation of the creative act within its cultural context, it is possible that the understanding of structural change over the history of art may, in fact, lead to an increased sensitivity to facets of particular changes in style. Although artists in a particular epoch struggle to establish changes in style as alternate

solutions to the problems posed by their predecessors and are unaware of the future direction of art, this does not preclude the possibility that their revisions follow a logical and natural order,
characterized by increasing differentiation, integration, complexity,
and abstraction. Changes in style as steps away from prior solutions
are not necessarily inconsistent with a natural developmental continuum in which the stages of solution, while distinct, are still interrelated, progressive, and hierarchical. Contextual forces within a
society can lead to stability, rigidity, flexibility, or chaos (Peckham,
1965). Certain periods in history provided the social freedom necessary for remarkable changes in style, others demanded stability instead of change, and the social upheaval of still other periods fostered
temporary setbacks and declines. Sensitivity to the fine balance between the forces for stability and for change within a culture enables
the creative artist to capture the moment and to contribute to constructive change and the development of artistic style. Artistic style is
the vector that results from complex and conflicting cultural pressures. Cultural values and technological skills determine the potential
range of artistic expression; individual artists explore the options
available within the range of an artistic style (Gay, 1974).

THE SEARCH FOR A "VOCABULARY OF FORM"
OR A "SYSTEM OF SCHEMATA"

Despite the reluctance of some art critics and historians to consider a
developmental progression in the history of art, there has been increasing call for a definition of a "vocabulary of form" or a "system of
schemata" (Gombrich, 1960) that can provide a matrix through which
changes in the modes of representation can be evaluated systematically. Most art historians stress the need to assess the formal, syntact-
ical, or symbolic dimensions, and the structural principles of form
and schemata through which elements are organized into a composition. The analysis of the formal or structural principles involved in
the representation of the form of objects and of space would be independent of judgments of aesthetic value and merit (Bell, 1913; Fry,
1927). These formal or structural dimensions are central to most
concepts of style. For example, Gombrich (1960, p. 87) stresses the
need to understand the "system of schemata" used to represent the

visual world and Ackerman (1960) considers the vocabulary of formal and symbolic elements, and the syntax by which they are organized into a composition, as central concepts of style. Riegl (1901/1927) considered artistic development as a single continuous process in which the transitions of major epochs are forged in the creation of new forms to solve specific problems (Schapiro, 1953). Riegl found that the definition of formal principles enabled him to appreciate each epoch and style in its own right, independent of aesthetic and value judgments, and to study the inevitable developmental progression in art. Riegl, Wölfflin, and Dvořák consider the history of art as the history of the development of the representation of space and the organization and composition of form. The definition of the form of objects and the integration, coherence, and harmony of pure form are essential dimensions in art (Fry, 1928).

One of the most articulate and extensive statements about the importance of the formal dimension in the study of style is the work of Henri Focillon (1934/1948). Focillon's work derives from Wölfflin's and Reigl's formulations of the autonomous development of form. For Focillon (1934/1948, p. 2) "a work of art is the measure of space" as matter, movement, and form. Form is the central modality of life, the essence of art is the "construction of space and matter." Form has an internal logic, meaning, and nature; the metamorphosis of form is endless—it is the essence of style. The formal dimension of style is comprised of elements (its vocabulary or semantics) and a system of relationships (its syntax). Forms have inherent rules that are determined by the nature of our mental apparatus. But for Focillon (p. 14) "style is not merely a state in the life of forms . . . it is a homogeneous, coherent, formal environment . . . [which] give(s) birth to . . . various types of social structure: styles of life, vocabularies, states of awareness." It is in the various conceptions of space that the art historian can observe the redefinition of form. The life of art is manifested in the metamorphosis and transformation of this central theme: the development of form. The development of history of forms, however, according to Focillon cannot be indicated by a "single ascending line" or constant, fixed, universal postulates, but rather by various new geometries.

The stress on the importance of form and the conception of space has persisted throughout art history and is a major emphasis in contemporary art historical analysis and criticism. Susan Sontag (1961,

p. 12), for example, states that, first and foremost, greater attention should be given to form in art. A descriptive vocabulary of form would serve to limit an "arrogance of interpretation" that occurs because of an "excessive stress on content" in the study of art.

While there are many elements that must be considered in the analysis of style, such as light, shading, color, and content, most art historians consider the analysis of form and of space a central dimension. The emphasis on the importance of the structural elements of form and space for the analysis of style has been a persistent theme for most art historians, but as noted by Kleinbauer (1971, p. 49), the complexity of 20th century art has made scholars acutely aware of the need to develop more subtle and refined analyses of a formal vocabulary. Read (1952) has stated this position most succinctly.

> I believe that among the agents or instruments of human evolution, art is supremely important. I believe that the aesthetic faculty has been the means of man's first acquiring, and then refining, consciousness. Form, the progressive organization of elements otherwise chaotic, is given in perception. It is present in all skills—skill is the instinct for form revealed in action. Beyond this physiological and instinctive level, any further progress in human evolution has always been dependent on a realization of formal values. (p. 13)

This emphasis upon the study of form is not only central to an analysis of changes in style in the history of art, but the development of spatial forms is a central dimension for understanding all of human cognitive activity. Throughout civilization the construction of concepts of space has been central to understanding nature. Thus, there must be a common structure to the artist's creation of spatial forms and the scientist's conceptualization of space. As discussed by Whyte (1951), there is a basic congruence in the expression of space and time in the various disciplines within the arts, the sciences, and the humanities.

The definition of a vocabulary of form can provide more precise specification of the relationships between various modifications and revisions of modes of representation. Considerable effort has been devoted to deriving a vocabulary of form from psychological theory and research including the study of the sequences through which children learn to draw, the nature of perceptual processes, and the development of cognitive schemata, mental representation, and symbol formation.

Psychological Criteria for a Vocabulary of Form

There are two major types of criteria for assessing changes in style. Some art historians utilize criteria essentially intrinsic to art, while others utilize criteria established in disciplines independent of art (e.g., theories of visual perception, child development). Kleinbauer (1971) discusses both these approaches to the study of style as "intrinsic analyses" because they study the work of art itself rather than the cultural-social context in which the art was produced. But within these intrinsic analyses, it is important to distinguish criteria inherent to art from concepts and constructs that have an independent validity. These latter types of criteria can be evaluated within their own domain as well as in the study of artistic style. Art historians whose formulations are primarily based on concepts internal to art itself include Schapiro, Ackerman, Wölfflin, Riegl, Dvořák and Hauser. Art historians who have used concepts external to art criteria based primarily on psychological theory and research include Gombrich (1960) and Arnheim (1954/1974) who use perceptual theory and research; Loewy (1900/1907), Britsch (1926), Schaefer-Simmern (1948), and Arnheim (1954/1974) who noted a correspondence between aspects of the history of art and the sequences through which a child learns to paint and draw; and most recently Burnham (1971), Edgerton (1975), and Gablik (1976) who, based on Panofsky's (1924/25) earlier formulations of perspective as symbolic form, have utilized the research and theory about the child's development of increasingly differentiated, articulated, and integrated modes of mental representation to analyze the development of artistic modes of representation in the history of art. Using the psychological research and theory of Jean Piaget and other developmental psychologists, Jack Burnham, Samuel Edgerton, and, especially, Suzi Gablik have stressed that the psychological theory of the development of mental representation, rather than a theory of perception, may have considerable value in the study of the history of art. The development of perception and representation is interrelated, but the development of representation (or symbol formation) is a more extensive process because it includes the development of perceptual processes. Formulations from a theory of mental representation will be compatible with formulations derived from a theory of perception, but will be more encompassing. Thus a theory of mental representation can provide a model to account for the development of perspective as well as more

recent developments in the history of art that go beyond the perceptual *trompe l'oeil* of linear perspective and include the more abstract
and formal expressions in contemporary art.

Perceptual Theory Gombrich, in numerous articles, discusses "the
riddle of style" (e.g., 1960, 1966) and the necessity for establishing
normative criteria in order to consider issues of style. For Gombrich,
the classic is the basic norm from which non-classical or anti-classical
variations and deviations in principles of composition and representation can be evaluated. Dimensions of style are specified by considering what has been excluded or sacrificed in comparison to the
classic rather than as the development of an evolving structure.
Changes in style reflect choices or preferences between alternatives.
The choices involve some sacrifice or exclusion of the classical, and
the nature of these exclusions provides an understanding of the entire cultural context. "Most stylistic changes have more to do with the
mutual adjustment of conflicting norms which can perhaps be understood but never measured by any objective formal criterion. . . .
Neither normative criticisms nor morphological description alone will
ever give us a theory of style" (Gombrich, 1966, pp. 97–98). For
Gombrich (1968), style can only be considered against a background
of choices of alternative forms of expression of the classical norm.

Gombrich (1960) believes that art develops by manipulating ambiguous cues until images are indistinguishable from reality. The
processing and integration of perceptual data lead to a progressively
more differentiated and integrated "making and matching" of visual
images. Agreeing with Malraux (1954) that artistic representations
are partly based on the conventions established by predecessors,
Gombrich stresses the role of perception and the need to understand
the psychological processes of image making and image reading. He
uses perceptual theory research (e.g., Gregory 1966; Hebb, 1949) to
understand central problems in the history of art and especially why it
has taken "mankind so long to arrive at a plausible rendering of visual
effects that create the illusion of life-likeness" (1960, p. 291).

But Gombrich (1960, 1971) also calls for the development of a scale
or spectrum of configurations within which one stage can be compared with its predecessor. Within the range of the scale of
configurations or the system of schemata, various works of art can be
described and plotted at "variable distances from the central point"
(Gombrich, 1971, p. 96). According to Gombrich, visual schemata are

invented and not discovered simply by looking intensively at, or copying, nature. Art develops by the progressive invention and development of a "vocabulary of forms." Alternative forms of representation enrich and extend prior forms of schemata. One learns how to represent an object by studying the schemata or representations of earlier artists and by extending the grammar or schemata of forms (Gombrich, 1960; Olson, 1970). New forms of representation are the end product of a constant interaction between established schemata and subsequent correction. The development of new schemata or modes of expression and representation is the creative process in art.

Gombrich (1960, p. 360) discusses remarkable "inventions in the history of art," such as foreshortening, linear perspective, tonal modeling, and highlighting for texture. He stresses that the arbitrary and subjective nature of the analysis of the history of art will be diminished if we attend to the "structural relationships within a scale or matrix," rather than to the "likeness of elements" (Gombrich, 1960, p. 370). The study of structural relationships offers control of arbitrary and subjective interpretations because it indicates the modes of rendering what the artist sees and has in mind. Thus Gombrich is interested in the artist's continuing need for a vocabulary of forms that widen the range of representational possibilities. The history of art is the study of the deviation of the artist's vocabulary and modes of representation from the traditions of the past. Gombrich views the history of art as a series of decisions between alternatives based on the complex and subtle interaction between the artist and the prevailing style. It is the artist's interaction with the prevailing style, and his deviations from that style, which indicate the move toward a new level in style—the development of a new language, schema, or matrix of form. Gombrich (1960) succinctly summarizes some aspects of the development of the vocabulary of form in the history of painting:

> The primitive artist used to build up, say, a face out of simple forms rather than copy a real face. . . . We have often looked back to the Egyptians and their method of representing in a picture all they knew rather than all they saw. Greek and Roman art breathed life into the schematic forms; medieval art used them in turn for telling the sacred story. . . . Neither was urging the artist to "paint what he saw." This idea dawned only during the age of the Renaissance. . . . Scientific perspective, *"sfumato,"* Venetian colours, movement and expression, were added to the artist's means of representing the world around him; but every

generation discovered that there were still unsuspected "pockets of resistance," strongholds of conventions which made artists apply forms
they had learned rather than paint what they really saw. The nineteenth-
century rebels proposed to make a clean sweep of all these conventions;
one after another was tackled, till the Impressionists proclaimed that
their methods allowed them to render on the canvas the act of vision
with "scientific accuracy." (pp. 393–394)

Gombrich (1960, p. 370) stresses the difference between artistic
representation and perception. Artistic representations are not dupli-
cations or replicas of visual experiences, but are renderings within a
medium acquired through "tradition and skill." The history of art is
the history of the artist's overcoming limitations and widening the
range of representational possibilities. The art historian evaluates
changes in modes of representation in terms of their revision of the
prior vocabulary of form and of the traditional modes of representation. Changes in the modes of representation and the grammar
of form must be evaluated within a scale or matrix of structural relationships. The definition of this matrix could provide the framework
for the understanding of revisions and extensions of prior modes of
representation. While we may never fully understand all the factors
involved in the construction and creation of individual works of art,
an articulation of the extensions and revisions of the grammar of
form within the matrix of structured relationships can provide an
understanding of the historical development of style and some of the
social, historical, and psychological factors that may have led to the
various revisions in the history of art. Despite Gombrich's stress on
the importance of considering the extensions of the grammar of form
and modes of artistic representation within a matrix of structured
relationships, his basic model for such an analysis, however, derives
primarily from perceptual theory and research and not from a theory
of representation and symbol formation.

One of the earliest contributions in the application of perceptual
theory to art historical analysis was the work of Emanuel Loewy
(1900/1907). Based on the work of Von Hildebrand (1893/1907) and
the theories of sense-data psychology, Loewy viewed art early in the
history of civilization as expressing vague images in which sensory
impressions were retained in memory as coalesced shapes. According
to Loewy, artists early in civilization, like children, drew objects in a
direct, literal fashion based on these memory images, representing

their most distinctive features concretely, as they exist; from several points of view.

> The aspect which is selected by the memory is that which shows the form with the property that differentiates it from other forms, makes it thereby most easily distinguishable, and presents it in the greatest possible clearness and completeness of its constituent parts: this aspect will certainly be found in almost every case to be coincident with the form's greatest expansion. (Loewy, 1900/1907, p. 12)

Loewy concluded that early artists, like the child, represented objects in their most distinctive form so they could be remembered. They represent humans frontally and animals from the side or from above, depending upon which view is most distinctive. The early modes of representation involved a few typical, singular forms schematized in regular linear patterns. Figures were outlined in their broadest aspects with little overlapping of parts and without gradations of color and light or the representation of depth. For Loewy, progress in the history of art involved the struggle to overcome the pressure to retain the literal memory image in order to create the illusion of reality. The development beyond these "archaic" modes involved a gradual adjustment of the concrete image to natural appearances (Gombrich, 1960, p. 118). Loewy explained the general principles of change in the style of representation in early art as a shift from a schematic representation based on the vivid memory image, to increasingly naturalistic representations that eventually included perspective that was derived from the direct perception of the object.

Both Schapiro (1953, p. 301) and Gombrich (1960) comment that despite the limitations of Loewy's concept of the memory image as the source of an early mode of representation, his account of the characteristic structure of these early representations is valuable. Gombrich, however, is critical of Loewy's suggestion of a developmental sequence in the history of art, especially because Loewy equated the art of early societies with the drawings of the child and concluded that these societies lacked either the skill and/or the motivation "to do anything else because they still had the mentality of children" (1960, p. 22). Loewy, however, was influenced by the conception of his time, a conception of ontogeny recapitulating phylogeny, rather than a conception of parallels among developmental sequences in independent processes (e.g., the individual and the culture) in which each stage contributes in turn to the developmental process. Schapiro

(1953) comments that Loewy's formulations do not help us to understand why some cultures develop more rapidly, while others, such as the Egyptians, retained an archaic mode for many centuries. Schapiro also comments that Loewy neglected to note the specific content of the representations and, therefore, failed to recognize that in archaic art emotional factors lead to an accentuation of parts and proportions of the object. Despite these limitations, both Schapiro and Gombrich stress the importance of Loewy's contribution to the understanding of the development from archaic to naturalistic art.

After Loewy, Gustav Britsch (1926) made the next major contribution to a developmental formulation of art history based on perceptual and psychological principles. His point of view, however, was more fully articulated by Schaefer-Simmern (1948). Britsch considered that children's drawings progress through a definite structural order, similar to the development of great works of art. Order in this development of "artistic form" proceeds from simple to more complex structures—a general developmental sequence that Britsch saw as providing the basis for the growth and development of artistic activity. Later, Schaefer-Simmern (1948) extended Britsch's formulation that development in the history of art follows sequences similar to the child's development of the capacity to draw. Schaefer-Simmern considered visual configurations in art to be the result of mental activity, of the transformations of sensory experiences into a visual entity. The form and the content of this visual entity or configuration are the artist's language for expressing experiences of nature. In children's drawings and in the history of art, visual configurations create constancies of form that provide the basis for artistic creation. Rudimentary configurations are succeeded by more complicated ones. Simple outlined figures emphasize the basic distinction between figure and ground, and subsequently the spatial configuration is extended vertically and horizontally. The line becomes a plane, and planes are then integrated into structural organizations of form based on horizontal and vertical order. The simple outlined figure becomes more fully defined in terms of the relationships among parts of the figure, and this part–whole relationship provides a new structural organization. The unity in direction and organization that governs the relationships among parts of a single figure is then extended to include a larger complex of figures.

According to Schaefer-Simmern, early forms often appear along with more developed forms during the transition to a higher level of visual configuration, both in children's drawings and in art history. Initially, figures are organized side by side and above and below, and spatial depth is defined by structural organization in one plane. Figures are not arranged one behind the other because this would distort the clear structural definition of the figure and the figure–ground relationship. Depth is indicated by figures organized one above the other or, later, "by a gradual diminution in the size of the figures toward the upper part of the picture" (p. 19). Depth is subsequently represented by a parallelism of lines and "slanted lines" that not only represent angles within a plane, but also, in combinations with rectangles, create the impression of spacious depth. The use of the slanted or diagonal line and the achievement of spatial depth is a complicated form of visual conception and a particularly important nodal point in the development of more complex artistic form.

With greater differentiation within figures as well as with increasing numbers of figures in the picture, figures begin to touch. New figure–ground relationships are defined, particularly between adjacent figures. The previous sharp delineation of a single figure is replaced by a new visual conception in which there is a more gradual transition between separate figures and between parts within figures. Overlapping adds to the representation of spatial depth, while shadow and light enrich and extend the overlapping. Shadow and light attain a functional value within a definitive relationship of form, a value enriched even further when shading is extended to gradual nuances of color tones. Schaefer-Simmern considers shadow and light a mature stage of visual conception and artistic ability. Color also comes to play an increasing role in the structural order of art. Similar to the early stages in the conceptualization of form and direction, color is initially used in its pure form with great contrast and only gradually is there more differentiated use of nuances of color. In the history of art, Impressionism achieved highly differentiated color schemes to express light, air, and atmosphere and this defined a completely new approach to the visual conception of light (see also Barnhart, 1942, for a similar analysis of children's drawings).

Schaefer-Simmern is aware that he presents a condensed and idealized version of a complicated process of development. Furthermore, he seeks to explain only the development of basic pictorial artistic forms, ignoring the psychological, historical, and cultural context of art. He is interested in the specific mental activity involved in the transformations that constitute advances in visual conception. For

Schaefer-Simmern, visual conceptions evolve from simple to more complex forms of organization. Each phase of development is the preparation for the manifestations of the next stage; thus there is an inherent principle of natural growth underlying the developmental sequence observed both in the development of the child's capacity to draw and in art history.

Rudolph Arnheim (1954/1974) extended the work of Gustav Britsch and Henry Schaefer-Simmern and elaborated the natural, logical sequences in the development of art from the perception of simple patterns to increasingly complex ones. For Arnheim, as Britsch and Schaefer-Simmern, the history of art reflects the struggle to achieve an orderly representation of reality. "Pictorial form grows organically according to definite rules, from the simplest to progressively more complex patterns, in a process of gradual differentiation" (Arnheim, 1954/1974, p. 171). Along with Britsch and Schaefer-Simmern, Arnheim believes that the sequences and stages in the child's development of the capacity to draw clarifies sequences in the history of art.

Arnheim notes that initially the child, like artists early in cultural development is more concerned with generalities than specifics, drawing a simple overall image. Initially simple and isolated, the image becomes more complex and aggregate. The pictorial forms proceed from a horizontal and vertical orientation to an inclusion of the oblique, from a simple and isolated figure to the complex and aggregate. Straight lines become right angles, providing symmetry and defining relationships between directions. The right angle is the basis for the articulation of the horizontal and vertical. All angular directions are represented initially by the right angle until obliquenes is mastered. Obliqueness creates a dynamic image because it is perceived as a deviation from the invariant dimensions of horizontal and vertical. When combined with the horizontal and vertical, obliqueness provides the third dimension of space and becomes the basis for the representation of three-dimensionality. The ability to represent volume is a late development. In children's drawings, there is a gradual development from a primordial ball, to the one-dimensional stick, to the gradual differentiation of flat from cubic bodies, to the real roundedness of three-dimensional space. The representation of perspective and depth proceeds from an initial representation of each view considered in isolation in horizontal stripes, one on top of the other, to an overlapping in which there is a three-dimensional stacking, to an integration of the entire picture plane from front to back and side to side. Eventually, various views are integrated into a single, cohesive, continuous space.

Arnheim, like Gombrich, considers the figure–ground relationship a basic dimension in perception. Figure–ground contours define flat two-dimensional space parallel to the frontal plane. This can give the appearance of objects at different levels of depth—usually, however, at only two levels. Thus, figure–ground relationships are a fundamental perceptual factor in defining levels of depth. The negative space between figures is important not only in defining the relationship between the figures but also in establishing depth. Development proceeds from the figure–ground relationship, to a "stacking of frontal visual objects," to overlapping and superimposition, to transparency, and to deformations involving perspective and the oblique. All these factors contribute to the creation of depth, volume, and three-dimensionality (Arnheim, 1954/1974, p. 245). Depth is facilitated further by the use of gradients of size, texture, shape, sharpness, and dimensions of color such as brightness, saturation, and hue. Arnheim (1954/1974, p. 283), however, in contrast to Gombrich (1960), finds it paradoxical that it took so long in the history of civilization to develop perspective, since the method is suggested "most naturally to everyone by the evidence of visual experience."

The three dimensions of space define the shape and location of objects in relation to each other. At first, space is limited to a linear track, without specification of shape. Two-dimensional concepts provide limited extension into space, with a restricted capacity to create varieties of shapes and sizes and differences in direction, orientation, and placement. Eventually, in three-dimensional space, shapes can have extent, direction, and a freedom of position. The representation of changes in both shape and location, however, requires the addition of the dimension of time to the three dimensions of space. According to Arnheim (1954/1974, p. 218) extension beyond the three dimensions of space can be achieved only by "intellectual construction" since visual imagery is insufficient.

Based on Gestalt perceptual theory, Arnheim discusses the child's development of the capacity to draw as the development or the recasting of schemata in which there is a correspondence between the progressive differentiation in the child's perceptual world and in the child's drawings. Progress is accomplished by further development of a vocabulary of forms and schemata. Development in the history of art does not occur simply by drawing what is perceived, but involves instead the development of new schemata. Though Arnheim stresses the importance of the development of new schemata, he discusses progress in art primarily in terms of concepts of visual perception. Rather than distinguishing between perception and representation, Arnheim (1954/1974; 1968) differentiates the perception of effect from the perception of form and concludes that it is the change in the perception of form that is essential for the development of new schemata.

Much of Arnheim's formulation of development in the child and in the history of art is based upon Gestalt perceptual theory. While Arnheim discusses the differences between perception and representation, between recognition and imitation, he, like Gombrich, uses a theory of perception rather than a theory of mental representation as his basic model. Though Arnheim (1954/1974, p. 170) does distinguish between the "perception of effect and perception of form, the latter being needed for representation," he does not elaborate a theory of representation. Instead, he is primarily interested in perceptual processes, in dimensions of visual imagery and "visual thinking" and their role in portraying the three dimensions of space. Arnheim utilizes Gestalt perceptual principles (e.g., Kohler, 1947; Wertheimer, 1945) such as perception of good form (pragnanz), figure–ground contours, and size and shape constancy, but he does not make the leap to integrate the development of visual imagery and perceptual processes into a broader model of mental representation or, to use Arnheim's (1954/1974, p. 218) term, "intellectual construction."

Arnheim, like Loewy, Britsch, Schaefer-Simmern, and others (e.g., Barnhart, 1942; Miljkovitch, 1979), found the study of the child's development of the capacity to draw particularly useful for studying the development of perceptual processes and applying them to changes in the history of art. But recent formulations of developmental psychological theorists such as Jean Piaget (e.g., 1937/1954) and others (e.g., Werner, 1948; Werner & Kaplan, 1963) indicate that while perceptual processes are an important developmental process, they are only part of a more extensive and comprehensive development of intellectual constructions, representations, and symbolic forms. These recent theoretical formulations in developmental psychology can provide a more comprehensive model for understanding

the complex development of modes of representation that have occurred throughout the history of art.

A Theory of Mental Representation   Piaget (1937/1954) makes a fundamental distinction between perception and cognition. He defines
perception as the process of clear-cut recognition and the immediate
reading of figurative aspects in the presence of available stimuli, and
he differentiates this from processes that involve constructions, operations, and transformations of absent objects. But perception and
representation (cognition) are also closely interrelated; perception
provides the basic information for the development of cognition, and
cognitive processes in turn enrich and extend perception. Though
representation is clearly based on perceptual input, representation
goes beyond perceptual processes. Because perception and representation are interrelated, analysis of the development of style in the
history of art from a theory of perception would be consistent with
insights gained from an analysis based on representational theory, but
representational theory provides a broader and more comprehensive
theoretical model. Perceptual theory has made important contributions to understanding the development of modes of representation
in the history of art, particularly the development of linear perspective—the process of creating the *trompe l'oeil*, the highly realistic representation of a three-dimensional reality on a two-dimensional surface,
and the representation of the manifest appearance of objects within a
unified conception of space. But perceptual theory is insufficient for
understanding the more conceptual modes of representation of contemporary art.

Bernheimer (1961, p. 2) notes that "beyond the range of recognizable and familiar subject matter lay another range of vaster proportions, but of baffling indeterminacy." As Janson (1961, p. viii–ix)
comments in his introduction to Bernheimer's provocative book, *The
Nature of Representation,* abstract works of art, "whether geometric or
biomorphic," are "nonobjective" and "postrepresentational" in that
they do not depict "recognizable objects, but they nevertheless refer,
however obliquely, to a reality separate from that of the work of art
itself. They still create an illusion, an image of some kind, and to that
extent retain representational significance." Janson (p. ix) calls for "a
framework theory," a "semantics of the visual arts," that will provide a
basis for art historical analysis. For Bernheimer (p. 25), a theory of

representation would be applicable to both "reproductive" art and the
"higher symbolic phases" and could provide a comprehensive
framework for the evaluation of the function and inner structure for
all of art. A theory of representation, for example, could provide
understanding of the development of modes to represent manifest
concrete features, the development of linear perspective, and the
establishment of a unified conception of space. But a theory of representation could also provide understanding of the development of the
representation of the more abstract, symbolic, internal structure of
objects. A theory of representation could encompass both the "optical" and "conceptual" modes of representation and even provide a
basis for understanding their interrelationship. A theory of representation allows for an extension of an analysis of the history of art
based on perceptual processes of image making and image reading
(Arnheim, 1954/1974; Gombrich, 1960) to an analysis based on cognitive processes and the construction of symbols. A theory of representation would consider the different modes of representation
throughout the history of art as various expressions of symbol formation.

Art historians, such as Gombrich and Arnheim, have used the term
representation as an expression for artistic performance in a particular medium. The term representation has been used by philosophers
(e.g., Cassirer, 1955) and in genetic epistemology (e.g., Piaget 1937/
1954) to refer to a conceptual, imagined, or internal event that lies
behind behavior. Representation in philosophy refers to both the
content and the structural form of an internal event. In psychology,
modes of representation refer to cognitive structures—the abstract
processes that mediate between perception and construction (Olson,
1970). The development of new cognitive structures (modes of representation) is a critical aspect of individual human development and a
crucial aspect of the development of culture. The development of
these cognitive structures is particularly apparent in the development
of modes of representation (construction) in the history of art.[2] The

---

[2] It would be more accurate to reserve the term representation for the
mental event and utilize the term construction for the artistic process. But in
order to maintain continuity and consistency with prior terminology, the term
representation is used to refer to the cognitive structure expressed in the
mental event (mental representation) as well as to the artistic product (artistic
representation).

artist learns how to render nature from tradition—from established modes of representation that must be extended and revised to create a new style. New styles and new modes of representation in art are grounded in prior modes and are the result of experiments with past and present achievements and motifs. The innovator must revise established cognitive structures and the mental set predominant in the culture and actively seek alternative interpretations and modes of representation. These revisions, however, are more than a simple rejection or revision of established modes, but involve creative extensions of prior modes of experience and representation. When viewed from this perspective, then, the history of art is a series of experiments to find new modes of representation that facilitate adding a new dimension to the experience of the reality that the artist seeks to communicate.

As discussed in Chapter 2, substantial research has been conducted on the individual's development of modes of representation and symbolic forms. This research can provide a theoretical model for the understanding of the progressive development of symbolic forms within the history of art, a model external to art itself and with considerable validity and scope in its own right. Application of such a theoretical model allows the successive transformations in artistic representation throughout history to be considered in relation to the broad topic of the development of cognitive processes. The vocabulary of form or the system of schemata sought by art historians, such as the development from haptic to optic (e.g., Riegl) or optical to conceptual or schematic to perspective to impressionistic (Fry, R. E., cited by Gombrich, 1960), can be considered as part of a general development of symbolic forms. Loewy's formulation of progress in the history of art as the overcoming of the pressure to retain the memory of the literal object to create the illusion of reality, for example, can be considered as part of the process in which there is a change in symbol formation from concrete, literal representation to those in which there is an integration of objective and subjective dimensions.

To study processes of representation in art history as forms of symbol construction shifts the focus from understanding art as an imitation of nature to an emphasis on the symbolic operations and conceptual schemata inherent in artistic representation. It diminishes the need to differentiate between imitation (perception) and representation (construction) and allows all art to be considered as conceptual. Like language, artistic styles differ in their articulation and in the number and types of questions they allow the artist to ask and answer (Gombrich, 1960). The study of artistic modes of representation as symbolic operations can provide a conceptualization of the grammar of forms and the schemata of representations that could facilitate the study of the longitudinal development of style (a diachronic analysis) and the identification of similarities in the symbolic form expressed in the multiple cognitive endeavors of the culture—in its art, literature, mores, philosophy, religion, science, and social order (a synchronic analysis) (see, e.g., Peckham, 1965; Praz, 1970; Ruskin, 1873; Schapiro, 1937; Sypher, 1955, 1960).

Erwin Panofsky (1924/25), in his seminal contribution that considers perspective as "symbolic form," was among the first to anticipate the importance of a theory of mental representation and symbol formation for understanding the development of style. Panofsky considered both the content and the formal dimensions of art in his formulation of style. In terms of the content of art, he differentiated between apparent meaning and the intrinsic or symbolic meaning. Apparent meaning is the primary or natural subject matter, the literal meaning of ideas, the stated facts and their interrelationships. Apparent meaning consists of the conventional subject matter, the larger themes and concepts of general cultural and historical knowledge. Yet another level of meaning, according to Panofsky (1955b), is a synthesis of the apparent meaning of the general cultural context with relevant ideas from other humanistic disciplines. On this level, evidence from other fields is integrated with the ideas expressed in art. The relationship of ideas among related fields is the intrinsic meaning of the subject. Panofsky contrasts the study of the intrinsic meaning of images (iconology) with the apparent and cultural meaning of art (iconography).

When considering the formal, or structural features of composition, Panofsky (1924/25) was particularly interested in the development of perspective as a symbolic form that reflected the general cognitive orientation of the Renaissance: Panofsky discussed the development of perspective primarily in terms of the development of symbolic forms and of modes of representational construction and not as a matter of artistic or aesthetic merit. He discussed the development of the representation of space as proceeding from a figure in isolation, to space as an aggregate of figures, to space as a comprehensive and coordinated system. According to his theory, the achievement of perspective during the Renaissance was only one ex-

pression of the developments in epistemology and science that occurred at this particular moment in history. The development of
perspective in art was part of the general repudiation of an Aristotelian world view, in which the cosmos was built around the midpoint of
the earth as the absolute center enclosed by outermost spheres of the
heavens as an absolute limit. This conception of the universe was
replaced by conceptions of infinity, defined both in terms of God and
nature.

Building upon Panofsky's formulations, several art historians
(Burnham, 1971; Edgerton, 1975; Gablik, 1976) began to consider
modes of representation in art. as a process of the development of
symbolic forms and cognitive schemata. They have begun to use the
development of representation, particularly as formulated by Jean
Piaget, as a broad theoretical basis for an analysis of the history of art.
Burnham (1971) discusses the importance of concepts of structuralism in the work of Piaget and Levi-Strauss for art historical analysis.
Edgerton (1975) bases his analysis of the development of linear perspective on Piaget's formulations of the child's development from an
initially egocentric viewpoint to a growing understanding of "space
structuration." Edgerton notes clear parallels between the development of linear perspective from the Middle Ages to the Renaissance and the development of the child in learning to perceive
abstract structured visual space and linear perspective (Ginsburg &
Opper, 1969; cited by Edgerton, 1975). In evaluating this developmental process, Edgerton stresses that one should not consider
early stages in the history of Western Civilization, such as the medieval
European period, as a regression but rather as "qualitatively different" and as "an entity in its own right," not in contrast to the eventual
or current level of function, but in contrast to the preceding stage.

The developmental model of representation based on Piaget's formulations, first introduced into an analysis of the history of art by
Burnham and subsequently elaborated by Edgerton, received fuller
consideration in the work of Gablik (1976). Gablik proposes that art,
like the history of science, develops and progresses in a continuous,
orderly process. She is particularly interested in the development of
form in the history of art and how it relates to the structure of mental
processes as articulated by Jean Piaget. Gablik considers developmental growth in the history of art as part of an integrated system that
expresses an unfolding of structure similar to the laws of development of cognitive processes in the child. Gablik (1976) agrees

with Piaget that the child's development of intelligence essentially defines a "genetic epistemology"—the study of the genesis of systems of knowledge in many different areas. The history of art reflects a distinctive cognitive process that has evolved through stages and fundamental transformations to increasingly more complex and logical schemata. Gablik (p. 12) stresses that there is a "clear and unbroken line of development" in the history of art expressed in the "transformations of space and the elements of geometric form: flat planes, deep space, proportion, regularity, symmetry, progression and the structuring of measured relationships." She discusses how the capacity to represent the human figure as a total volume developed as a continuous process in which new strategies continually emerged and led to a greater synthesis, proceeding from a semi-static, semicontinuous configuration to configurations that are continuous and kinetic.

Basing her work on Piaget, Gablik discusses the development of cognitive structures or schemata, and how they provide the basis for the organization of knowledge progressing from relative globality and lack of differentiation to stages of increasing differentiation, articulation, and integration. Gablik delineates three stages in the development of mental schemata and demonstrates a similar sequence in the history of art. First in a preoperational stage the basic mode is enactive and the spatial concepts are topological. This stage is expressed primarily in ancient and medieval art. The second is a stage of concrete operations in which the mode is iconic and the concepts of space are projective and Euclidean. Gablik (1976) sees this stage of mental schemata as occurring primarily from the Renaissance to the modern period. In the third stage, one of formal operations, the mode is symbolic with an indeterminate concept of space. This stage is expressed primarily in the modern period. For Gablik, the history of art is a slow, laborious liberation of forms from content and a move away from the iconic modes of representation to the expression of formal logical systems dealing with pure abstract relations. Contemporary art moves toward formal operational thought and away from the "grip" of the concrete image. Although she discusses these separate stages, Gablik (1976, p. 46) stresses the continuity between them—"Each stage carries the seeds of the next phase, and each new cognitive structure includes elements of earlier structures but transforms them in such a way as to represent a more stable and extensive equilibrium." Spatial conceptions cannot be reduced to "pure perception, or to a system of images" (1976, p. 73), but are based on cognitive operations in which eventually there are transformations and coordinations of multiple dimensions in operational thought. Gablik, like Piaget, stresses the difference between perception and representation and notes that perception is literal, direct, and immediate, while representations involve transformation, integration, and coordination of perceptual experiences. Representation thus transcends perception. The mental image of an object is not a simple copy of the object, but rather a mental construction and representation, a series of transformations and operations that organize and integrate perceptual experiences and coordinate different dimensions and aspects of objects. In applying Piaget's developmental concepts of representation to an analysis of art history, Gablik considers the development of art from classical to contemporary times and demonstrates the shifting and evolving schemata in three major epochs. She discusses extensively the shift from iconic to formal modes of representation and its implications for understanding modern art. The analysis of the history of art to be presented in this book is in the tradition of Panofsky, Bernheimer, Burnham, Edgerton, and Gablik.

A STRUCTURAL ANALYSIS OF A
VOCABULARY OF FORM

The persistent call in art history for the identification of a "vocabulary of form," "a system of schemata," "a matrix or scale of structured relationships" is consistent with the recent attempt in a number of disciplines to define the principles and cognitive structures that underlie all human intellectual endeavors. Structuralists (e.g., Chomsky, 1968/1972; Jakobson, 1960; Lacan, 1977; Levi-Strauss, 1963; Piaget, 1970b; Werner and Kaplan, 1963) in a variety of different disciplines have sought to identify organizational principles and structures that provide rationality and order for human behavior. This search for the underlying, unverbalized (unconscious) order in cognitive endeavors is a quest for the identification of the basic constructs through which individuals understand and organize their universe. Structuralists seek to identify and define the innate (deep) cognitive structures and the rules through which these cognitive structures evolve and are transformed (Lane, 1970). The interest in inner form and structure rather than manifest form and content allows for the possibility of specifying the basic cognitive structures that occur in all spheres of human intellectual endeavor. The underlying hierarchical organization of forms, patterns, and structures in general systems—the innate mechanisms and rules of transformation, the similarities in organization and origin that are below apparently similar or dissimilar surface qualities (Overton, 1975)—can provide homologies which can be applied to intellectual activity in a diversity of contexts. Basic to the identification of form, configuration, pattern, and structure is the concept of an ordered complexity governed by underlying principles that define the development and transformation of the forms of manifest shape (Whyte, 1951).

The basic relationships of form and their processes of transformation, discussed as "cognitive schemata," patterns, or gestalts, have been used to understand neurological processes (Head, 1920), memory (Bartlett, 1958; Paul, 1959), perception (Koffka, 1935; Köhler, 1947; Wertheimer, 1945), information processing (e.g., Miller, Galanter, & Pribram, 1960), linguistics (e.g., Chomsky, 1968/1972; Jakobson, 1960; de Saussure, 1959), social order (e.g., Levi-Strauss, 1963), and the development of children (e.g., Piaget, 1929/1965, 1970b; Werner & Kaplan, 1963). In psychoanalysis, Guttman (1973) has also discussed concepts of structure in personality organization (e.g., id, ego, superego) as the mechanisms and processes that are relatively stable (Hartmann, Kris, & Loewenstein, 1946) or develop at a slow rate of change (Rapaport & Gill, 1959). The definition of structures in psychoanalysis as the relatively stable organizations of mental functions is consistent with the concept of structure in contemporary theories of art and science. A structural analysis identifies the formal connections that define a system—the elements in their own right and the relationships and interrelationships among the elements. Guttman (1973) sees the search for the concept of structure in psychoanalysis and in other areas, such as art and science, as an attempt to understand the cohesive, or organizing, forces that maintain individuals in an integrated state, enabling them to relate successfully to their environment.

Cognitive organization is clearly more than a simple accumulation of individual elements of sense data, but is a function of a coordinated network of patterns determined by structural laws. Modern concepts have moved away from a simple emphasis on individual elements of sense data, to a much higher order of complexity in which elements are placed in a hierarchy of relations and interrelations. Structuralists believe that understanding the patterns of interrelationships is the key to understanding all intellectual endeavors. The understanding of structure and structural principles is more than defining independent parts. It is an understanding of the interconnections and interactions of complex elements in which parts interact with one another within a hierarchy of substructures proceeding from relatively low levels of structure to superordinate structures (Guttman, 1973). In contrast to outer form, structure is the "form seen inside, as the definitive arrangement, static or changing, of localized parts" (Whyte, 1965, p. 21). The specification of the actual and potential transformations of elements and their interrelationships leads to the identification of a variety of levels of interaction within a hierarchy of substructures that continue to interact to form superstructures. The evolution of these organizing structures can be considered in all cognitive endeavors—in art, literature, mathematics, philosophy, science, and in concepts of time, space, and causality (Cassirer, 1946).

The invariant forms and their rules of transformation are regularities that specify the basic principles of organization and structure. For example, despite the apparent diversity, instability, and disorder of multiple languages, customs, and rituals in a wide range of cultures, structural anthropologists (Durkheim, 1912/1976; Hertz, 1909/1973; Levi-Strauss, 1963; Mauss, 1950/1954; Needham, 1973) have discussed a set of invariant forms, such as binary opposition (right–left, up–down, etc.), and transformational rules that are expressed in kinship patterns, customs, myths, and language of all cultures. They have identified some of the relationships of surface manifestations of the society to the basic principles of social organization and of the structure of the mind. They have identified "binary opposition" as a fundamental cognitive structure that appears in myth and kinship formations in primitive and civilized societies. The universal tendency to develop dichotomies and to perceive opposites suggested to Needham (1973, p. xxxiii) that "human beings all over the world tend to order themselves and their environment in remarkably similar ways, and by implicit recourse to classificatory principles so general and adaptive as to appear natural proclivities of the human mind." In similar investigations, linguists (e.g., Chomsky, Jakobson) have also sought to identify a set of invariant forms and transformational rules that are the basic syntax of all language. Jakobson and Chomsky identified structural dimensions in linguistics and demonstrated how these structural properties in language are similar to principles in visual perception (Tynianov & Jakobson, 1928/1972). Concepts of differentiation and integration, binary opposition, structured stages, and developmental progression are present in individual cognitive development and are expressed in a multitude of cultural processes including language and social organization.

In their investigations of basic structures in individual development of cognitive processes, Piaget (1937/1954, 1970) and other developmental psychologists (e.g., Werner & Kaplan, 1963) define a number of levels of cognitive structures ranging from sensorimotor, to preoperational, to intuitive, to concrete and, eventually, to formal, operational thought. These structures organize and direct behavior in an increasingly comprehensive and effective fashion. Although individuals are unaware of these underlying structures, they are the basic coherent principles that determine human behavior and experience. These underlying elements of form—their relationships and transformations—are reflected in a multitude of overt forms in individual thought and action, and in the basic structure and organization of society (Rosenwald, 1975).

In a structural analysis, the primary emphasis is upon holistic conceptions in which there are attempts to define the underlying structures, the relation and organization of elements into forms and patterns, and the transformation of these patterns into more complex levels of organization. The formal systems can be placed in a hierarchy of relative "strength and weakness" (Piaget, 1970b, p. 33). Evolution of structures is a continuous process of transformation and construction. These "operational" structures are transformational and result in higher, more formal systems that allow for the testing of earlier presuppositions and propositions. A higher level of abstraction is needed to test a proposition of an earlier and lower level system (Godol, 1965, cited by Piaget, 1970b). A procedure, or a conceptualization, cannot be used to assess its own validity—one needs an external methodology or a higher order of generality to assess the validity of propositions within a given system. An understanding of the development of structures in one area, for example, could provide an independent model for studying the development of structures in another area.[3]

Structuralism derives in part from Kant and from Cassirer's neo-Kantian views, which stress that knowledge of nature is a function of the categories we utilize to organize experiences. Kant and Cassirer were interested in the innate capacities and structures of the human mind, the unformulated modes of organization that form the basis of a person's cognitive constructions. Cassirer sought to unify the sciences by articulating the forms and functions of cognition into a universal order. He sought to define the symbolic forms inherent in all human endeavors that allow for the transformation of impressions into a world of knowledge. The problems of representation and the structure of consciousness, specified in various kinds of temporal, spatial, and causal relationships, are central to all symbolic activity. A system of "transcendental logic" enables individuals to construct subjective schemata that organize experience and knowledge. The schemata, in turn, influence the perceptual experiences in both the selection and processing of sensory information into systematic forms of knowledge. Thus, these schemata have an important role in constructing an understanding of nature, and they are expressed in art, literature, and science. Symbolic forms and the development of meaning are creative cognitive constructions that organize and shape understanding of, and interaction with, nature. Time, space, and causality are intuitions and symbolic constructions that order experience and provide the basis of knowledge. The range of available symbolic forms is determined by our sensory apparatus and neurological structures, and the innate conceptual structures already available within the society. The characteristics of our sensory ap-

---

[3]Structuralism, of course, as a theory and a method, like all intellectual endeavors, reflects the cognitive structure (episteme) of our time—the search for internal structure and organization and for abstract principles. This contemporary emphasis on underlying structure and principles of organization is like the search for subatomic particles, the interest in abstract art, and the emphasis on relativity and a holistic field. Structuralism, as a theoretical model, dominates current modes of investigation in numerous disciplines. Numerous areas search for the stable principles of internal organization that underlie variations of surface manifestations. The entire movement of structuralism is our contemporary mental construction through which we attempt to bring order and organization to our experience.

paratus and neurophysiological and psychological processes both facilitate and limit our conception of the universe and determine all our observations, including our scientific concepts and theories. Representations and cognitive schemata are the mental structures through which we observe, organize, understand, and appreciate nature. The structural organization of these modes of representation evolves over time, both within the individual and in the history of civilization. We continually construct the cognitive schemata we apply to nature.

For Kant (1871/1929) and Cassirer (1946), the universe does not have objective properties such as finitude or infinitude. Space is not an inherent dimension of reality that must be learned in experience, but a particular construction of the human mind. Space, time, and causality do not exist as dimensions in external reality that are perceived and learned; they are constructs imposed on experiences to establish order and organization. They serve as the basis for all understanding and knowledge. The cognitive schemata reflect the various ways experiences are processed, retained, organized, stored, and transformed (e.g., Falmagne, 1975; Miller, Galanter, & Pribram, 1960; Newell & Simon, 1972). Predominant cognitive schemata indicate the range of cognitive processes available within a culture, as well as an individual's preferred cognitive modes—the way one experiences, knows, remembers, and thinks about the world. The construction of representations is a process of establishing formats for the encoding of information and experiences so they can be retained effectively in memory. Representation, like memory, is an active, constructive process (Loewald, 1976) that bears the stamp of the situation, the individual's prior experiences, and his level of cognitive development.

Modes of representation evolve within the life cycle of the individual and through the history of civilization (Piaget, 1970b). Scientific conceptions of the universe, for example, illustrate how cognitive constructions and representations have evolved over time. And likewise, in the history of art, the modes of representing a three-dimensional reality on a two-dimensional surface have become increasingly differentiated, articulated, and integrated. These modes of representation are not inherent in reality. Rather, they are constructions by individuals within a culture through which they attempt to bring organization to their experiences.

Piaget (1971) asserts that his study of the cognitive growth of the individual essentially defines a genetic epistemology that can be applied to the study of the development of cognitive stuctures in the history of civilization. According to Piaget, cognitive structures in the history of civilization have evolved through the same major stages of development that he observed in individuals–stages of sensorimotor-preoperational, intuitive, and concrete and formal operational thought.[4] Piaget (1970b) asserts that there is a basic parallelism between the developmental processes in the individual and in the history of civilization. The study of these parallel forms in the individual can provide guidelines for understanding the development of cognitive schemata in cultural history. The fact that the development of cognitive schemata in the history of civilization parallels the development of the individual need not demean or depreciate earlier stages in the history of civilization. Rather, it only implies that people and civilizations learn from each other and, therefore, the forms of cognitive structures early in a developmental sequence will be less differentiated, articulated, integrated, and complex than cognitive structures that occur later.

Symbolic constructions evolved developmentally over the major epochs in the history of civilization and are expressed in multiple ways in the culture. Panofsky (1924/25), for example, discussed how the concepts of infinity, homogeneous space, and linear perspective were all part of the same conceptual structure that began late in the Renaissance and continued through the 17th and 18th centuries and was expressed in a variety of endeavors in art, science, literature, and theology. Impressed with the structural similarity that appears simultaneously in a large number of different disciplines, Foucault (1970) sought to characterize the nature of cognitive structures in order to construct a theory of scientific change and epistemological causality. He believes that a hidden network determines the way various areas interact—an inherent inner law or fundamental code of a culture that governs language, schemes of perception, techniques, values, practices, mores. Foucault (1970, p. xxii) refers to this underlying order as epistemes, in which knowledge is not related to rational value or

---

[4]Concepts of the deity, for example, early in civilization, were primarily based on concrete physical events and nautral phenomena and cycles. Subsequently, there was a personification of the deity into specific individual(s); later the concept became more abstract, involving something unseen and unknown, and, even later, a set of formal ideals and principles.

objective forms, but rather to "configurations within the *space* of knowledge which have given rise to the diverse forms of empirical science," (Foucault's italics). Piaget (1970b, p. 132), however, is critical of Foucault for simply defining Kantian "historical apriorities" and conditions for knowledge, without adequately discussing or explaining the sequences in which they occur. Piaget comments that Foucault's cultural epistemes are described as simply following one another in the course of history, without defining the fundamental principles or the epistemological structures of the period or how these principles relate to those of the periods that precede and follow. Also Foucault fails to define the conditions necessary for the emergence of a new episteme or to evaluate its validity. Piaget (1970, p. 132) is also critical of Foucault's attempt to describe the cognitive nucleus common to "all subjects at the same level" and at the time, without relating this synchronic analysis to the epistemes of other periods, either developmentally or historically. Piaget (1970b) goes on to argue for the importance of a diachronic analysis in the study of cognitive structures because it is only through the subsequent development of "stronger" or more comprehensive structures and systems that the validity of an earlier, more elementary structure (Godol, 1965) can be ascertained. This criticism was actually inherent in the comments of Tynianov and Jakobson a number of years earlier when they noted that the distinction between diachronic and synchronic relationships may be partly illusory because each synchronic system had a past and a future, and these are essential structural elements of the system— "the history of a system is in turn also a system . . . each synchronic system contains its past and future as inseparable structural elements of the system" (Tynianov & Jakobson, 1928/1972, p. 82).

Cultural history is often characterized by sudden and thorough reorganizations in which similar changes occur at the same time in diverse disciplines. These changes are governed by revisions in the basic cognitive schemata or epistemes of a culture—the set of unconscious (unformulated)[5] presuppositions about the nature of the universe. Revisions of these presuppositions reflect a fundamental change in the conception of the world and of nature. Kuhn—(1962/

---

[5] Foucault, like Lacan, defines the unconscious descriptively, as the unformulated and unverbalized. This is in contrast to the psychoanalytic concept of the unconscious that is dynamic rather than descriptive.

1970) discusses major shifts in the conceptual structure and rules of discourse in the history of science. These changes involve an entire constellation of related ideas in science, art, philosophy, and religion. These "paradigmatic" shifts in conceptual structure occur with a beginning awareness that some aspect of nature has been either ignored or violated in current understanding and representation. The new awareness brings with it a more or less extended exploration to correct the anomaly or inconsistency. Exploration ends when there is a paradigmatic shift in cognitive structure that, for the time, resolves the problems and inconsistencies. Subsequent research attempts to articulate the paradigm, examine its implications, and increase its precision until another inconsistency or anomaly is noted. The identification and solution of the anomaly results in another universally recognized reorganization and the cycle repeats itself. Thus, theories in science do not develop through gradual, steady accumulation of individual discoveries and inventions, but by drastic shifts—revolutions—that alter the currently acceptable conceptualizations as well as the historical perspective of scientists regarding past accomplishments. The scientific revolution produces a shift in the problems available for scientific scrutiny and transforms the very nature of scientific inquiry. There is a reconstruction of prior theory, "an intrinsically revolutionary process that is seldom completed by a single man and never overnight" (Kuhn, 1962/1970, p. 7). Paradigmatic shifts are "non-cumulative developmental episodes in which an older paradigm is replaced in whole or in part by an incompatible new one" (Kuhn, 1962/1970, p. 92). These scientific revolutions are initiated by the growing awareness that an existing paradigm is no longer adequate for explaining and facilitating the exploration of nature. Successive stages in the developmental process are marked by significant shifts in the definition of both potential problems and possible solutions, and this process occurs without benefit of a goal or a permanently fixed scientific truth (Kuhn, 1962/1970).[6]

According to Kuhn, the succession of tradition-bound periods punctuated by discontinuous, noncumulative breaks describes not only scientific development but also the history of literature, music,

---

[6] As discussed earlier, several art historians (Ackerman, Gombrich, and Hauser) make a similar point in discussions of development in the history of art when they insist that art does not move toward a predefined or ideal goal, but rather progresses by revisions of prior modes of representation.

art, and political development. The history of Western Civilization is often separated into major epochs and periods in terms of revolutionary stylistic revisions. Difficulties in the conceptualization of style in the history of art could be resolved if the development of painting could be seen in terms of paradigmatic shifts rather than abstract canons of style. Major figures in the history of art, such as Michelangelo, Leonardo, Rembrandt, and Cézanne, invented solutions for inconsistencies and anomalies they sensed in the existing modes of representation. Their revisions of the modes of representation, much like the contributions of Aristotle, Copernicus, Newton, and Einstein in science, constitute paradigmatic shifts—revolutions in the history of art. Continuity and change in art, like in science, can be understood and conceptualized by examining the major developments and paradigmatic shifts that occur within particular dimensions.

Art is an aesthetic expression of the symbolic system of a culture, and as such it is an integral part of the culture's predominant mode of representation—its contemporary conceptual and symbolic construction. The procedures artists invent for representing aspects of nature on a two-dimensional surface are expressions of the particular conception and organization of reality available within the society. When a new conception or level of representation is implicit within the culture, artists develop procedures for representing that conception of reality. Conversely, pressure for stability within a culture discourages the exploration of new modes of conceptualization and representation in all cognitive endeavors including art. Thus changes in modes of representation occur at a variable rate, but when changes do occur they follow a logical developmental sequence. These symbolic systems are transmitted from one culture to another and they evolve and develop as extensions of the accomplishments of prior cultures. But the artistic style of each culture expresses the culture's predominant symbolic conception of reality and the universe. As Clark (1969) has asserted, artists have always responded intuitively to the culture's latent assumptions about the nature and shape of the universe.

Cognitive structures evolve in open systems such as in subject–object and social interactions. Individuals as well as cultures establish and revise levels of cognitive schemata when inconsistencies and anomalies are encountered. The anomalies are expressions of an egocentrism and the process of "decentration" from this egocentricity is the "generator" of new structures (Piaget, 1970b, p. 66). Decentration involves establishing new coordinations and reciprocal relationships that resolve prior inconsistencies and anomalies (Olson, 1970). For Piaget (1970b), the construction of new cognitive structures is an unending process that proceeds by reflective abstraction from one structure to a higher, more comprehensive structure. Since structures are open systems of operational transformations, there can always be a more encompassing structure. Thus, the ascertaining of the ultimate structure of all structures is an unobtainable ideal.

Mental constructions or cognitive schemata are attempts to organize the individual's personal relationships with reality (Bion, cited by Home, 1966). These symbolic constructions are expressed in the multiple cognitive endeavors of the culture and they are transmitted and expressed in multiple ways in the basic fabric of the culture, including its child-rearing practices. They are transmitted to the child in an interpersonal matrix, in the relationship between a child and its caring agents, and in the child's relationship to its culture at large (Blatt, 1974; Parsons & Bales, 1955; Vygotsky, 1962). Vygotsky (1962) discusses the ontogenesis of regulatory processes, of all specifically mediated human mental processes, and how they arise only in the course of social interaction—in the process of cooperation and social intercourse. Psychological functions are at first shared between two people, in particular between a child and an adult, and later become the internalized psychological processes of one person (usually the child, but not exclusively so). Thus, cognitive structures are present in external social activity and are internalized by the child as the structures of mental processes. The development of language is an example of the child's progressive internalization of the cognitive structures that exist within the culture. From numerous theoretical perspectives, the social or interpersonal interaction between caretaking agents and the child provides the basic experience necessary for the establishment of mental structures. Structuralists (e.g., Lacan, 1968; Levi-Strauss, 1963; Piaget, 1937/1954, 1970b) stress the importance of object relationships—the intimate experience of the other—as essential for the development of all human cognition and mental activity. The child acquires these basic cognitive structures in direct interpersonal relationships; structures are transmitted through language, custom, ritual, and knowledge within the culture. The development of these basic cognitive structures (schemata), however, can be acquired by the child only to the highest level of cognitive structures available within the society. Members of the society can utilize cognitive structures only as far as they have been articulated and evolved within the society. With the discovery of new knowledge or with a change in social conditions, the society may establish a new level of cognitive schemata, which will then be transmitted through the interpersonal, parent–child relationship and the cultural matrix. Thus, while cognitive structures of the culture facilitate the understanding of reality, they also place limits on the capacity of the human mind to make finer differentiations and more complex integrations. While individuals possess the inherent potential to develop more complex, integrated and abstract cognitive structures, the development of new cognitive structures is dependent upon their being articulated initially within the culture at large.

Recent cross-cultural research by Abel (1981) indicates that there are major cultural constraints placed upon the cognitive structures available to individuals within that culture. Abel studied the cognitive processes of Navajo and Pueblo Indian adolescent boys and girls who were 16 to 18 years old, of at least average intelligence, and enrolled in a Catholic high school. Abel's data clearly indicate that utilization of cognitive schemata is determined by cultural traditions and not by capacities or potential of the individual. Navajo and Pueblo native art is flat and two-dimensional. In studying Indian adolescents, Abel found that when they were working with the two-dimensional mosaics of the Lowenfeld Mosaics Test, they made designs primarily from the Indian culture, such as ritual figures and symbols, a hogan (a native hut), rug designs (Navajo), or implements of importance in the Pueblos and Indian reservations such as a truck. When working with three-dimensional geometric forms of the Lowenfeld Kleidoblocs Test (e.g., cubes, rectangles, rods, and arcs), the Indian adolescents made themes primarily from the urban, non-Indian culture such as apartment complexes, shopping centers, oil derricks, "houses of the future." The data indicate that while these children were capable of three-dimensional representations and constructions, items from the Indian culture were represented only in the culturally determined and approved two-dimensional structure. Thus, the utilization of particular cognitive schemata appears to be determined primarily by cultural tradition rather than individual capacities. These findings are consistent with earlier reports by Segull, Campbell, and Herskovitz (1963) and Scribner (1974) that suggest that cultural and environmental factors strongly influence learned visual habits.

New and advanced cognitive structures are articulated in paradigmatic shifts. When these cognitive structures are consolidated as a mode of thought within the culture, they then can be transmitted to the developing child. Earlier phases of the child's development reflect less developed forms of the culture's cognitive structures, while the most advanced cognitive structures of the culture are internalized as a general mode of thought by the most able members of the culture. And it is this group of individuals who possess the potential to revise the current cognitive schemata for the culture's next paradigmatic shift in cognitive structure. Adolescents and young adults in a society often provide the impetus for change and revision of the current, established modes of thought. Creative and talented adolescents are often those members of the society who have usually adequately internalized the cultural values and the contemporary cognitive schemata of the society, but are still sufficiently open and uncommitted so that they can recognize anomalies and inconsistencies and consider revisions of contemporary social norms and modes of thought. This capacity to consider revisions of the basic cognitive structures of a society is the most mature and creative expression of the more general task in which adolescents seek to define themselves as separate and individuated from their parents, while still retaining ties to their cultural heritage. On an individual basis with their families, as well as on a cultural level, adolescents and young adults seek to revise, modify, and refine contemporary values and modes of thought. For this revision to be effective it must maintain, to some degree, a continuity with the past. It is this process of modification, revision, and extension of contemporary schemata that makes cultural development a progressive process with a developmental history.

Obviously, we cannot anticipate the next level of cognitive development until it is expressed within the cultural matrix. Once it has been articulated within the cultural context, it is communicated to the members of that culture as a new form of cognitive schemata. Thus we possess both the collective inheritance and current cognitive limitations of our culture. Every individual participates in the "cultural collective consciousness," but the "profound collective passage" of individuals in the development of this collective consciousness is "beyond our comprehension" (Huyghe, 1974, p. 32). Observations of the child's development of cognitive schemata, however, may provide some guideposts to an understanding of how this process has evolved in the past.

The child's evolving conception of reality provides a model through which we can more fully understand the formal and structural dimensions of attempts to render experiences of nature onto a two-dimensional surface. It should be stressed, however, that this is a model of the development of the formal or structural aspects of the concept of the object and of space. These structures, rather than content, can contribute to establishing a basis for articulating a language and grammar of forms, the matrix or system of schemata, which many art historians consider necessary for a systematic evaluation of the modes of representation in the history of art. The child's evolving capacity to construct mental representations of the world, particularly its spatiotemporal dimensions, provides a model that can facilitate further understanding of developments in the history of art. In both the development of the child and in the history of art, representations progress from concrete, literal depictions of the most distinctive, manifest features of objects and events, to more subjective representations of reality based on foreshortening, perspective, and subtleties of nuances of color and shading to express affect and feeling; to representations of nature that are abstract and express the underlying, internal structure of a flexible, mobile universe in unending flux.

Hauser (1953/1959), Friedlaender (1958), and Giedion (1941/1967, 1962), discuss the importance of changes in the representation of the form of objects and of space for understanding developments in the history of art. Friedlaender, for example (1958, p. 8), comments on "the struggle between the picture surface and the presentation of depth in space which is of such vital importance throughout the whole history of art." For Giedion (1962), the all-embracing quality of art is the experience of space. All artistic utterances reflect spatial conceptions and thereby conceptions of the world and nature. Space, for Giedion, portrays the unconscious relations with the environment. The spatial

> conception of a period provides . . . an insight into its attitudes toward the cosmos, mankind, and external values. . . . [These] attitudes toward space change continually, sometimes in very small degree, sometimes basically. But there have been very few space conceptions throughout the whole development of man. Each has covered long periods of time. Within each of these epochs, however, many variations and transitions have occurred; for man's attitude toward space, always in a state of suspension, can shift almost infinitely within the framework of the overriding concept. (p. 516)

Probably the most extensive and eloquent statement about the importance of the representation of space in the history of art has been the work of Henri Focillon who discussed at length the life of forms in the representation of objects and of space. For Focillon, the mind seeks to create forms out of its experiences in nature, inventing new forms by revising and extending prior forms. Focillon (1934/1948) is convinced that it is possible, and would be highly useful, to build up a "psychographic method" based on the tendency of the mind to create new forms. The creation of forms is a basic aspect of human consciousness so that "even at levels far below the zone of definition and clarity, forms, measures, and relationships exist" (p. 44). Form mediates between individuals and nature; nature is experienced in and conceived of through form. Focillon believes that a psychology of art requires a definition of "the processes whereby the life of forms in the mind . . . taking natural objects as the point of departure, makes them matters of imagination and memory, of sensibility and intellect" (p. 47). Forms are for Focillon, "the very substances of art . . . at the crossroads of psychology and physiology." They are "the concrete and active forces powerfully at work among the things of matter and space" (pp. 49–50).

Focillon draws a parallel between the world of forms in the artist's representation of space and matter and the world of forms in the mind. They are identical in principle and "differ only in plan or, possibly, in perspective." The activity of the artist and of the mind is to create a world of forms that are "complex, coherent, and concrete" (p. 44). Focillon stresses how each of us in our night dreams, daydreams, and memories constructs images and forms of beings and nature in a space of "illusory authenticity" (p. 45). Artists struggle to use these mental forms "to free themselves from the tyranny of the model" of prior forms, in order to construct new forms. The life of forms "in the mind is simply a preparation for its life in space" (p. 46). The development of forms is guided by a process of "metamorphosis" that "go[es] forever forward, by its own necessity, toward its own liberty" (p. 64). While the development of forms may follow a progression, the life of forms is not governed by a strict, flawless, predestined constancy. While there are limits imposed on potential metamorphosis of form that can occur at a particular time by nature, by our minds, and by the cultural context, within these broad limitations, there is a wealth of alternatives that can be introduced into this order by individual artists.

Focillon notes that there is a basic correspondence between certain orders of form which can define the relationship among works within particular periods. The representation of the form of objects in space provides the essential point of departure for the classification and definition of works of art and of individuals. "The life of forms establishes an intimate relationship" (p. 52) that can exist between individuals within a culture independent of the extent of their active personal contact. Focillon emphasizes that it is critical to study "the various stages of artistic behavior in the plainest and most intelligible words" (p. 45), to build a "psychographic method" based on the tendency of the mind to create new forms, and to define the families of forms that characterize particular periods.

Art historians have frequently called for the development of a vocabulary of forms or a vocabulary of schemata to provide a theoretical model for the analyses of changes in the formal structure and composition of painting. A basic hypothesis of this book is that developmental psychology can provide such a theoretical model for art historical analysis—a theoretical model that has definition and validity external to art itself and therefore can provide an objective metric for the systematic assessment of a wide range of changes in the formal or structural qualities of style. This book will explore the extent that knowledge about individual development of the capacity for mental representations can provide a model for conceptualizing and studying the development of modes of representation of the forms of objects and of space in the art of Western Civilization. As postulated by Werner and Kaplan (1963), Brunswik (1959) and others, there is a formal parallelism between the processes of differentiation and integration observed in individual development and the development of modes of representation in the history of art. In both the individual and the history of art, changes in the modes of representation occur through extensions, revisions, and refinements of prior modes of representation. Both in individual and cultural development, appropriate conditions at appropriate moments facilitate development of new modes of representation while untoward social conditions can produce a reversion in modes of representation.

The development of modes of representation in art is an integral part of the society, and major factors can facilitate or impede the development of representations. Art is defined by a cultural norm and standard, and the artist who attempts to change the content and form of the prevailing modes of representation is, to some degree, violating the standards of the culture. Since there may be social sanctions and prohibitions against major revisions of the modes of representation, each step in the sequence of development often has to maintain vestiges of prior modes of representation. Artists who contribute to major revisions in modes of representation must resist the societal pressures to maintain stability (Riegl, Hauser) and must find support for their creative endeavors both within themselves and in segments of the society. Significant changes in modes of representation occur when a particular artist or group of artists is sensitive to the inadequacy of prevailing modes of representation because they, and the society, have the psychological freedom to consider revisions and can struggle to achieve a new mode of representation. While the manifest content of art is determined by the preoccupations of each epoch and by the personality characteristics and interests of the individual artist, the structure of the composition is determined primarily by the level of structural organization. It is this structural organization that must change if a new mode of representation is to be achieved. Creativity in art is an expression of individual spirit as well as a simultaneous expression of the basic cultural context in which the artist lives (Huyghe, 1974). A psychological theory of the individual's development of mental representations allows us to articulate major dimensions of the underlying structural organization of visual art and the sequence through which these dimensions have evolved. A developmental psychological model enables us to systematically assess the relative contributions of different artists in different epochs to the development of modes of representation in the history of art.

2
The Development of Modes of Representation

INTRODUCTION

Central to the study of cognitive processes is the understanding of the development of modes of representation, especially the construction of the concept of the object and the concept of space. Developmental psychologists (e.g., Piaget and Werner) have described cognitive processes as developing through five fundamental levels of organization: sensorimotor, preoperational, intuitive, concrete operations, and formal operations. Cognitive functions, including the development of the concept of the object, space, time, and causality, all proceed through these five basic levels. From this basic theoretical model of cognitive development, Piaget and his colleagues have articulated three types of spatial concepts: topological, projective, and Euclidean. At the earliest levels of cognitive organization (sensorimotor, preoperational, and intuitive) the concept of space is primarily topological and involves an emphasis on features such as proximity, boundary, contour, and surround. More advanced levels of cognitive organization (concrete and formal operations), beginning around the age of seven, are associated with the development of projective and Euclidean concepts of space in which there is increasing coordination of the three basic spatial dimensions of above–below, right–left and before–behind. While Piaget and Inhelder (1948, 1967) have discussed at length the development of topological, projective, and Euclidean concepts of space, contemporary physics and mathematics alert us to an even more advanced level of spatial concepts: a relativistic four-dimensional, spatiotemporal field as articulated in the contributions of Bernhard Riemann and Albert Einstein. Riemannian concepts of space serve to integrate and extend projective and Euclidean concepts of space.

This chapter presents a theoretical model of cognitive development, primarily the development of modes of representing concepts of the object and of space, derived from the formulations of Jean Piaget and his colleague Bärbel Inhelder, and Heinz Werner and his colleague Bernard Kaplan. Subsequent research and formulations in these areas by David Olson (1970), Jean-Marie Dolle (1973, 1974, 1975), Melvin Feffer (1959, 1967), Howard Gardner (1972), and Monique Laurendeau and Adrien Pinard (1962, 1970), and others have clarified and extended the formulations of Piaget and Werner. Some of the basic assumptions of this developmental model include the distinction between perception and representation, assimilation and accommodation as processes of internalization and equilibration, and their role in the development of concepts of the object and of space.

The study of the development of modes of representation by developmental psychologists, particularly Jean Piaget, has been based primarily on the study of children as they interact with inanimate objects (e.g., toys) in relatively neutral conditions (Wolff, 1967). Investigators of developmental processes from a psychoanalytic orientation (e.g., A. Freud, 1965; Jacobson, 1964; and Mahler, 1968) have also studied the child's development of the concept of the object, but primarily as it evolves within an interpersonal matrix and particularly under different states of arousal. Psychoanalytic investigators have been particularly interested in the integration of affective and cognitive experiences in the development of the concept of the person including the concept of the other as well as of the self. The integration of the formulations of the developmental psychologists with psychoanalytic formulations provides a model which describes affective as well as cognitive development and the central role that reflective self-awareness has in developmental processes, particularly in the phase of concrete operations and the development of projective concepts of space.

THE DEVELOPMENTAL MODEL

According to cognitive developmental psychology and psychoanalytic theory, the individual, throughout psychological development, constructs increasingly differentiated and integrated cognitive schemata. Increasingly complex principles of cognitive organization enable the individual to become more effective in coping with the complexities of reality. Cognitive structures are maintained until the individual becomes aware of further complexities of the environment—when current cognitive structures are no longer experienced as being fully effective. The individual attempts to accommodate to inconsistencies and inadequacies (perturbations) experienced in understanding reality. Subsequent levels of cognitive organization are developed in an attempt to resolve the contradictions inherent in less differentiated and integrated schemata. Cognitive structures change as the individual attempts to achieve more penetrating and effective understanding. When an individual encounters inconsistencies or contradictions between his modes of organizing experiences and the inherent nature of reality, he seeks a cognitive reorganization that achieves a new level of understanding. The individual then uses this new level of cognitive organization until subsequent contradictions are experienced and the process repeats itself once again (Piaget, 1927/1930, 1950, 1937/1954, 1968). There is a constant transaction between increasingly differentiated behavior patterns and increasingly complex levels of cognitive organization. A dialectic exists between the individual and the environment; the relationship between the individual and the environment changes as a function of this interaction, and initial forms of cognitive organization are reintegrated into higher ones. Lower levels of cognitive organization are relatively unarticulated, global, lacking in differentiation and integration, and are, therefore, relatively unstable. Higher levels of organization have greater stability. Cognitive development at the early stages proceeds relatively rapidly, while in later stages, progression and development are somewhat slower. For Piaget (Piaget, 1956, 1926/1963, 1968; Piaget & Inhelder, 1966/1971) knowledge is gained through the process of assimilation and accommodation (integration), in which, through a series of transformations, knowledge about reality becomes part of the individual's interaction with the world. Knowledge is acquired through the internalization of the results (i.e., information) of action and the development of operational sequences, rather than through a more differentiated perceptual registration of reality.

Werner (1948) and Werner and Kaplan (1963) also discuss the developmental progression of "genetic levels" of increasing differentiation and integration. Diffuse, global, fragmented, concrete, and unstable levels of organization become increasingly articulated, integrated, abstract, flexible, and stable. Higher levels of organization modify and integrate, rather than simply supersede, prior levels. Modes of representation proceed through normal increments in structure and organization from an initial reflexive (sensorimotor) level to a more reactive (perceptual registration) and eventually to a reflective (conceptual) level. Thus, there is a developmental progression from sensorimotor action, to perception, to conceptual levels of organization. An initial fusion of doing and perceiving is subsequently integrated into a concrete conception of "objective" objects in reality and eventually integrated into symbolic processes in which there is both a differentiation among, and an integration of, the signified object, the symbolic referent or signifier, and the symbolizing agent (the self).

In contrast to Piaget and his colleagues, who have studied cognitive development in children as they respond primarily to inanimate objects, usually while the children are in states of relative comfort and quiescence, psychoanalytic investigators (e.g., Anna Freud, Edith Jacobson, Selma Fraiberg, Sybil Escalona, Thérèsa Gouin Décarie, Margaret Mahler) have considered the complex interplay between the child's affective and cognitive development, primarily in interpersonal contexts and in states of affective intensity, such as pleasure, hunger, fear, or general discomfort. According to psychoanalytic theory, the primary factors in cognitive growth and development are the interactions between the child and significant people in the environment around need-gratifying experiences. In the basic caring relationship, the child learns to make significant differentiations within the environment and to integrate these differentiations into increasingly more complex conceptions of the universe. Contemporary psychoanalytic theory (e.g., A. Freud, 1965; Jacobson, 1964; Mahler, Pine, & Bergman, 1975) stresses the role of the mother–child interaction, particularly around issues of pleasure and pain, as providing the most important experiences for cognitive growth and development. Just as experiences and information about reality from interaction with inanimate objects become internalized as cognitive structures

(Piaget, 1937/1954), so do experiences and information from inter-personal transactions become internalized as cognitive structures. These cognitive structures develop sequentially and achieve stability or equilibrium at different levels of organization (Blatt, 1974; Fraiberg, 1969; Jacobson, 1964; Mahler, 1968; Mahler et al. 1975).

Each stage of cognitive development has particular characteristics of thought that become relatively stable and well structured. The principles of cognitive organization achieved at each of the major developmental stages serve to organize, guide, and direct behavior in both interpersonal and impersonal situations. Thus, cognitive de-velopment evolves in the child's interactions with the animate and inanimate world, and the cognitive structures that are established as a result of these interactions are then utilized subsequently to organize and direct behavior in both realms. As indicated by the research of Ainsworth (1967), Bell (1970), Clarke-Stewart (1973), and Décarie (1965), the development of the concepts of the person and of the inanimate object are interrelated and develop simultaneously. The various levels of cognitive development are expressed in concepts of people, including the self, and inanimate objects, as well as in more general concepts about the structure of nature such as space, time, and causality.

Piaget (1961/1969b) makes a fundamental distinction between per-ception and intelligence (i.e., cognitive processes). In innate percep-tion there is an immediate, clear-cut recognition and simple reading of "figurative aspects" of a stimulus field, while intelligence (cogni-tion) involves cognitive operations such as construction, deduction, and transformation. Transformation includes operations such as or-der, combination, generalization, synthesis, and integration of com-ponents of objects and their actions. Piaget, like Cassirer (1955), considers many aspects of perception a basic, primary, innate, and immediate presentation of an undivided total experience that cannot be broken down into different elements. But perception soon be-comes integrated with cognition and they become a unified cognitive-perceptual process. Knowledge is gained in symbolic systems not immediately given in innate perception. Concepts are not copies of immediate, sensory material but are symbolic systems based only par-tially on concrete, perceptual data. Percepts occur in the presence of a physical stimulus, whereas cognition involves a mental image (a repre-sentation) in the absence of the object. The mental image is con-structed on a different level than its corresponding percept (Piaget & Inhelder, 1966/1971).

Piaget (1937/1954, 1927/1962a, 1961/1969b; Piaget & Inhelder, 1948/1967, 1969, 1966/1971) maintains a fundamental distinction between perception (figurative aspects) and intelligence (operative and constructive aspects) throughout all levels of development. The figurative aspects of knowledge are the effects of perceptual centering, while the operative aspects of knowledge, ranging from rudimentary, sensorimotor, prerepresentational activity, to complex and formal levels of operational thought, are the effects of actions or of operations performed for the mental construction (or representation) of the object. According to Piaget, cognitive structures develop out of a functional and reciprocal interaction between perception and intellectual operations. Perception provides the basic information for intellectual operations, and in turn, cognitive operations enrich and extend the flexibility of perception. Even though perception and intellectual operations are related and develop in a complementary fashion, they are also distinctly different aspects of a knowledge of reality (Laurendeau & Pinard, 1970).[7]

Imitation and play make important contributions to the development of cognitive processes, ranging from sensorimotor activities to the development of representations. Both involve the introduction of symbols and the coordination of a signifier for a

---

[7] Olson (1970), in contrast to Piaget, stresses the continuity between perception and representation; in both types of processes stimuli are experienced as a function of alternative (or contrast) sets (Garner, 1962) that differentiate alternatives for actions to be performed on objects (Gibson, 1966). Olson (1970, p. 185) emphasizes that the development of perception is not simply a matter of perceiving increasingly large and more complex sets of features of objects and events, but rather "images are the information accumulated in the course of various performatory attempts in various media." Based on these formulations, Olson stresses that cognitive schemata are more than the internalization of action sequence; action sequences simply provide the occasion for apprehending information from the perceptual world. It is this new information, not the action, that is internalized in cognitive structures or schemata. Perceptual activity detects distinctive features that reduce uncertainty and serve to differentiate an object or event from alternatives (Garner, 1962) and to direct subsequent perceptual analysis. Action in various media provides the individual with the occasion for confronting alternative, invariant cues about the perceptual world. It is the elaboration of the perceptual world in a variety of media, including language, that leads to the development of representation and conceptual intelligence. Actually, Piaget (1974, p. 141) also emphasizes the importance of information "abstracted from the actions or operations performed by the subject on the objects."

signified object. In the early stages of imitation, the child mimics either immediate movements or sounds or those based on a memory of an actual recent event. In this process, the external model has been replaced by an internal one (Werner, 1948; Werner & Kaplan, 1963). The sensorimotor schemata, the ways in which the infant reacts to an object, become memory images and these eventually become the evocative representations of the object that indicate the development of symbolic activity (Piaget, 1945/1962b). Play provides the opportunity to develop different meanings for the symbolic representation of the absent object. In this process there is an increasing coordination of signifiers for the signified, absent object. Initially, in the sensorimotor stage, the signifier is a signal that is part of the action sequence; later, the signifier is a static image—a sign derived from a concrete, perceptual totality—and, with the development of operational thought, the signifier becomes more abstract and symbolic.

Each of the stages in the internalization of action (or information gained from performatory acts) corresponds to a stage in the development of the image. There is continual development and transformation of the signifier (i.e., the image) and the signified (i.e., the information and the operations abstracted from actions performed on the object). Objects come to exist independently of the subject and the subject's action, and this independent existence is revealed by a series of causal reactions or operations (classification and inclusion, partitive addition, conservation, seriation, transitivity, etc.) that can be performed on the concept of the object. The image of the object is, however, only a way-station in the coming to know an object. Images develop through a continued assimilation of external factors, but images are an intermediate stage between perception and representation (mental construction). Although the image is essential as a symbol, it is only part of the conceptual relationship. Initially, the concept of the object is based solely on brief, irreversible, memory images of previously performed actions (reproductive images) (Piaget & Inhelder, 1966/1971). There are two major points in the development of images: at the end of the sensorimotor stage with the formation of reproductive images and, again, at the beginning of concrete operations with the emergence of anticipatory and transformational images. Images at the end of the sensorimotor period are essentially static, while anticipatory and transformational images evolve from causal (transformational) reactions and are involved in the development of operational thought with its reversibility and conservation. As the actions that the child recalls become more complex and as these actions begin to be coordinated, thought becomes increasingly independent of the image. Though the image continues to function as an "essential auxiliary," it is replaced to a considerable degree by the coordination of action in transformational schemata. At the stage of concrete operations, and, later, at the stage of formal operations, thought is becoming sufficiently logical and precise, that isolated images play an increasingly subordinate role and are replaced by coordinated sign systems of images, language, and symbolic relationships. Thus, the image performs a different function at the various developmental levels. In the later stages of development, the image acts as an auxiliary symbol in which, for example, an entire class may be envisioned by the image of one of the members of the class (Piaget & Inhelder, 1966/1971).

Stages of Cognitive Development

According to Piaget (1937/1954, 1962a) and Werner (1948), cognitive schemata develop through a complex sequence ranging from sensorimotor activity to formal operations. The first level of cognitive schemata is achieved at the end of the sensorimotor stage (at approximately eighteen months of age); higher and more complex levels of cognitive schemata are achieved in subsequent developmental sequences (at preoperational, intuitive, and concrete and formal operational levels). At each developmental level, cognitive schemata are revised; each of these revisions achieves stabilization ("equilibration") in the establishment of a new level of cognitive schemata (Piaget, 1977). In "vertical decalage," cognitive schemata are extended and reorganized at successive levels of development. According to Piaget (1954, 1962a), the development of cognitive schemata is an actual constructive deduction that integrates current experiences with earlier cognitive schemata so that current experiences are understood in greater and fuller form. The development of cognitive schemata progresses to increasingly stable, cognitive structures that have greater stability, generality, flexibility, constancy, and complexity.

Sensorimotor Level. The forms of cognitive organization are established from early childhood on through adulthood. The first forms of cognitive organization develop in infancy, from birth through approximately one and a half years of age, in a sensorimotor stage in which the child knows the world primarily in terms of immediate actions focused primarily around sequences of need gratification. The object is known only through its actions (Elkind, 1974) and primarily those actions that provide the child with experiences of pleasure and pain. The child is unable to differentiate and coordinate a number of different aspects or dimensions and consequently focuses on only one gesture at a time. Thus, the child is inordinately influenced by particularly vivid single elements in the environment. At this early stage, the child does not appreciate the totality of a situation and the interrelationships among the different parts and features.

Piaget (1954) distinguishes several phases in sensorimotor development that lead to an initial grasp of the permanent existence of external objects. Initially, the child has no concept of himself or of others; he is aware only of action sequences and sensations and does not differentiate objects from the action sequences. When an object disappears, the infant continues to stare at the place where the object was last seen. Subsequently, the infant extrapolates beyond his immediate experience and seeks to maintain contact with the object by following and anticipating the movement of the object. The infant searches for a lost object rather than immediately giving up. But the search is still an extension of the action sequence and not a conception of the object as a separate entity. The search for an object becomes more extensive in subsequent phases in sensorimotor development; for example, the child will search for an object observed being hidden behind a screen. While the child's conception of the object is still dependent on the action sequence in this stage, the concept of the object is becoming increasingly independent of the action sequence. The child is first able to infer visible, and later invisible, displacements behind a screen. With the capacity to infer invisible displacements, the child has become capable of representation or symbolic activity and is able to begin to appreciate that objects have stable and consistent properties and an existence, separate and independent of their specific and immediate activity.

Initially in the sensorimotor stage, the child responds to the action of objects and not to the object as an independent entity. The cognitive schemata at this stage are immediate, direct, and have only minimal permanence. The cognitive schemata link perceptions and movements as if they were "static images" and there is little overall understanding of a total situation. Sensorimotor schemata are prerepresentational and are based on activity, and—as stressed in developmental psychoanalytic theory—this activity occurs initially around sequences of the gratification of sensuous bodily needs and the alleviation of pain and frustration. Experiences of pleasure and pain, hunger and satiety, and apprehensions about annihilation and survival that an infant can experience when feeling abandoned by the need-gratifying object are often central to the definition and experience of the object during this early developmental phase. The cognitive schemata of the sensorimotor stage form the nuclei for subsequent constructions. Eventually the object is identified independent of its need-gratifying action. The development of symbolic processes begins in this differentiation of the object from its action.

Preoperational Level. Slowly, children free themselves from the specific action sequences and single perceptual features. The child begins to consider objects through their part properties in a specific, fixed context and to have images of previously experienced actions and of objects no longer present in the physical environment. Objects begin to have an existence independent of their actions; they are experienced as a general, global, perceptual totality with some sense of constancy and permanence beyond the immediate perceptual field and sensory experience. At this preoperational stage, the child has only a general, overall conception of substantial and permanent objects. This conception is relatively fixed, concrete, and literal.

According to Piaget (1928/1962a, p. 282), the preoperational stage (extending from the appearance of language to the age of four) is the "first form of conceptual thought" which, as a result of language, is superimposed on sensorimotor schemata. Initially, words are personal symbols that refer to actions, not to objects. Eventually, words take on more general meaning and begin to refer to objects as well as to actions. As discussed by Werner (1948), gradually there is a shift from the proprioceptive, sensorimotor experience to cognitive schemata that merely signify the object by images and semi-individual verbal expressions. These cognitive schemata are representations of only momentary situations and partial elements and lack conservation and constancy beyond the immediate perceptual field. The representation of the object is relatively fixed, concrete and literal, and there is little capacity to tolerate transformations of the object or changes in the context and still maintain the identity and definition of the object. These cognitive schemata are not expressions of general classes or relations, but are simple correspondences between pairs or small sets of objects that still lack a differentiated conception of the total object and its relationship to the context (Piaget & Inhelder, 1969).

Intuitive Level. The preoperational or preconceptual stage is followed by a stage of intuitive cognitive schemata (ages four to seven) that serve as a transition to the stages of conceptual operations. In this intermediate, intuitive phase, the static and fragmentary schemata formed by sensorimotor activity become increasingly flexible and structured. Gradually in the intuitive stage, the child moves beyond the simple, semi-individual, cognitive schemata and begins to construct cognitive schemata of the object within a total situation or global configuration. Cognitive schemata are no longer based on a comparison between part properties or small sets of component features, but rather the schemata begin to integrate an entire series of part properties into a total configuration. At this time, mental representations and the concept of the object are primarily reproductive images. The object is represented as a concrete, fixed, idealized, perceptual totality. The basic organizational principle is external form: the concrete, manifest features of the object as a perceptual totality. The child becomes increasingly aware of the totality and the interrelationships of the isolated, specific, concrete parts of the object; the concept of the object becomes increasingly coordinated and integrated.

Knowledge of part–whole relationships develops slowly. The representation of part–whole relationships of the intuitive stage is quite different than the preoccupation with fragmented, isolated part properties during the earlier sensorimotor and preoperational phases. During the earlier phases of development, the part is equivalent to the total object. Now, in the intuitive phase, part properties are defined in relation to the total object; they elaborate and enrich the representation of the object and eventually come to serve as signifiers for the object. The separate part properties are integrated into a total conception of the object that is initially concrete and global but eventually become increasingly diverse, integrated, conceptual, and symbolic. In the intuitive stage, the child becomes increasingly aware of the various complementary dimensions that constitute an object and a situation. There is a coordination of several dimensions, but the cognitive schema are still linked to a particular image and context; an

operational schemata with a capacity for reversibility and transformation is still lacking.

The apprehension of the configuration and part properties of objects leads to the creation of operational schemata in which there are
transformations with conservation and reversibility. Initially, in the
sensorimotor and preoperational phases (until the age of four), action
is recalled concretely and always subsequent to being performed.
Slowly, the recollection of actions just previously performed becomes
the anticipation of potential actions to be performed. Eventually (beginning around the age of seven), several cognitive schemata can be
activated for the same object and the resulting schemes can be coordinated into new operations; several alternative actions can be simultaneously considered in reversible combinations within an operational
system.

Concrete and Formal Operational Levels. Slowly and intuitively, the
child has begun to differentiate a number of complementary dimensions that constitute the object. As the child becomes aware of a number of dimensions and their interrelationships, he or she can begin to
manipulate and transform these various dimensions while still being
able to maintain the basic identity and definition of the object. The
object, for example, is no longer conceived of as a general, undifferentiated perceptual totality, but instead different features and
functions or appearances in different contexts can be integrated and
the basic identity and definition of the objects still maintained. At first,
the more concrete and manifest dimensions of objects are manip-
ulated and transformed. The shape of a pliable object, for example,
can be altered, or water can be moved from a tall, thin container to a
short, wide one and still be conceived of by the child as the same
object or the same amount of water. The child is able to coordinate
two or more dimensions (or operations) into a structural whole and
through the process of transformation and reversibility is able to establish "conservation" of an object. The concept of the object has
permanence and can be represented independent of a particular context and as more than a single, concrete, literal, perceptual totality.
With the development of concrete operations, the child's cognitive
schemata include reproductions of movements (changes in positions),
transformations (changes in form), and anticipatory schemata of
things not previously perceived or experienced. These cognitive
schemata are no longer tied to certain global configurations and to

specific and static experiences, but are now concerned with concrete and, later, symbolic transformation.

The concept of the object becomes less dependent upon external manifest concrete form and begins to involve signs and symbols that represent the inner functions, forms, and properties of the object. There is a steady progression from the manifest and concrete to the abstract, from the external to the internal, and eventually to the coordination and integration of these various dimensions. Cognitive development involves a progression from operations automatically applied by the subject to objects, to an awareness and differentiation of properties and operations inherent within the object, to an awareness that one is selecting among and balancing the properties and operations that one applies to objects. The initial differentiation of subject from object leads to an articulation of aspects inherent within the object and the self, and finally to a reflective self-awareness of the relativity of one's cognitive operations. The elaboration and articulation of aspects inherent within the object, the self, and the operations applied to the object are initially defined in terms of external manifest properties and later in terms of abstract and internal (structural) properties. During the stage of concrete operations (beginning around the age of six or seven) the child can consider different actions, operations, and transformations of the object and, through a process of reversibility, maintain a conservation of the basic identity of the object. Concrete operations and transformations are replaced by transformation of more abstract dimensions in a stage of formal operations (beginning around the age of eleven) in which the child is able to identify inner meaning and structure, and coordinate and integrate these more abstract dimensions with more manifest and concrete features.

The period of concrete operations is an "unfolding of a long, integrated process that may be characterized as a transition from subjective centering in all areas to a decentering that is at once cognitive, social, and moral. This process . . . reproduces and develops on a larger scale at the level of thought what has already taken place on a small scale at the sensori-motor level"—the representation of an object independent of its immediate, physical presence. The "decentering [is] based on the general coordination of action, and this permits the formation of operatory systems of transformations and constants or conservations which liberate the representation of reality from its depictive figurative appearances" (Piaget & Inhelder, 1969, p. 128).

The child initially is able to establish an individual point of view but egocentrically assumes that it is the only point of view. Subsequently, the child becomes aware of having different points of view at different times, and later recognizes that others may have different points of view. The child is now capable of recognizing and distinguishing that people can each have different points of view and that these are different from his own.

In summary, the child's intellectual development is first based on the nature of the child's actions upon the world and the degree of coordination of these actions. Early on, the child is able to integrate a set of actual actions to achieve a specific goal and later on the child synthesizes potential actions toward an object. With the capacity to anticipate potential actions, there is the beginning of representational thought. Until this point in development, the child's representations are reproductions of objects and events previously experienced. Now it is possible to evoke memories of objects and events outside the perceptual field by means of signs, images, and symbols. With the development of the capacity for evocative memory and anticipation, the child can begin to represent objects and events that are transformations and extensions of objects previously experienced and, eventually, of things not previously experienced or perceived. Different actions can now be coordinated and the child is capable of the cognitive operations of reversibility and conservation in which two operations or dimensions are coordinated. Concrete operations lead to more abstract and formal operations in which operations can be performed upon abstract propositions as well as upon concrete objects. With the development of formal cognitive operations children have access to and the capacity for abstract mathematical reasoning. Piaget states that all knowledge proceeds from an initially inseparable relationship between subject and object. The individual defines objects and develops operations (e.g., transformations) through actions. The operations are based on the child's actions and the objects affected by these actions. The resultant operations enable the individual to construct an even fuller understanding of the object. There is a formalization of the general coordination of actions and operations in which the object is defined independently of the action. The coordination of actions and operations is expressed in a multilevel, hierarchically organized series of prelogical and logical cognitive schemata that can, in turn, result in the development of higher order operations.

CONCEPTS OF SPACE

Piaget maintains a sharp distinction between perception and representation (intellectual constructions) and considers representation as the central process in cognitive development. This distinction applies to all aspects of knowledge, and particularly to the development of the representation of space. There has been a great deal of research in the perception of space (Gibson, 1950, 1966; Ittelson, 1960; Koffka, 1935; Wapner & Werner, 1957), but there have been relatively few studies of the representation of space (Laurendeau & Pinard, 1970). While innate perception undergoes a developmental sequence similar to the development of representation, the developmental processes involved in perception are relatively brief. Innate perceptual processes interact with the development of cognitive schemes and become an integrated cognitive-perceptual process. The innate perception of space (e.g., depth perception) according to Piaget, involves relatively fixed, irreversible structures, whereas the representation of space involves the development of reversible structures based on topological, projective, and Euclidean relationships (Olson, 1970; Piaget, Inhelder & Szeminska, 1960). Concepts of space are initially undifferentiated and become increasingly structuralized; they develop from relative globality to increased differentiation and hierarchical integration (Werner, 1957). Topological relationships of proximity, boundary, separation, enclosure, order, and continuity develop first, and projective and Euclidean relationships derive from them. Spatial knowledge and the representation of space are not based on concrete, perceptual data alone, but involve symbolization in which differentiated spatial features are organized into conceptual systems. "What we call 'space' is not an independent object that is mediately represented to us, that presents itself and is to be recognized by certain signs; rather, it is a particular mode, a peculiar schematism of representation itself" (Cassirer, 1955, p. 149). The individual's representation of physical space is defined by the operational structure that develops in a transaction between the cognitive operations available within the subject and qualities that are inherently part of the object.

The representation of space follows the same basic developmental sequence as the development of cognitive processes—that is, through sensorimotor, preoperational, intuitive, and concrete and formal operational stages. The representation of space in the early stages of cognitive development is relatively static and fixed. It is primarily topological in nature and concerned with qualitative features inherent in an isolated figure. The representation of space in the later stages of cognitive development, in the concrete and formal operational levels, is primarily based on projective and Euclidean concepts. The progression from topological concepts of space to projective and Euclidean concepts involves increasingly complex coordination among the three dimensions of space and the development of conceptual systems to express this coordination. Piaget's formulations of the child's construction of concepts of space is most fully articulated in the book written in collaboration with Bärbel Inhelder (Piaget & Inhelder, 1948/1967) and subsequently confirmed and elaborated by the research of Monique Laurendeau and Adrien Pinard (1970).

Topological Concepts

Piaget and Inhelder (1948/1967), basing their argument on their general theoretical model, discuss the child's sense of space as proceeding through three levels: a topological, a projective, and a Euclidean level. Topology is based on purely qualitative relations inherent in a particular figure. The primary properties of topological space are proximity, boundary, contour, and separation rather than size, distance, or angularity. Topological concepts are initially limited to the inherent properties of the particular object (e.g., figure–ground) without the requirement that the object be located in relation to other objects, neither in terms of a particular perspective or point of view (projective concepts of space) nor in terms of a system of axes or coordinates (Euclidean concepts of space) (Laurendeau & Pinard, 1970).

In the development of perception, the dimension of boundaries, contours, and outlines is a basic process that occurs spontaneously and very early in development. Experimental research in the development of perceptual processes (Kagan, 1971; Karmel, Hoffman, & Fegy, 1974; Kennedy, 1974) indicates that early visual orientation involves scanning at the boundary of figures, where the contours are most vivid. Research with neonates indicates that the response to contour and outline is a very early developmental process. Study of perceptual processes subsequent to the removal of congenital cataracts (von Senden, 1932; cited by Osgood, 1953) and considerable developmental research on visual orientation (Berlyne, 1958; Carpenter, Tecce, Stechler, & Friedman, 1970; Fantz, 1963; Fantz & Nevis, 1967; Haith, 1966; Karmel, 1969; Salapatek & Kessen, 1966; Wilcox, 1969) and neurophysiology (Hubel & Wiesel, 1959; Karmel et al., 1974; Kuffler, 1952) indicate that high contrast of edges and boundaries is a primary factor in the earliest forms of visual orientation. Likewise, in the development of representation, Piaget (1954) and Werner (1948) discuss the first perceptual-cognitive differentiation as the representation of a boundary occurring in an initially undifferentiated field. The capacity to experience, perceive, and represent the contour and the boundaries of an object constitute some of the earliest and most basic developmental steps (Blatt & Wild, 1976).

Piaget and Inhelder consider topological relationships as an essential preliminary step, prior to the development of projective and Euclidean relationships. Topological relationships are primarily qualitative and are concerned with intensity rather than with quantity. Initially, the child has no concept of continuity, only a qualitative sense involving the intrinsic relationships of proximity, separation (edge), order, and simple enclosure in the spatial relations of a single configuration. Figures are defined in terms of separation and contour, with no account of relative dimension, distance, or position in space. Only the inherent properties of the object are considered, based entirely on the relations of boundary or enclosure of elements of a single figure. There is no integrated sense of space and little appreciation of the relations among objects. Rather, the emphasis is primarily upon the homeomorphic relations within the configuration of a single object—its shape, outline, surround, and continuity–discontinuity. There is no appreciation of depth or of the space between objects. Space is always part of an object and there is no definition of space beyond the inherent relations within a single object. Regardless of how complex it may be, topology is always limited to elements of a single configuration and does not constitute a total space in which several objects are located in relation to one another according to a framework "which takes objective distances and possible points of view into account . . . Piaget conceives of the child's topological space as a mosaic of fragmentary and distinct spaces whose respective borders are fixed by the continuity of a given perceptual field or by the functional unity of each of the child's particular experiential fields" (Laurendeau & Pinard, 1970, p. 167). In the development of topological space there is a progressive dichotomous "subdivision of the object, first into a few elements, continuous and isomorphic with the whole, then their further subdivisions into points, still finite in number; and lastly, the subdivision of these points into an infinite number of points having neither shape nor size" (Piaget & Inhelder, 1948/1967, p. 459).

The relations of proximity, separation, order, enclosure and continuity are built up empirically between the various parts of figures or patterns which they organize. They are independent of any contraction or expansion of these features and are therefore unable to conserve features such as distances, straight lines, angles, etc. during changes of shape. Hence it is impossible for relationships of this type to lead to comprehensive systems linking different figures together by means of perspective or axial co-ordinates, and for this reason they are bound to remain psychologically primitive.

This primitive topological space is purely internal to the particular figure whose intrinsic properties it expresses, as opposed to spatial relationships of the kind which enable it to be related to other figures. (Piaget & Inhelder, 1948/1967, p. 153)

Proximity is a given in topological space and serves as the starting point for the construction of new levels of concepts and operations of topological space. At first, objects are differentiated from the field (figure–ground) and later differentiated from other objects. Separation is experienced when two objects have no point in common and is further facilitated as the child develops the concept of surround or boundary (enclosure). Piaget and Inhelder (1948/1967) discuss three types of enclosures that provide the simple intuitive definition of boundary: a one-dimensional system having a non-dimensional point as a boundary, a two-dimensional system having a one-dimensional line as a boundary, and a three-dimensional system having a two-dimensional surface as a boundary. The development from singular to plural dimensional systems leads to groupings that likewise proceed from singular to multiplicative groupings of elements or objects or relationships.

The notion of order is constructed from a linear series of elements or enclosures. The concept of continuity develops in a "form intermediate between perceptual and mathematical continuity" (Piaget & Inhelder, 1948/1967, p. 462). At about the age of six or seven, as the child begins to develop concepts of projective space, the whole is broken up into neighboring elements and then reintegrated again into a continuous whole. These elementary preoperational groupings are then related to one another and give rise to the concepts of "extension" and "intention" (Inhelder & Piaget, 1955/1958, 1964). Extensive preoperational groupings refer to the spatial configuration of a series as a whole—that is, the elements are arranged in a quantitative order such as along the dimension of size. Intensive, qualitative preoperational groupings refer to the repetition of a size relationship between the pairs of elements within a series (e.g., $a < b < c$, etc.). The continuous extension and intention of proximities forms the highest level of topological concepts "which foreshadows the projective and Euclidean system" in which extension and intention become more integrated and coordinated. The child masters intensive topological relationships of proximity, separation, enclosure, order, and continuity by the start of concrete operations and this provides the basis for developing quantitative concepts. Topological spatial concepts express general properties of space that are dependent on the child's action and have nothing to do with either the coordination of viewpoints or with metrics. The early conception of continuity (preoperational extensive and intensive groupings) constitutes the final synthesis of topological relationships (Piaget & Inhelder, 1948/1967).[8]

Topological relationships are merely the continuous series of individual elements that can be expanded or contracted at will and, there-

---

[8]Laurendeau and Pinard (1970, p. 423) systematically studied the development of spatial concepts in children from ages two through twelve and found that "the earliest behaviors depend on spatial relations which are limited to internal elements of a single perceptual configuration (or image representation)," independent of any other system of viewpoints or coordinates. Their findings emphasize the importance of topological relationships of neighborhood, surround, or enclosure (e.g., localization of topological positions), and of continuity and discontinuity. The relations of separation and order constitute the elementary topological concepts that precede the development of projective and Euclidean levels of spatial conceptualizations.

Laurendeau and Pinard (1970) also found that children around the age of three and a half to four can perceptually recognize familiar objects and discriminate certain geometric forms based solely on topological relations. From ages four to seven years, children begin to discriminate curvilinear from rectilinear shapes and finally, around the age of seven years, the child can recognize most complex shapes. In the study of spatial representations, they found that children's conceptions of space begin with a reliance on elementary topological aspects such as neighborhood, surround, enclosure, without any account of projective coordination of above–below, left–right, before–behind, or elementary Euclidean estimates of distance. The early stages rely solely on topological cues furnished by the elements of the perceptual field or on cues of simple symmetry. Subsequently, the child begins to recognize projective dimensions and comes to coordinate them when the concomitant topological cues are clear and available. These first projective coordinations remain basically egocentric, and the child is unable to make reversals. Later on (around the age of seven), the child frees himself from his own point of view and is able to make simple reversals. Eventually (at the age of ten or eleven years), the child is able to make reversals and locate positions without the assistance of well-defined topological cues.

fore, are unable to contribute to the conservation of straight lines, distances, or angles. Topological concepts are not based on a stable system that defines positions of objects or the shape and orientation of objects relative to various planes and points of view. In topological space "each continuous domain constitutes a space and there is thus no universal space operating as a frame and enabling objects or figures to be located relative to one another" (Piaget & Inhelder, 1948/1967, p. 467). There are as many spaces as there are objects themselves and the intervals between objects either belong to the objects themselves or are not spatial at all.

Proximity and separation lead to an appreciation of enclosure (or surrounding), order, continuity, subdivision of lines and surfaces, and, ultimately, into an awareness of points. This development of topological space is essential for subsequent development of projective space, which includes an appreciation of perspective and a coordination of multiple perspectives, and for the development of Euclidean space, which involves the conservation of parallels and the integration of different systems of reference including horizontal and vertical coordinates and scales. The concept of the straight line is the basis for projective spatial relationships, and the possibility of transformations ensures equivalency of figures. Euclidean or metric space is based mainly on the concept of distance in which the equivalence of figures depends on mathematical equality. While projective and Euclidean concepts of space are distinct and we discuss their development separately, it is important to keep in mind that they actually develop as integrated projective-Euclidean concepts throughout the concrete and formal levels of operational thought. Each phase in the development of projective concepts of space achieves stability and equilibrium in the quantified coordinates of Euclidean concepts.

Projective Concepts

The elementary relationships in topological concepts of space (separation, order, enclosure, etc.) serve as the basis for the structural relationships that persist as the concepts of space until the first period of operational thought is established (around the age of seven). Projective concepts of space add to topological concepts the capacity of "locating objects or elements of a single object in relation to each other within a given perspective". The child has already learned certain elementary projective relations (e.g., size and shape constancy) at the level of perceptual activity during the sensorimotor and preoperational phases. With the advent of the representation of images at the intuitive level, "coordination of fragmentary projective relationships progressively acquires more and more flexibility and efficiency." Eventually, an operational system of projective relations is organized that coordinates perspectives and the reversibility of points of view. In the elaboration of projective space and perspective, the topological concept of simple linear sequence is eventually transformed into concepts of rectilinear coordinates, and the reciprocity of neighboring regions from one perspective is eventually transformed into the reciprocity of perspectives (Laurendeau & Pinard, 1970, pp. 16–17).

Projective concepts involve the development of a specific point of view that can account for internal topological relationships of each individual element as well as the shape and relative position and distance of figures. The development of perspective permits the definition of the reciprocal relationships among the parts of an individual figure, and among separate, completed figures, both in relation to one another and to the entire scene. In contrast to topological concepts, projective concepts involve a reference system that allows for the coordination of viewpoints and the coordination of planes on which figures are projected. According to Piaget and Inhelder (1948/1967), projective space defines

> the relative positions of parts of figures, or figures relative to one another, and the whole in relation to an observer or the plane corresponding to his visual field. From the psychological stand-point, the essential feature of this process is the entry of the observer, or the "point-of-view" in relation to which the figures are projected. (p. 467)

The development of elementary projective concepts involves the same operations as the development of topological concepts, only with the addition of a viewpoint or frame of reference (Piaget & Inhelder, 1948/1967). For example, the addition of a particular viewpoint allows topological order to be constructed as a projected straight line that can be reduced projectively to a single point. The topological dimensions of a simple linear series, a notion of inside and outside a closed linear boundary, or a closed two-dimensional boundary (surface), can be defined in projective space in the relative orientations of left and right, above and below, and before and behind, denoting three-dimensional space. Projection and sectional planes are two fundamental operations in projective space. The major task in projective relationships is the coordination of successive or multiple viewpoints by means of elementary projections cut along various sectional planes. As with topological relationships, projective relationships are at first only "intensive," qualitative, sublogical operations that later acquire quantitative, mathematical form.

The addition of the projective dimensions (before–behind, left–right, above–below) to the internal topological relations within a single object or configuration radically transforms the concept of space. A series of elements are arranged from the viewpoint of a single observer, such that one object partially hides another (before–behind) and this constitutes the first basic dimension of projective space: the straight line. Similarly, the addition of left–right or above–below relations to the before–behind dimension converts a surface or projective plane to create volume and three-dimensional space. Projective concepts conserve relative positions of objects in relation to the observer's projective plane, but they do not account for objective distances and the actual dimensions of objects. Projective concepts are based on transformations of apparent size and shape that place objects in relation to one another from a single vantage point. With subsequent development of projective concepts of space, this coordination of perspectives increases in complexity, flexibility, and stability and enables the child to have an awareness of multiple points of view instead of the "egocentrism of a single and momentary viewpoint" (Laurendeau & Pinard, 1970, p. 169).

Development in projective relationships involves the overall coordination of points of view that initially result from taking account of interposed objects or parts of objects. Order in projective space takes on the unique function of a straight line; enclosures and groupings in projective space are not confined to inside or outside, but rather involve relationships that correspond to concepts of left–right, above–below, and before–behind. These relations result in the concept of a plane or set of planes (as distinct from a surface) in three-dimensional space. The multiplication of planes and reference systems creates a set of planes in three-dimensional space. These planes play a fundamental role in the representation of perspective in which height and width of the background are related to the dimensions of the foreground. Multiplicative groupings of relations in three dimensions facilitate the understanding of foreshortening and projective decreases in length. The coordination of successive perspectives provides the starting point for the development of an orthogonal system of one-to-one correspondences along two or three dimensions, and this enables the child to recognize equivalent elements among varying perspectives. One–many correspondences describe triangular structures such as a pair of perspective lines meeting at the horizon. While initially this system is two-dimensional, the one–many correspondences of decreasing distance between the two perspective lines that form the relationship of the horizon to the foreground brings the child close to the "extensive quantification" of Euclidean space—the mathematical treatment of perspective (Piaget & Inhelder, 1948/ 1967).[9]

Projective space adds a new element to spatial conception because different elements of a single object are no longer considered solely in terms of the relations between elements of the object (topological space), but now an object is considered in relation to an external observer. The change from topological to projective spatial concepts

---

[9] In a series of studies designed to investigate the development of projective spatial concepts, Laurendeau and Pinard (1970) first investigated the child's capacity to construct a straight line. While the child is able to perceptually identify a straight line at a fairly early age, the mental representation and the ability to construct a straight line do not occur until at least the age of six or seven years (beginning of concrete operations) when the child is able to utilize rudimentary projective or Euclidean spatial concepts. Before that age, the child is able to distinguish a straight line from a curved or broken one and can draw a straight line provided it is done in a single stroke, but is unable to construct a succession of elements in a straight line. The construction of a straight line involves the projective operation of constructing before–behind relations (depth) without requiring the coordination of the two other directions of projective space—width and height. Initially, the child must depend upon perceptual indices (e.g., follow the edge of a rectilinear table) to construct a straight line. Because of a lack of projective or Euclidean constructs, "the preoperational child must rely solely on topological relations of neighborhood and order. He . . . is not able to coordinate . . . successive movements in a single total structure in order to maintain a constant direction and reach his goal" (Laurendeau & Pinard, 1970, p. 113). He lacks the internal structures (constructs) necessary to guide his constructions and must rely on perceptual straight lines present in his visual field. When the child can construct a straight line without the perceptual support of rectilinear contours, we can assume that he has achieved projective or Euclidean operations (Laurendeau & Pinard, 1970). In utilizing projective operations, the child initially attempts to differentiate and coordinate the multiple points of view of visual space. The child must select from all possible perspectives the preferential position in which he places himself in the extension of the straight line.

derives from the subordination of objects to the observer and this radically transforms the basic dimensions of space. The observer's "infinitely variable perspective produces a network of new relations (e.g., projective transformations, multiplication of perspective, etc.) between the observer and the object" (Laurendeau & Pinard, 1970, p. 247). With the addition of a point of view external to the object, objects can be considered as to the left or right (width), below or above (height), or in front or behind each other (depth). All three dimensions of space are created with the establishment of the individual's perspective (Laurendeau & Pinard, 1970). A central aspect in the construction of projective concepts of space, therefore, is the establishment of the sense of self as a stable, enduring, unique reference point. As we discuss subsequently, the sense of self has not been discussed extensively by Piaget, but he has discussed the development of three levels of egocentrism and the "decentering" from each of these egocentric levels as an important aspect of the development of projective concepts of space.

The development of the concept of left and right has been studied extensively and the complex sequence involved in its development is an integral part of the long and complex process involved in the construction of projective concepts of space. Laurendeau and Pinard (1970, pp. 250–251) describe the development of the concept of left and right as proceeding through three successive stages following a progression of "decentration going from pure egocentrism to complete relativity." During the first stage (ages five to eight years) left and right are distinguished egocentrically, solely from the child's own point of view. This initial differentiation of left and right is based on a "relation of internal opposition." The second stage (ages eight to eleven years) corresponds to an early form of relativity ("reciprocity of viewpoints") in which the child, through a process of simple reversals, becomes able to recognize the left and right of a person opposite the child. This is the beginning of the establishment of the variable, or multiple, viewpoint. Finally (around eleven to twelve years), there is "complete objectification and reciprocity . . . and the child . . . is then able to consider concepts of left and right from the point of view of the objects themselves." At this highest level, the viewpoint of the subject is integrated with the viewpoint of the object in a single system. In this stage, the child becomes capable, for the first time, of a general coordination of viewpoints that is a synthesis of two distinct groups of relations. The coordination of viewpoints and the integration of two groups of relations are the beginning of formal operations. Relative concepts of time, speed, movement, and the comprehension of proportions require the coordination and integration of several relations into a single general system in which all constituent elements of the relations are considered simultaneously (Laurendeau & Pinard, 1970). According to Piaget, these formal operations do not bear directly on the relations between objects but rather on the relationship among relations. Piaget attributes the relatively slow development of projective concepts of space to the fact that a given object is no longer considered by itself but is now considered in relation to an external observer, and these perspective relationships are based on "a complex system of relative viewpoints." There is an integration of a succession of partial perceptions and perspectives into "a general system which includes simultaneously all the relationships existing between the observer and each of the objects as well as between the objects themselves" (Laurendeau & Pinard, 1970, p. 310).[10]

_____

[10] Laurendeau and Pinard (1970) systematically studied the child's ability to coordinate simultaneously left–right and before–behind relations in reproducing the perspective of an observer variously located around a block of miniature mountains. They investigated the child's ability to integrate a system of perspectives and coordinates that facilitates the maintenance of the relations of order and distance, despite reversals in perspective experienced in the rotation of a model landscape. Thus the task required an integration of topological concepts (neighborhood) with projective (before–behind and left–right) and Euclidean concepts (distance and angles). The subject was required to manipulate simultaneously two dimensions (left–right and before–behind) and to coordinate the relative positions of several objects in relationship to a single observer occupying several successive positions or in relationship to several observers in different positions. Earlier research with this procedure (Piaget & Inhelder, 1948/1967) found that the coordination of perspective develops about the same time as the ability to deal with simple representations of various perspectives potentially available on a single object. Piaget concluded that the major issue in this task appears to be the child's capacity to disengage from an egocentric perspective. The decentration from this egocentricity is basic to the development of various perspectives of a single object and the coordination of projective relations among several objects. Representation of any perspective, including creating a general system that coordinates all perspectives, requires an awareness of the uniqueness of one's own point of view and consequently of other potential viewpoints as well. Thus Laurendeau and Pinard (1970) propose that the capacity to localize positions is a function of the child's capacity to become free from egocentric attitudes. Initially the child lacks the ability for decentration from an egocen-

In addition to the concepts of up and down and of left and right, another major aspect in the development of projective space is the concept of the diagonal. Recent research (Dolle, Bataillard, & Guyon, 1973–74; Dolle, Bataillard, & Lacroix, 1974–75; Dolle, Vinter, & Germain, 1974–75; Olson, 1970, 1975) indicates that the attainment of the concept of the diagonal is a central aspect of the development of projective concepts of space. Horizontal and vertical, in contrast to the diagonal, are invariant dimensions with specific and fixed images and are therefore easier to discriminate and represent than diagonal or oblique lines. There is considerable evidence indicating that up and down is easier to discriminate than left–right, and that both of these are significantly easier to discriminate and conceptualize than the diagonal (Goldmeier, 1972; Olson, 1975). Olson (1970) in studying the child's capacity to construct the diagonal concludes that the diagonal is an essential dimension of projective space because it requires more than just an appreciation of an invariant dimension, such as horizontal and vertical, but also the projection of a straight line using the self as the reference point. The construction of the diagonal requires an appreciation of the properties of sequences and the extension of sequences through space. Once the concept of diagonality is achieved, it is a conceptual structure that has stability, generality, and reversibility—in Piaget's terms it has equilibrium at an operational level. In order for the child to construct the diagonal at the appropriate age (around the age of nine), the component forms and features of the diagonal must be differentiated from other concepts.

---

tric position, but in a second, transitional stage there is a partial decentration and an oscillation between egocentric behavior and partial and complete decentration. Eventually, the child establishes an operational coordination of projective relations and can adopt a specific reference point and contrast it with other perspectives. Projective space has become a system of possible viewpoints subject to laws determined by relative transformation. This process develops slowly, and the ability to coordinate perspectives occurs in only a small portion (28%) of children by age twelve. The failure of most children to master the coordination of perspective by this age suggests that operational coordination of perspective may derive from the formal level of operational thought. While the test of the coordination of perspective does not have the complexity of proportions, it does have "a degree of complexity which places it in the last period of the concrete operational stage" (Laurendeau & Pinard, 1970, p. 401). The coordination of perspective involves issues of relative perspective but not quantification or the mathematical structures for this coordination.

The construction of the oblique is only achieved by the complex coordinated representation of asymmetrical deviations from both the vertical and horizontal, the differentiation of the diagonal from other relevant schemata, and the transformation of perceptual images of the diagonal into non-linguistic conceptual categories and schemata (Olson, 1975). The schema involves, in its early form, defining oneself as a reference point and establishing the diagonal as an extension from this reference point into space. The establishment of the self as a stable reference point enables the child to begin to deal with variable dimensions that are more complex and unstable than the invariant dimensions of horizontal and vertical (Witkin, 1965).

The important role of the concept of the diagonal in the development of projective space is indicated in the studies of Dolle and her colleagues (Dolle, Bataillard, & Guyon, 1973–74; Dolle, Bataillard, & Lacroix, 1974–75; Dolle, Vinter, & Germain, 1974–75) on the mental and graphic representation of three-dimensional space.[11] Dol-

---

[11] In a detailed analysis of children's ability to understand and learn how to depict a cube, Dolle and her colleagues found three major developmental stages in the child's acquisition of perspective. Before the age of six or seven, in the preoperational levels, the child can correctly describe a cube when it is perceptually available, but the ability for the mental construction and graphic rendering of the cube proceeds through a lengthy and ordered developmental sequence. In the first stage, from six to nine years of age, the child is unable to reproduce graphically a three-dimensional cube and is usually content simply to enumerate the various properties of the cube. Although the child has a perceptual understanding of the cube, graphic productions are restricted to the "perceptually visible." The child simply enumerates the faces of the cube by surrounding the frontal square with rectilinear deformations of the other sides. The child's verbal descriptions and graphic renderings emphasize topological characteristics of separation, juxtaposition, surround, and continuity of separate elements of the total figure. While children recognize the cube and can describe it, they have not yet formed a mental representation of it and cannot graphically reproduce it, despite the numerous suggestions by the experimenters.

In the second major phase in the development of the concept of the diagonal, from age nine to twelve, the child's first representation of three-dimensional space is indicated by the use of an oblique or diagonal line that connects two parallel planes and indicates a recession of a lateral surface from the vantage point of the child's visual angle. Dolle and her colleagues labeled this stage "empirical perspective" because the perspective was constructed exclusively from the viewpoint of the subject. The child's discovery of the oblique line seems to be based on the perceptual discovery of the recession of one angle from the frontal face of the cube. The production of one oblique

le's findings indicate that the child, in learning to represent volume and perspective, proceeds through the three major phases articulated by Piaget: the topological, projective and Euclidean concepts of space. The representation of volume appears to be quite independent of perceptual processes and much more contingent upon the development of cognitive schemata at appropriate times after more limited techniques and concepts have been well established. Dolle's findings are consistent with the findings of Olson (1970, 1975) and indicate that the concept of the diagonal or the oblique is a major developmental step in the development of projective space and the capacity to represent perspective and volume. These research findings also support the contention that the development of projective space requires the development of the sense of self as a stable and unique point of reference.

Though Piaget does not discuss the concept of the self in the development of projective and Euclidean concepts of space, he does discuss the role of various levels of egocentrism. Egocentrism was a central construct in Piaget's early formulations of the development of space, but eventually he found the concept ambiguous and used it less

---

edge is subsequently coordinated with a second oblique edge. The two oblique lines are initially produced in divergent directions so that the point of recession into the picture plane is centered within the subject. The lateral faces spread out from the frontal plane. Only slowly does the child begin to use symmetry and eventually the second oblique edge is reciprocally coordinated with the first. With this coordination of the oblique lines, the first and second planes are constructed as parallel. Later, the two upper obliques are drawn in coordination with lower obliques. The coordination of the upper and lower obliques integrates the two parallel frontal planes with two adjacent lateral sides giving the appearance of a volume slanting away from the position of the child. Thus, in this stage of empirical perspective, the child is beginning to integrate operations in a limited system of reversible and parallel symmetry, but these are not yet coordinated into a general system. It is only in the third stage of "causal perspective," beginning at the age of twelve, that the child begins to be able to envision every element of the cube in relationship with every other element, based on parallelism, reversibility, and reciprocity. At around age twelve the child is capable of a graphic representation of a cube in frontal presentation with recession going either to the right or left; later the child can graphically represent the cube from different positions. The child has integrated the various properties of volume into an organized schemata based on propositional combination and double reversibility.

and less frequently. In his introductory comments to Laurendeau and Pinard (1970), Piaget notes that there are positive and negative aspects to egocentrism. Piaget discusses three levels of egocentrism, and at each level of development egocentrism plays a constructive role in the child's early attempts to understand reality by relating aspects of the immediate situation to prior experiences. This aspect of egocentrism is an inherent part of the process Piaget calls assimilation. While an egocentric primacy of the child's actions and point of view are initially useful to the child in the process of assimilation, eventually several levels of egocentrism must be relinquished in order for the child to appreciate actions and perspectives of others and to integrate and coordinate them with his own viewpoint. Difficulty appreciating another's perspective is the negative aspect of egocentrism. Though Piaget (1970a) continues to have reservations about the value of his concept of egocentrism, Laurendeau and Pinard (1962, 1970) found the concept essential for understanding the child's development of projective space and concepts of causality.

Piaget, in his developmental theory, articulated three levels of "egocentrism" and demonstrated how the child, in relinquishing succeeding levels of egocentrism, comes to appreciate actions and perceptions different from his own and is able to integrate and coordinate them with his own viewpoint. Each succeeding level of egocentrism is relinquished through a gradual process of "decentration." There are three successive levels of egocentrism—from an initial state of total egocentrism to full objectivity (Inhelder & Piaget, 1955). At first, the child has no image of himself or of the external world; the two exist as one undifferentiated reality. Gradually, he becomes reciprocally aware of himself and of others. Throughout the sensorimotor and preoperational stages, there is an initial decentration in which the child learns to distinguish his own activity from that of others.[12] He assumes, however, that his immediate viewpoint is the

---

[12] Werner (1948) also discusses the importance of the child's relinquishing an initial egocentric position in the development of cognitive structures. Cognitive development is the result of the progressive differentiation of the ego from the external world. The first sense of reality (and of space) begins with practical concepts that are centered mainly in physical actions related to one's own body. Werner discusses cognitive development as proceeding from a primitive type of practical, sensorimotor intelligence focused around one's body to a steady development characterized by an increasing differentiation between self and object.

only possibility and that it is shared by others; e.g., if he covers his eyes he assumes that not only can he not see you, but also you cannot see him. This initial stage of egocentrism, in which the child confuses his actions and views with those of others, is finally resolved by the time the child begins the period of concrete operational thought (ages six to seven).

A second decentration begins to occur as part of the development of concrete operational thought, from about the age of six to seven to the age of eleven to twelve. Initially, the child is able to recognize and appreciate only his own perspective, but gradually he begins to recognize that his own displacement results in a changed point of view. He then becomes aware that if different positions are held by different people, different perspectives result. Thus he becomes aware of his subjective existence and of the multiplicity of other possible viewpoints. He becomes aware of himself as a unique object among other objects and of the relativity of his personal perspective. He is able to maintain his unique perspective while appreciating and understanding the viewpoint of others (Laurendeau & Pinard, 1962).

Finally, at the level of formal operations (beginning around twelve years of age), there is a third decentration in which a final form of egocentrism is relinquished and the child differentiates his perspective from the reality to which he must adapt. He becomes aware not only of the independent existence of objects but also of the independence of his cognitive processes from the environment. He becomes aware that he is responsible for his construction and understanding of reality. With this reflective self-awareness and appreciation of the nature of his own thought processes, as well as the viewpoints of others, the child can develop genuine social reciprocity in which he can maintain his own subjectivity while appreciating the subjectivity of others and differentiating it from the more objective dimensions of reality. As Piaget notes (Laurendeau & Pinard, 1970), at the highest level one recognizes that there is always a subjective, relativistic dimension in the understanding and interpretation of nature.

Feffer (1959, 1970) considered the implications of Piaget's formulations of the development of egocentrism for social behavior. Using concepts of social psychology, particularly the work of Solomon Asch, Feffer discusses how effective social interaction requires the capacity to consider oneself simultaneously both as subject and object and to take the viewpoint of the other while maintaining one's own viewpoint. Complementarity in social interaction involves being able to take the viewpoint of the other, to be simultaneously the experiencing subject and the object being experienced by others. Feffer postulates that, like impersonal conservation based on the coordination and reciprocal correlation of complementary physical dimensions, interpersonal conservation can be viewed as requiring the coordination and reciprocal correlation of complementary roles represented within the self-organization. Feffer and his colleagues (Feffer, 1959, 1970; Feffer & Gourevitch, 1960) found parallels between the development of cognitive decentration (the ability to relinquish egocentricity) and the child's capacity for role-taking in an interpersonal context. At first the child is able to take only a limited perspective, but later (after nine years of age) he is able to achieve the simultaneous coordination and synthesis of a number of different perspectives and roles. Feffer (1959, 1970) found that the differentiation of one's own viewpoint from that of others and the ability to coordinate and integrate these multiple perspectives correlated significantly with age, with an appreciation of aspects of interpersonal relationships including the capacity for role-taking (Feffer, 1970) and empathy (Lohman, 1969), and with the cognitive capacity for conservation, class inclusion, and cognitive decentering (Feffer, 1970). As part of the development of conservation and reversibility of operational thought, the child becomes increasingly aware of subtle subjective experiences within both himself and others (Feffer & Suchotliff, 1966).

The self becomes stable and defined as a unique object among many other objects. The child becomes aware of his own continuity with his past and his potential extension into the future. With the development of the self as a unique and stable reference point, a wide range of subjective experiences becomes available. Subjective experiences, such as affects, emotions, values, and personal meanings, become increasingly differentiated, integrated, and symbolic. There is increased recognition and appreciation of one's own personal reactions, feelings, and values, and an increased awareness of the perspectives, feelings, and values of others. The development of the self leads to greater differentiation of affective nuances and the capacity for fuller interpersonal relationships characterized by reciprocity and mutuality. At each stage of development, subjective aspects are coordinated with concepts of the external world. At the lower stages, affects are part of sensorimotor activity and impel the individual toward action and discharge. At the higher stages, one's understanding of reality is integrated with the recognition of personal meanings, affective experiences, priorities, and values. With the development of a stable concept of the self and the capacity for reflective self-awareness, affects and emotions assume a signal (Freud, 1923) or an informational (Blatt & Feirstein, 1977) function. Thought and action are based on self-awareness and reflectivity.

Reflective self-awareness (Schafer, 1968), the establishment of the self as a unique and stable reference point, is an essential part of the development of operational thought and projective concepts of space. It is an essential part of the development of an appreciation of subjective aspects of experience. Understanding of reality is more differentiated and articulated because it is integrated with the recognition of the importance of personal meaning, affective experience, priorities, and values. The highest levels of operational thought are based on self-awareness and reflectivity.[13] The establishment of a stable, constant self-reflective awareness of experiences and thoughts is a major developmental milestone according to cognitive psychology and psychoanalytic theory (e.g., Bettelheim, 1967; Federn, 1952; Jacobson, 1964; Mahler, 1968; Schafer, 1968). It is integral to the development of concrete operational thought; of projective concepts of space including the capacity to represent foreshortening, the diagonal, depth, volume, and perspective; to the capacity to utilize affects and emotions to enrich one's understanding of reality;[14] and to develop an appreciation of interpersonal relations, empathy, and social mutuality and reciprocity (Blatt, 1983).

---

[13]Inhelder, Sinclair, and Bovet (1974), for example, contrast an earlier form of thought, homological thinking, based on perceptual experiences and isolated bits of information, with more conceptual, analogical thinking based on alternatives not physically present. Cocking and Segal (1975) in a discussion of Inhelder, Sinclair and Bovet's distinction of homological and analogical thinking, stress that the symbolic functioning of analogical thinking requires self-awareness, self-reflectivity, and the establishment of the self as a stable and important reference point.

[14]Clinical and experimental evidence indicates a correlation between preferred modes of spatial representation (topological and projective) and levels of personality organization (Blatt, Quinlan, & D'Afflitti, 1972; Blatt & Ritzler, 1974; Blatt & Wild, 1976; Roth & Blatt, 1974). These studies indicate a particular relationship between the representation of depth and volume (projective concepts of space) and the nature of affective experiences.

Euclidean Concepts

Euclidean concepts of space also derive from topological concepts and are constructed in parallel with the development of projective concepts of space. Projective and Euclidean concepts of space are distinct, but their development is closely intertwined. Projective concepts coordinate different perspectives of an object and adjust to variations in apparent size. Euclidean concepts coordinate objects within the total framework of a stable metric reference system that facilitates the conservation of surfaces and objective distances. Conservation of distances and surfaces in Euclidean space, based on the reciprocity or symmetry of perspectives, is an essential aspect of the development of a quantified concept of space (Laurendeau & Pinard, 1970).

Topological concepts consider only the inherent relations of a single object, without external reference, and ignore the features and dimensions of objects and the relations between them. Topological concepts of space are essentially limited to a concern with a single configuration. An object is defined without regard for the interval between separate objects. The concept of distance is reduced to "topological intuitions" about separation, discontinuity, and continuity, without reference to a point external to the objects themselves. Projective and Euclidean concepts of space are established with the beginning of concrete operational thought. Projective concepts form a comprehensive system that coordinates several different objects within a projective plane in relation to the viewpoint of an external observer. A projective system of perspective is eventually formed which allows for the coordination of objects from all possible viewpoints. The coordination of the relations of left–right, before–behind and above–below from an observer's viewpoint forms projective concepts of space and establishes the first level of Euclidean metric operations (Laurendeau & Pinard, 1970).

The child does not organize spatial position or orientation in terms of horizontal or vertical dimensions until about nine years of age. Position and orientation are initially represented with topological concepts of adjacency and order, or later in terms of the projective frame of reference that organizes the salient properties of the visual field. Around the age of nine or ten, the child develops the concept of the horizontal and vertical coordinate axes and this is the beginning of Euclidean concepts of space (Piaget & Inhelder, 1948/1967). The discovery of the horizontal and vertical axes and the subsequent capacity to represent the diagonal provide the basis for Euclidean concepts. The progressive coordination of the three spatial axes and the discovery of the equivalence of the three perpendicular geometric coordinates create the general referential system that become the dimensions of Euclidean space and the first level of Euclidean metrics. The referent axes represent ordered sequences of potential positions; within this general metric referential system objects can be located in relation to one another without undergoing distortion in objective size and distance. The qualitative reference system for the coordination of space that was based on early projective concepts of space and begun during the intuitive phase has gradually developed into a more quantitative system in which the relations among objects in space are defined mathematically. The three dimensions of space have become equivalent coordinate axes. The space between objects as well as objects themselves become part of a homogeneous field in which there is an appreciation and conservation of distance.

According to Piaget and Inhelder (1948/1967) the final achievement of spatial constructs is based on the coordination of partial spaces within a total homogeneous space. Based on a system of perspectives (projective space), objects are coordinated in a variety of potential or actual positions in relation to one another. The coordination of the three geometric axes provides a matrix through which objects are located in a single comprehensive, quantitative structure. In this stable reference system, objects are located in homogeneous space in their actual and potential positions. Euclidean concepts conserve size, distance and position within a diversity of viewpoints or projective planes. Projective concepts alone do not conserve these real dimensions and distances; this is achieved only with Euclidean concepts in the coordination of objects and their actual and potential positions in an integrated quantitative system. As the intervals separating objects are considered as potential positions, space becomes a stable structure in which distance and size are conserved, and measurement becomes possible. This transformation progressively leads the child to begin to consider space as a homogeneous "container" in which objects are no longer situated in space but rather are themselves part of space (Garcia & Piaget, 1974). Establishing a system of fixed reference points or geometric axes creates a network of possible directions and positions in which objects can be coordinated in space, distances can be conserved, and "elementary Euclidean concepts of parallelism, slope, similarity, proportion, etc. can be consolidated" (Laurendeau & Pinard, 1970, p. 170; see also Piaget & Inhelder, 1948/1967).

In Euclidean space there is conservation of parallels, angles, and distances. Objects retain their shape and relative position in Euclidean space according to a relation of proportionality, despite changes in size and distance. Similarity among figures is no longer established on the basis of contour alone, but by means of the parallelism of the corresponding sides and the equality of angles. The operations of the Euclidean system go beyond dealing with objects relative to a point of view, but are now relevant to issues of "placements" and "displacements." Euclidean concepts of space pertain not only to the relative location of objects, but also to the coordination of the location and the movement of objects. The relationship between the displacement of an object and its successive positions leads to the development of conservation of distance. Conservation of distance and length is an essential part of the development of an overall quantitative frame of reference. From a psychological standpoint, it is the degree to which the individual can coordinate different viewpoints and can construct projective relationships that allows for the conservation of distance and the construction of Euclidean relationships. Thus, while projective and Euclidean relationships are separate systems, they are interdependent. Projective and Euclidean relationships both lead to objects being related to one another within an overall frame of reference. The development of the projective system leads to the coordination of changes in position of objects in relation to the observer; the development of the Euclidean system leads to the coordination of the various positions and displacements within a unified coordinate system. Most developmental psychologists (e.g., Dolle, Bataillard & Guyon, 1973–74; Dolle, Bataillard, & Lacroix, 1974–75; Dolle, Vinter & Germain, 1974–75; Laurendeau & Pinard, 1970; Piaget, 1962b; Piaget & Inhelder, 1967; Olson, 1970, 1975) consider the coordination of three-dimensional space, not as innate, but as a mental construction that is the culmination of complex psychological development. Ultimately, the various multiple perspectives, the view from one's own vantage point and the multiple potential vantage points of others are integrated within a single, comprehensive, quantified, referential system.

Each phase in the development of projective concepts of space achieves stability and equilibrium in the quantified coordinates of

Euclidean concepts (Piaget, 1977). As projective concepts of space become more extensive, the Euclidean system becomes a more comprehensive, quantified system. Eventually, in the projective-Euclidean phase, concepts of movement and distance are achieved and integrated into the comprehensive system. The Euclidean coordinate system is a hypothetico-deductive, quantified, proportional system in which multiple, actual and potential, placements and displacements can be represented. It involves a conception of distance, angles, reciprocity, symmetry of perspectives, and a conservation of parallels. The integration of the three perpendicular geometric coordinates into a unified quantified system allows for the representation of order, sequence of positions, and relative locations without requiring changes in apparent size or distance. Space is conceptualized as a homogeneous container with a fixed, arbitrary reference point and coordinated axes. Equal intervals in the metrics of the coordinate system allow for the representation of potential positions in space. With the representation of actual and potential displacements in space there is an integration of movement and distance, and this introduces, for the first time, the potential for the articulation of the concept of time (Piaget, 1927/1969a). Time becomes a fourth coordinate; above–below, right–left, front–behind are supplemented by before–later.

Eventually the three spatial coordinate system is elaborated in a conception of a fourfold spatiotemporal field in which knowledge of reality is recognized to be a function of the relative position and movement of the observer. The concept of space has evolved from a Cartesian coordinate system to a Riemannian system that includes the fourth dimension of time and the observer as integral aspects of the spatiotemporal field. The Riemannian system involves an appreciation of the self as part of a complex field and an awareness that one's conceptions of the universe are products of one's own mental constructions. The fixed rectilinear concepts of space of the Cartesian coordinate system are now supplemented by alternative non-rectilinear geometries. New conceptions of space are derived from various non-Euclidean, non-rectilinear and equally valid geometries. The equal interval scaling of rectilinear space is now extended to include the possibility of proportional and ratio scaling of hyperbolic space. These new conceptions of space involve a more abstract and comprehensive system than was possible with the three rectilinear Cartesian coordinates. In developmental terms, the "decentration" from the egocentrism of the Cartesian coordinate system led to the next level in the development of concepts of space—a level that includes concepts of relativity and the four dimensional spatiotemporal field. The relativity expressed in spatial constructs is also expressed in conceptions of personal, social and cultural relativity.

Riemannian Space

By the end of the 19th century, most physicists agreed that there was no evidence to support Newton's concept of absolute space and, even further, that a concept of absolute space was no longer needed to explain the centrifugal forces of rotational motion. Ernst Mach (1905), for example, discusses space as relative, but he still assumed that space was essentially Euclidean in nature. The discovery of non-Euclidean geometries (e.g., Gauss, Bolyai, Lobechevski, and Riemann) led to the elimination of the last traditional characteristic of absolute space, and modern physics moved to a concept of space based on the Riemannian n-dimensional manifold (Jammer, 1954/1969). This new theory of space is based on the continuity principle in which all laws are formulated on a concept of a field and not on actions at a distance. In a field theory it is possible to designate position in space without using a material coordinate system. As Jammer (1954/1969) notes, until the Renaissance, space was defined in reference to objects, but in modern physics the concept of space triumphs and objects are defined in reference to a hyperbolic conception of space (Grünbaum, 1963).

The contemporary conceptual construction of space in modern physics is based on the assumption that objects can have both a change of position and a change of state. For Einstein, it is the alteration of position that is of fundamental importance for the concept of space. There is no action at a distance, as there was in the finite geometry of Euclid and in the Newtonian inertial system. The inertial system was replaced by the adoption of the concept of a field expressed in the four parameters of space-time. Einstein's revision of the Newtonian concept of space placed an emphasis on the relativity of the role of the observer and on the integration of the dimension of time with the three dimensions of space. Einstein's formulation of the four-dimensional space-time continuum is more conceptual, abstract, and less intuitive than the immediately perceptible and concrete conception of three-dimensional space. The revised concept of space is now based on the quantification of the relativity of space-time and the role of the observer in defining space. The Euclidean quantification of the three spatial coordinates is now integrated with the dimension of time and the concept of the relativity of the spatiotemporal field. Riemannian concepts of space are an elaboration and an extension of projective and Euclidean concepts of space.

Projective and Euclidean conceptions of space have been revised and extended to include more fully the relativity of the observer. Physical properties of length, distance, and duration, and all properties derived from them, are now defined relative to the observer. As Eddington stressed (1922, p. 14) we must "realize the distortion imported into the world of nature by the parochial standpoint from which we observe it," and also recognize that we can never completely eliminate this distortion. The human element in our conception of space can never be eliminated, but we can recognize the distortions imposed by our particular spatiotemporal frame of reference (Perry, 1968/1970). What is common to all observers is a fourfold spatiotemporal framework. Observation of objects in three dimensions is only an illusion; observations change with the motion of the observer and there is a "super-object in four dimensions." Einstein defined the relations between frames of space and time for observers with different motions, and Minkowski demonstrated that "these frames are merely systems of partitions arbitrarily drawn across a four-dimensional world which is common to all observers" based on a fourfold order of right–left, before–behind, up–down, and sooner–later (Eddington, 1922, p. 15). Nature is a world of events based on a common fourfold order that, especially because of the temporal dimension, is represented differently by each observer. Time is a dynamic process and the concept of the now or the instant is an artificial partition of a chain of events. In addition, each object has its own space-time reference frame that must be appreciated and acknowledged if objects are to be described in comparable terms. Einstein's special theory of relativity stresses that there is no privileged space-time framework and there is no basis for establishing a priority for any one particular observer, observation, or framework. The integration of the three spatial dimensions into a more general, relative, fourfold spatiotemporal field requires an alteration and an extension of Euclidean concepts of space. Jammer (1954/1969) refers to this

TABLE 1
Individual and Cultural Development of Concepts of the Object and of Space

Individual Development		Cultural Development		
Concepts of Space	Concept of the Object	History of Art	Cosmological World View	Concept of Scaling (Stevens, 1951)
I. *Topological Concepts of Space* 1. Objects in isolation. 2. Proximity, separation, surround, contour, enclosure (boundary). 3. Space is fragmented and defined by contour of the isolated, single configuration. 4. Two-dimensional plane (without depth) with only a global sense of space. 5. Simple ordinal qualitative coordination of two-dimensional space. 6. Simple linear order and continuity.	I. *Sensorimotor—Preoperational Levels* 1. Experiences of action sequences around need gratification of basic polarities of pleasure-pain, hunger-satiety (life and death). 2. Isolated, segmented, momentary experiences without overall understanding of object, context or sequence. 3. Subject and object poorly differentiated. 4. Schemata develop around partial elements and momentary situations. 5. No schemata of general classes, serial correspondence, or conservation and constancy beyond the immediate situation. 6. Objects signified by static, fixed reproductive images and verbal expression of semi-individual, semi-general relations and partial elements without appreciation of context. 7. Simple correspondence between pairs or small sets of objects. 8. Transition to intuitive integration of object and context.	Paleolithic Art Egyptian Art	Animistic	Nominal (Classificatory) Scale. Mutually exclusive, discrete objects in a reflexive, symmetrical, transitive relation to each other. Designation of a class or type. Ordinal (Ranking) Scale. Comparative, monotone, qualitative, irreflexive, asymmetrical, transitive ordering of objects or groups.

Projective-Euclidean & Intuitive Levels		
II. Intuitive (Perceptual) Level		Aristotelian
1. Beginning integration of pairs or small sets of objects into total, general configuration of object and context (object constancy).	Greco-Roman Art	
2. General schemata of total situation or configuration.		
3. Perceptual totality of concrete, literal configuration of manifest features which transcends specific context.		
4. Intuitive (empirical) sense of perspective.		
5. Schemata based on total, fixed, constant, non-contradictory, ideal, general, universal image of object.	Middle Ages	
6. Some relations of manifest, concrete, part properties within total object.		
7. Beginning of relations between elements and independent objects in a total context.	Early Renaissance	
8. Transition to the beginning of cognitive operations with transformation, reversibility and conservation.		

II. Projective-Euclidean Concepts of Space

1. Space as defined by the straight line and projective-sectional planes.
2. Relationships between objects defined in relative terms based upon apparent size and distance in space.
3. Several interrelated objects in a qualitative organization of three-dimensional concept of space.
4. Differentiation among various alternative viewpoints.
5. Projective dimensions can be coordinated without the support of concomitant topological cues.

TABLE 1 (Continued)
Individual and Cultural
Development of Concepts of the Object and of Space

Individual Development		Cultural Development		
Concepts of Space	*Concept of the Object*	*History of Art*	*Cosmological World View*	*Concept of Scaling* (Stevens, 1951)

6. Geometric coordination of three-dimensional space.
7. Measurement in three-dimensional space by means of a coordinate system.
  a) Linear perspective in symmetrical, pyramidal structure.
  b) Linear perspective in asymmetrical, diagonal structure.
  c) Diagonal structure to organize space.
8. Space as homogeneous container, as stable, coordinated structure which allows for expression of actual and potential positions and movements in a coordinated, quantitative spatial system.
	III. *Concrete Operational Level*
	1. Transformations, reversibility and conservation of manifest, external features.
	2. Relationships of manifest part properties within total object (part/whole relationship).
	3. Relationship between different objects, and between objects and the context, based on manifest, concrete features.
	4. Concept of self and increased coordination of subjective and objective dimensions.
	5. Conception of objects no longer fixed, rigid, generalized, idealized image.
	6. Variations (transformations) of external attributes of both objects and context with conservation.
	7. Objects in dynamic, reciprocal interactions.
	8. Appreciation of unique perspective of self and of others.
	  a. Capacity of identification with perspective views of others.
	    1) Interpersonal relations.
		Late Renaissance
		
		Mannerism
		
		Baroque
			Copernican
			
			Newtonian
				Interval Scale.
				
				Quantified distance between points based on common, consistent, but arbitrary units of measurement and reference point.

9. Conservation of distance, angles and parallels, reciprocity, symmetry of perspective, proportionality.			
10. Multiple perspectives.			
III. *Riemannian Concepts of Space*			
1. Hyperbolic conception of space.			
2. Observer is an integral part of field.			
3. Time as a fourth coordinate.			
4. Four fold, spatiotemporal field.			
5. Relativity of position and movement of observer.			

	Art	Physics	Scale
2) Empathy (shared affect).			
b. Increased recognition of importance of personal perspective and meaning.			
9. Transition from emphasis on manifest features to recognition of internal structure.	Impressionism		
IV. *Formal Operational Level*			
1. Emancipation from concrete, manifest object for more abstract, inner form and structure.	Cubism		
2. Transformation, reversibility and conservation of abstract, inner features, dimensions and processes.			
3. Abstract symbolic concepts and basic structural principles of organization.	Modern Art		Ratio Scale.
4. Hypothetico-deductive, logico-mathematical, and propositional systems.			
5. Relations of relations (relations among structural dimensions and principles).			
6. Observer is an integral part of the field.			Precise scale values established on a defined scale in which there are specified ratios between all scale values and a numerically and experientially relevant reference point.
7. Full integration and coordination of subjective and objective dimensions.		Einsteinian	
8. Awareness that thoughts are not fully determined by nature, but are mental constructions.			
9. Cultural and interpersonal relativism.			
10. Appreciation of indeterminancy.			

new level of spatiotemporal conceptualization as Riemannian space, a concept of space that encompasses the observer and the components in a field in the fourfold parameters of time and space.

Table 1 presents a schematic overview of the developmental psychological sequences discussed in this chapter. The first two columns of Table 1 present a schematic summary of the sequences in the development of the concepts of space and the concept of the object. The last three columns of the table present an overview of the issues to be considered in Chapters 3, 4, and 5—the relationship of the psychological developmental concepts to the analysis of cultural development as seen in the history of art and science, and in the basic mathematical structures that have evolved in major epochs in Western Civilization.

3
From Topological to Projective Space: Painting in the Ancient, Greco-Roman, and Medieval Periods

ANCIENT ART

Among the earliest works of art in Western Civilization are the cave paintings discovered at Altamira in Spain, at Lascaux in the Dordogne region of France, and at other sites along the Northern Mediterranean, all dating from the last stage of the Paleolithic Period (12,000–10,000 B.C.). The Ancient period begins with these paintings and includes all the art produced before the Greeks began their quest for naturalistic representations. Schäfer (1919/1974, p. 84) called this art "pre-Greek" and included in this designation the art of the great pre-Greek cultures, such as Paleolithic, Mesopotamian, and Egyptian art. In her incisive epilogue to Schäfer's book on Egyptian art, Brunner-Traut (1974) argues for the use of the term "aspective" (or "pre-perspective") to describe the art of this period.

The earliest forms of Paleolithic art are simple hand prints and "meanders" created by fingers drawn through soft clay (Breuil, 1952; Sieveking, 1979). Although the dating of this prehistoric art is ambiguous and controversial, it is believed that these productions predate the representation of animal forms. The hand prints and meanders emerged as an extension of the artist's action that led directly to the construction of a rudimentary symbol. The artistic symbol directly expresses the artist's action—it is a sensorimotor–

preoperational construction. Subsequent representations are primarily of animal forms that proceed from simple to more complex figures, from simple silhouettes to a combination of profile and frontal views (profile body and frontal face), from single figures in isolation to more complex animal forms in aggregates.

The representation of space in the animal drawings of the Paleolithic period emphasize the boundary or contour of the figures, and this serves to define the separateness of the object from the surrounding void. The nearly life-size paintings primarily depict familiar animals (horses, bison, and wild boar) in outline form and in vivid colors (red, brown, black, and blue). Each object is clearly separate from, and independent of, any other object, and there is no concern with composition. The occasional representation of closely knit groups such as the foal and mare are still basically single forms (Gioseffi, 1965, 1966). Emphasis is on the figure–ground relationship and the articulation of the object as a definitive figure independent of other figures and the surrounding ground (Gombrich, 1960; Frankfort & Ashmole, 1971; Ivins, 1946). The figures are placed randomly and without direction. As illustrated by Fig. 1, Paleolithic art lacks order and direction, and is without combination and composition (Giedion, 1962). The basic principle is "the single form . . . simply set off against chaos" (Frankfort, 1951, p. 15). Giedion (1962), Leroi-Gourhan (1967) and others, however, do not consider primeval art as occurring in a context of chaos, but instead view Paleolithic art as indifferent to direction. The line and orientation of prehistoric cave paintings (e.g. Fig. 1) have no relation to horizontal or vertical—the paintings are completely free of any directional surface. For Giedion and Leroi-Gourhan the basic principle is the representation of objects

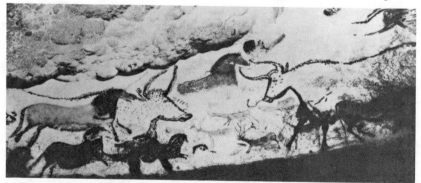

FIG. 1 *Hall of Bulls at Lascaux* (Early Magdalenian, c.15,000–10,000 B.C.) Dordogne, France. (Archives Photographiques).

in isolation, free of immediate surround, background, or direction. Giedion (1962) marvels at this "undisciplined freedom" that is lost in subsequent civilizations, never to be achieved again in the history of art.

In developmental psychological terms, Ancient art was initially sensorimotor—it expresses directly the action of the artist placing his hand print on the wall or drawing fingers through clay. Subsequent representation of animal forms involves an emphasis upon early topological principles of the simple boundary or contour of a single, isolated configuration. Each object is presented as an isolated experience without context or sequence. Images are randomly placed without orientation and coherence, often superimposed, inverted, and unrelated. The representation is a concrete, literal, life-size image with little concern other than the fundamental definition and identity of the object. Art was utilized in magical, ritual functions concerned with the basic struggle for life and survival. It expressed the cycle of creation—the hunting and killing of animals necessary for the sustenance of life, the struggle to adapt to the environment and to sustain life. The animals most frequently portrayed were those that were used for food or those considered most dangerous. The most frequent themes were about copulation and reproduction (Graziosi, 1960). Modell (1968, p. 14) concludes, based on Rochlin (1965), that "cave art served a religious function arising from this primitive society's proximity to death." The cave paintings were life-size, objective depictions that strove to create an image of the object and, in that way, to conserve it. The representations are primarily on a sensorimotor-preoperational level. Their purpose was to evoke an image of the object in order to preserve it from loss. "In soft, flickering light the animals take on an almost magical movement" (Giedion, 1962, p. 528) in which the continual appearance and disappearance gives them a vital, dynamic quality. As discussed by Bernheimer (1961, p. 18), representation in primitive art had an "apotropic function"; it is "a magical defense against the inexorable passage of time and the menace of demonical powers," a "desire for order, measure and stability" that expresses "man's power over the unknown . . . and help him acquire confidence in his own continuity and provides him with the means through which this continuity can be assured."

The Paleolithic cave paintings were attempts to create the hunted animal within the confines of the cave. Gouge marks suggest that spears may have been thrown at the images and that these images were treated as if they were alive; death of the image was equivalent to the death of the prey. Painting the animal on the cave wall gave the cave dweller power and control over the animal; animistic thinking assured the capacity to find and successfully kill the animal so that the food supplies could be maintained (Frankfort, Frankfort, Wilson, & Jacobsen, 1949).

The image of the animal was captured in the representation of only the most essential details. Its perfected form was portrayed in isolation and in profile. The delineation of contours and the structural relationships among the essential part properties were carefully maintained in a highly stylized fashion. The emphasis upon the relationships among the most essential features of the animal (Hagan, 1979) gives these works an immediate and direct appeal (Levy, 1948). The freedom from direction and orientation and the sense of continuous change experienced when these paintings are viewed in the flickering light of a fire within the cave creates a sense of "eternal present," in which there is a "perpetual interflow of today, yesterday and tomorrow" (Giedion, 1962, p. 538). Animals were also occasionally represented in motion which, when seen in firelight, created a powerful experience of remarkable beauty.

Although the cave dwellers could represent an animal in action, they were uninterested in the narrative function of art and were much more concerned with the sanctity and constancy of the animal form, the "recreations of abiding form" (Levy, 1948, p. 41), in order to control basic life processes of fertility and death and to attribute power to the image. Human figures were rare in cave art, and, when introduced, it was usually in some fusion of human and animal forms as part of a ritual act.

Subsequently, in the Mesolithic period (8000–3000 B.C.), art progressed from the depiction of the outline of a life-size animal in isolation to a diminutive representation of animals and men organized in scenes of a hunt, harvest, battle, or ritual dance. For the first time, human figures appear in aggregate, coherent groups and an interest in the narrative depiction of an activity replaces the emphasis on the naturalistic qualities of an object in isolation. (See Figs. 2 & 3). Human figures in isolation and in large integrated groups occurred often in the Mesolithic rock paintings discovered in North Africa and on the eastern coast of Spain. Like the earlier Paleolithic art, these paintings appear to have served a magical-ritual function, but they have greater vitality and movement and the figures are represented in a variety of

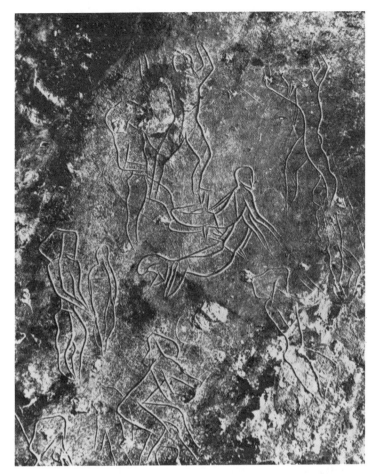

FIG. 2 *Engraved Rock with Human Figures* (Mesolithic, c. 8000 B.C.), Addaura Cave, Palermo, Sicily. (P. Graziosi, *Paleolithic Art,* New York: McGraw-Hill, 1960).

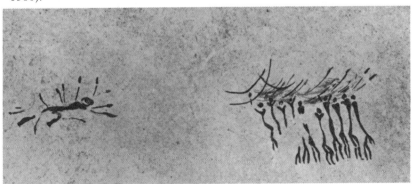

FIG. 3 *'Execution Group'* (c. 5000–2000 B.C.), Remigian, Castellón, Spain (Mr. Robert Erskine, London).

different contexts. Gardner (1975) notes a similarity between these rock paintings and pictographs and even phonetic hieroglyphics and comments that these early rock paintings are a major step in the development from literal, pictorial to abstract symbolic representation. Mesolithic art was narrative and anecdotal, commemorating a specific event such as hunting or fighting in comparison to the timeless, static, monumental stereotyped Paleolithic figures in isolation. Space was first represented in Mesolithic art in the distance established between the figures.

Major changes in social organization in the subsequent Neolithic period had an important impact on art. Nomadic hunters began to form food-producing villages, animals were domesticated, and stable communities of farmers and herdsmen were formed in both Mesopotamia and Egypt. Patterns of social order emerged with clearly defined divisions of labor and conceptions of deities were established either around the king or the cycles of nature. Growth and life were experienced in the seasonal renewal of crops and in the birth and death of animals. Eventually man's existence was no longer considered to be dependent upon ritual. The concept of the divine was not expressed in natural and animal form but in individual, social, and ethical form (Levy, 1948, 1963). There was also an emerging sense of self-awareness and identity that developed further in Egyptian culture and eventually reached a zenith in Greek civilization. With the change from a Paleolithic and Mesolithic hunting of animals to the development of Neolithic agricultural communities in Egypt, Mesopotamia and elsewhere, art began to reflect a new interest in "order, measure and relation." This interest was expressed in geometric ornamentation used to enhance functional objects such as vases and water jars (Frankfort, 1951). The function of art slowly began to change from primarily a magical-ritualistic role, to ornamentation, to a narrative, historical record.

One of the earliest examples of Egyptian painting is the predynastic mural at Hiereonpolis (c. 4000–3500 B.C.) of randomly placed men, animals, and boats in a narrative scene without a context, setting, an organizing ground or baseline, or depth (Fig. 4). As noted by Frankfort (1951, p. 16), "the boats, animals, and humans . . . are vertically arranged in groups . . . without the slightest consideration for logical coherence. . . . None of the figures are . . . spatially related . . . in a few instances, the human figures are joined by contact in a schematic action. . . . Their vertical orientation gives . . . the back-

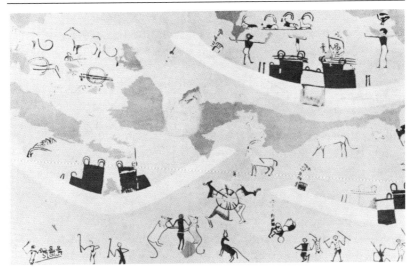

FIG. 4 *Men, Boats & Animals* (Predynastic Egypt, c. 3500 B.C.) Hieracon-polis. (L'Art et l'Homme, Larousse) (after Quibel).

ground the quality of depthless, undifferentiated space." The empha-sis is still upon the single figures and not upon the total composition.

Subsequent to the pre-dynastic period, individual figures in Egyp-tian art began to be placed on a baseline and these baselines defined different areas of the picture. The picture surface was articulated into zones that provided a clear organization for the picture. Objects and figures were no longer presented in isolation or randomly placed, but now were precisely located and aligned in space. Yet the figures were not coordinated within a unified conception of space. Egyptian art is fundamentally a two-dimensional art with a unique representation of space that lacks any indication of perspective and spatial depth (Schäfer, 1919/1974). In Egyptian art there is a beginning organiza-tion, spatial direction, and context, but subordinate to an overriding relationship to a single direction: the vertical. Several different as-pects of the same object are depicted on a vertical plane and although there is the representation of the horizontal, the ninety-degree angle, the axis, and bilateral symmetry, they are all outgrowths of the em-phasis upon the vertical as the basic compositional spatial principle (Giedion, 1962).

Throughout Egyptian art, figures continue to be presented primar-ily in profile, but include all the essential features and details of the frontal view. Highly stylized figures are carefully placed on horizontal baselines without overlap or superimposition. A fixed, stylized blend of profile view and frontal features emphasizes the major properties of the human figure and identifies the stable and fundamental facts of nature. Sharply drawn outlines of individual figures are presented primarily in profile. Egyptian art, as all pre-Greek art, had a primary emphasis upon the boundary or contour of the figure. According to Schäfer (1919/1974, p. 79), "there is scarcely any other art where everything is so much subject to the all-important outline."

Schäfer discussed Egyptian art as "pre-perspective," composed of images that present the predominant features of an object as they exist in nature, not as experienced or perceived. There is a "fixed character of the forms" used repeatedly for the representation of animals, plants, people, and inanimate objects (Schäfer, 1919/1974, p. 149). The total, concrete, whole object is portrayed as flat in the picture plane, without reference to either a spatial or temporal context. The goal is to capture the most essential and typical features of the object. Thus a frontal eye, or eyes, appears on a profile head. This "image-based" frontal-profile blend is faithful to the object as a concrete literal entity rather than to its visual appearance (Levy, 1943; Loewy, 1900/1907). The object is depicted part by part as it exists in reality with no attempt to create an illusion of depth. In a similar way, related objects appear together but without a defined spatial relationship: for example, a cobbler will have his tools in mid-air surrounding him (Schäfer, 1919/1974). The size of the figure is determined by its importance and not by its position in the scene.

For three thousand years little change took place in the formal, stylized, "two-dimensional" mode of representation in Egyptian art. The *Palette of Narmer* (3000 B.C.) serves as an excellent early statement of the mode of representation that was to dominate Egyptian art for 30 centuries. In the *Palette of Narmer* (Fig 5a, b) the figures are without perspective and are a presentation of essential profile and frontal details. The eye is shown frontally in a profile face, the head, legs, and arms are in profile; the torso is presented frontally. Shoulders, shown in profile, are joined with frontal torsos. The size of the figure is commensurate with its rank. Thus in the *Palette*, the King towers over his own men and his enemies; he is isolated from and surpasses all ordinary people. The picture plane is systematically subdivided into horizontal zones, and pictorial elements are placed in these zones in a precise and orderly fashion. The horizontal lines that separate the zones also provide the ground level upon which the figures are placed. The introduction of a groundline provides a degree of or-

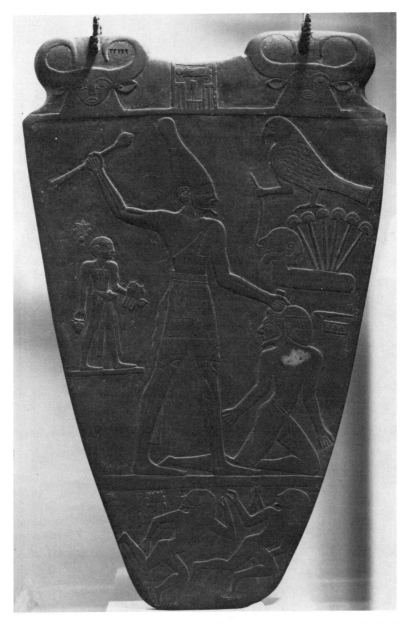

FIG. 5a *Palette of Narmer* (obverse side) (First Dynasty, c. 3000 B.C.)
Hieraconpolis. Cairo Museum (Hirmer Verlag).

107

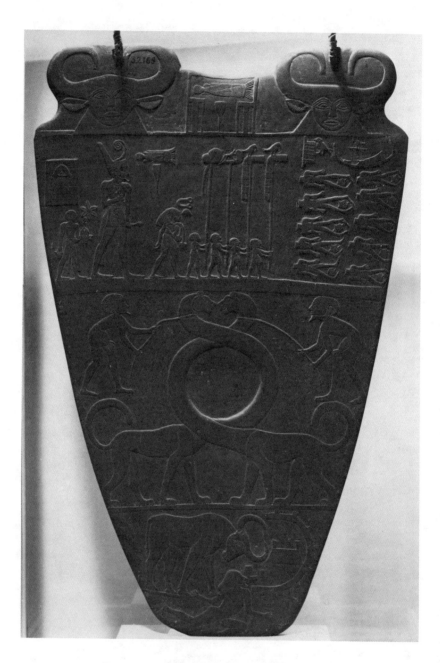

FIG. 5b *Palette of Narmer* (reverse side) (First Dynasty, c. 3000 B.C.)
Hieraconpolis. Cairo Museum (Hirmer Verlag).

ganization and coherence that places each figure in a definite, but unspecified, locality. Objects are no longer placed in a random or confused order, but are now restricted to a single plane on a single level. There is no spatial relationship possible between figures on separate groundlines, but figures on the same groundline are joined together through a "tenuous spatial link" (Frankfort, 1951, p. 20). No representation of spatial depth exists; figures are primarily organized only in a simple sequence of figures or actions. The painting is not about realistic acts performed at a particular place and viewed from a specific angle but of "a timeless act" (Frankfort, 1951, p. 21).

New subjects and more differentiated gestures and postures were introduced into Egyptian art; however, they did not portray human figures as more functional and realistic. Gestures and postures were not designed to express human emotion but primarily to indicate a status or an action. The static world of Egyptian art shunned naturalism, emotion, and spatial illusion. The mode of representation established in the *Palette of Narmer* was the standard for all subsequent Egyptian art, except for a brief period in the New Kingdom during the dynasty of Akhenaton in the 14th century B.C. This unchanging, formal, static, stylized mode of representation in art was consistent with Egyptian philosophy and social order in which kings were deified and their attributes made eternal. Frankfort (1951, p. 23) speculates about the relationship between "the strict dogma of divine kingship, which . . . did not allow of any tension between factual and ideal power" and the rigid modes of artistic representation in which human figures are not rendered as alive, vital, and emotionally involved in a network of relationships. An overwhelming preoccupation with the dogma of a divine and perfect kingship in the early Old Kingdom and with the representation of the king in "static perfection" (Frankfort, 1951, p. 51) is also expressed in a carefully prescribed formula for the representation of figures based upon a precise concept of proportions (Panofsky, 1955a). The major figure appears rigid, in a "robot-like" pose, in a state of static perfection. Illusionistic tendencies and dramatic scenes are shunned so that the timeless perfection of a divine king may be represented. At the same time, food, property, and other necessities of life are depicted with some kind of magical intent to ensure provisions for the deceased king (Frankfort, 1951).

The fixed and unchanging mode of representation established in the *Palette of Narmer* can be seen in the paintings and reliefs of the Old Kingdom, such as those from the tomb of Ti at Saqqara (Fig. 6). In a

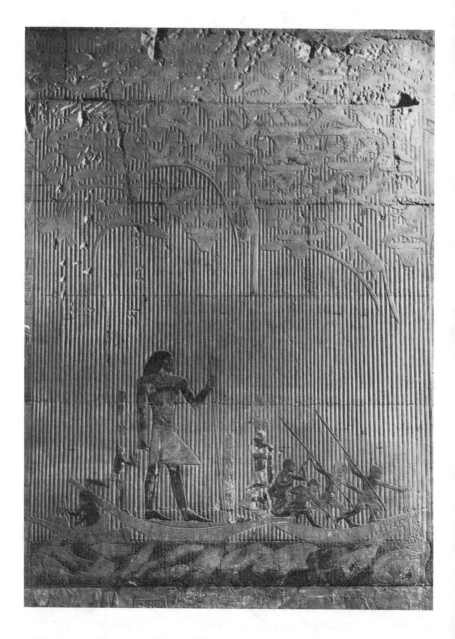

FIG. 6 *Hippopotamus Hunt* (c. 2500 B.C.) In the Tomb of Ti at Saqqara, (Hirmer Verlag).

relief of Ti on a hippopotamus hunt or in his household, Ti's rank is expressed in his disproportionate size and highly conventional pose. In the hunt the king towers over his warriors, and in his household the master of the house stands over his kneeling wife and his son, who has his hand on the lower part of Ti's staff. The son, although upright, barely reaches his father's knee. This relief also illustrates how the figures are represented in isolation, without a sense of relationship between them. Also, all three figures face to the left with their faces in profile, but their shoulders and chests are shown frontally. Ti is presented with two right feet with a big toe and an open arch. Often (although not here) the open arch is an important way of showing that someone or something is behind the figure in the foreground (Schäfer, 1919/1974). The isolated figure with a static stride leaning on his staff is a typical stance of the tomb owner in Egyptian funerary art (Frankfort, 1951).

This basic mode of representation continued to dominate Egyptian art of the Middle Kingdom but with a somewhat greater naturalism and monumentality. Figures began to be drawn in more realistic proportion and with a greater elaboration of detail in the figures; but there is still a combination of profile and frontal views and, particularly, no attempt to present the shoulders and back as foreshortened. Side and front views are simply joined together without the illusion of foreshortening and perspective. However, at this time the first deliberate attempt to break the rigidity of parallel registers appears. Contours of hills and mountains are presented without a baseline and are placed at various levels and "boldly joined by diagonals," which makes the higher contours appear as more distant, thereby achieving some kind of recession in depth (Frankfort, 1951, pp. 70–73).

In the art of the New Kingdom the basic formula for representation persisted as established in the *Palette of Narmer*, some 1500 years earlier. The size of figures is still defined by their rank, and horizontal registers can still be rigidly separated. Although the wall paintings in the tombs of the New Kingdom adhere to these basic principles of representation, they contain innovations in detailing and a new liveliness and vitality within clusters of interacting figures. Eventually Egyptian painting became somewhat more naturalistic and realistic. A New Kingdom painting of *User-her Hunting* (Fig. 7) illustrates the vivid liveliness, dramatic movement, and naturalistic features that supplement and enrich the highly stylized form of representation. Depth is depicted by overlapping and layering and

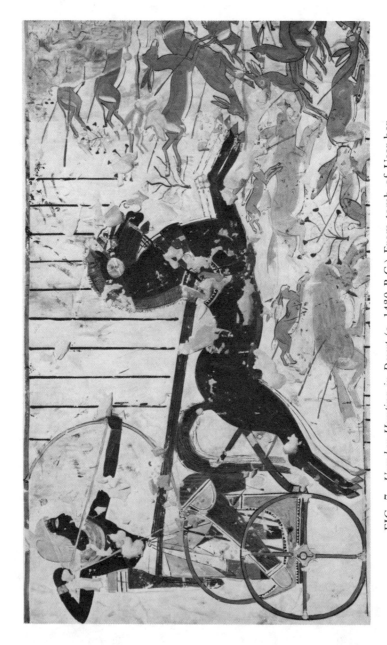

FIG. 7 *User-her Hunting in Desert* (c. 1430 B.C.) From tomb of User-her, Royal Scribe to Amenophis 11, in Thebes (The Metropolitan Museum of Art, New York City).

some beginning attempts at foreshortening appear, particularly at the shoulder and in the integration of the profile head with the frontal or three-quarter view of the torso. Small groups of figures appear natural and deliberately arranged. A lively and transient quality is combined with the static perfection of the old pattern (Frankfort, 1951). Hunting scenes contain more vigorous movement of hunters and animals both attacking and being attacked.

The innovations in details and liveliness in 15th century B.C. wall paintings of the New Kingdom continued into the 14th century in the reign of Akhenaton. But in the social revolution of Akhenaton that occurred at Amarna, artists also broke away from the old preoccupations that sought to transform ephemeral life into an eternal timelessness. The concept of the king, for example, changed from a figure with mythical qualities to a single human person with supreme and divine power. Akhenaton also tried to remove an anthropomorphism from religion and develop a more conceptual form of religion. In Egypt there had been a perennial worship of the sun in which various phases of the sun were recognized as distinct gods instead of aspects of a single god. Akhenaton's deity was also the sun whose rays emitted brilliance, warmth, and life. But Akhenaton deified Aton, the physical disc of the sun, as the single universal force that produced and sustained life (Wilson, 1956). This conception of the deity was maintained without a visual image and "was a genuine monotheism" (Gardiner, 1961, p. 227). Akhenaton's universal monotheism was part of a new social organization that included the personal conduct of the pharaoh and an emphasis on an appreciation of nature, life, truth, and candor (Aldred, 1968). Language and literature were colloquialized (Wilson, 1956) and, in art, a "sensuous treatment of surface texture, a tendency to greater 'realism' through softer, more voluptuous contours, slightly less rigid postures" (Frankfort, 1951, p. 96) was part of a new interest in the observation of nature and an increased emotional sensitivity. Art was more naturalistic and realistic and it often represented the warmth and intimacy of contemporary family life.

In the *Cairo Stela* (Fig. 8), the family of Akhenaton and Nefertiti are portrayed in affectionate interaction under the rays of Aton in a garden pavilion of reeds and rushes. The naturalism and realism create a contemporary family scene in time and space with which the viewer can empathetically identify (Aldred, 1968). These changes in art, as well as changes in literature and social order, evolved over

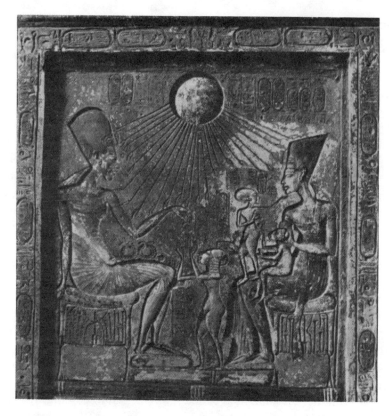

FIG. 8   *The Solar Disc of Aton Blessing Royal Family of Akhenaton, Nefertiti and Three Daughters* (14th century B.C.) Tel-el-Amarna (Cairo Museum).

several generations, but they were fully expressed and consolidated only with the change in religion from the anthropomorphic deity of Amon (the Hidden One) and the "mortuary" religion of the God Osiris to the monotheistic, natural, life-giving forces of Aton, the sun disc. God and the pharaoh were no longer remote and secretive but now viewed as creative, nurturant, and benevolent.

The art of Amarna has greater realism, soft contours, and a dynamic sense of action. For the first time in Egyptian art there is a differentiation between left and right hands and feet (Aldred, 1968). While groundlines are still used, and occasionally horizontal registers, there are important changes. Isolated, static, rigid figures are replaced with intricate arrangements of interacting and overlapping figures in small, self-contained groups. There is "a new relationship between scene and spectator" and a sense of naturalism and realism in a "coherent event in a definite spatial setting" (Frankfort, 1951, p. 105). Buildings are no longer rendered as a schematic outline or facade but as a combination of features to represent a specific building. The renderings are still highly stylized, yet they are intended to depict a particular building and to designate a specific place in which the action occurs. For the first time, the horizontal registers are ignored, and the distance between figures becomes significant, but the use of fragments of groundlines preclude "an illusionary relation in depth" (Frankfort, 1951, p. 106).

The Amarna revolution was a brief break in the great and lengthy continuity of the basic modes of representation of Egyptian art. It was a temporary relaxation of the preoccupation with death and timeless eternity; an increased interest in natural life and the expression of movement and emotions are expressed in flowing curvilinear forms. After this brief revolution in philosophy, social order, and art, Egyptian society returned to its long tradition and continuity. The Amarna revolution began to disintegrate and eventually Tutankhaton, Akhenaton's son-in-law, rejected the monotheism of Aton, changed his name to Tutankhamen, abandoned Amarna, and returned to Thebes, the city of Amon 300 miles to the south. The Amarna revolution gave way to the old reactionary forces that were to dominate Egyptian life once again. In religion, there was a return to mystical, hidden, malevolent deities who had supreme power, even over the god-king of the pharaoh. Individuals were no longer strong within themselves but once again needed the support of gods to counteract the fatal ephemeral quality of life (Wilson, 1956). The fluid, curvilinear artistic forms and the liveliness and movement of the art of Amarna were continued to some degree in the art of Tutankhamen. But, as illustrated in Fig. 9, a detail from the *"Book of the Dead" of Naun* (c. 1000 B.C.) there was an eventual return to the original mode of representation of the rigid, static, formal, flattened forms first expressed in the *Palette of Narmer* and the art of the Old Kingdom.

Brunner-Traut characterizes the basic mode of representation in Egyptian art as "aspective" as opposed to "perspective" (Bunim, 1940, calls these two modes "conceptual" and "optical"). These two modes are a fundamental distinction in the history of art, reflecting different attitudes toward the world. Brunner-Traut chose the term "aspective" to suggest a number of things: "*aspect* viewing"—a delimited and detached object; "a-spective"—a mental image independent of sight or visual appearance; and an alternative to "*per*spective." According to

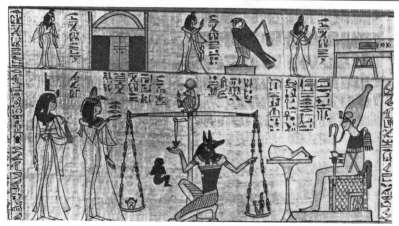

FIG. 9   *The Court of the Dead, detail of the "Book of the Dead" of Naun* (c. 1000 B.C.) Deir el Bahari. (Metropolitan Museum of Art, N.Y.).

Brunner-Traut (1974) the Egyptian aspective method of representation is

> a mode of seeing opposite and in the presence of the object, not forwards or backwards in time, and not moving outside its boundaries. . . . It does not relate the object, which it has separated in this way in space and time, to the totality of elements that constitute its real existence, and it does not link it functionally to another object, even in a causal relationship. (p. 430)

The Egyptian aspective mode of representation is based on a rendering of the object, part by part, as it existed in reality. "A square surface is shown as an equal, right-angled quadrilateral" (Brunner-Traut, p. 424). The object is an absolute entity, represented as a concrete, literal reality (Levy, 1943; Loewy, 1900/1907). In aspective art, each individual part of the object is viewed separately and each individual trait is represented in the same way according to a fixed formula, always independent of the viewing subject. The focus is fully on the concrete reality of the object instead of on its context. Its position in the spatiotemporal environment is ignored. Individual figures are sharply drawn and stand on a baseline. The baseline organizes the picture, often into registers, but this ultimately places a limit on the unification of the picture plane. Objects are clearly detached from their surroundings; each is a self-contained and independent structure with no expression of the relation between objects or between the object and its context. Objects are presented as flat and in isolation, usually in profile or in frontal view and not extended in space. Objects are neither seen from a certain distance in a functional relationship to the whole nor presented against a background or foreground. "The boundary is the first and last criterion of aspective" art (Brunner-Traut, 1974, p. 430; cf. Schäfer, 1919/1974, p. 79).

Frankfort (1951, p. 7) calls pre-Greek art "nonfunctional" because it does not adapt solid or three-dimensional forms to two-dimensional surfaces. For the Egyptians, space was indicated not by perspective and foreshortening but by either juxtaposing associated objects or depicting more than one side of an object as if both sides were in front, or using vertical or horizontal overlapping and layering (Frankfort, 1951). Time, as a succession of events, did not exist in aspective art. A sense of time requires some differentiation and distance between the observer and the event. Aspective time revolves around cyclical seasonal events and ritualistic eternal recurrences (Eliade, 1971), and, therefore, appears timeless in comparison with historical or astronomical time. To the ancient Egyptian, for example, there was no difference between cyclical and historical time. Egyptian chronology was periodic; each king marked anew the beginning of time. History, as linear succession, did not begin until the XVIII Dynasty with its extended frontiers, foreign influences, and serial lists of kings. Even the Egyptian language reflects the sense of perpetual present (Brunner-Traut, 1974).

The emphasis on the perpetual present is reflected in the funerary art of Egypt. The content of the art depicts the various forms of the seasonal and life cycles. The depiction of themes of life and death are an attempt to deal with the threat of death. Windows and eyes are placed on the tombs so that the deceased can view the world. Art in the tombs ensured the deceased a posthumous existence and immortality. The dead are portrayed alive, watching over the activities of life (Frankfort, 1951), often with these activities being performed by named members of their household. Frankfort states that while we may interpret a painting as a tomb-owner visiting his peasants on a farm, the Egyptians saw this depiction as two distinct and concrete realities: a portrayal of the deceased and a portrayal of a farmer tilling the fields. With our post-Greek orientation, we tend to misinterpret the painting as an illustration of an actual prior or imagined event, such as the man visiting his peasants. However, for the Egyptians, these may have been two separate images from two very different time periods. Also, the Egyptians rarely recorded a bygone reality in their art; rather, in the painting, the deceased is still "watching" the work on his estate (Gombrich, 1960). This "rendering of a typical timeless event meant both a potent presence and a source of joy to the dead" (Frankfort, 1951, p. 34). Scenes of activities of daily life are not meant to be a resumé of the events of the deceased, but a depiction of the deceased observing life. The deceased is usually depicted as inactive and in isolation, remote from considerations of space and time, and devoid of affect, but seeing or watching the daily activities of life. Often there are depictions of "a large, inactive figure bracketing a number of incoherent groups" and a consistent and deliberate rejection of functional human forms and illusionary space (Frankfort, 1951, p. 36). The unforeshortened Egyptian rendering of nature, the avoidance of affect, the lack of any reference to dimensions of time and space, and the avoidance of indications of functional relationships with other figures should not be seen as a desire to remove the represented figures from life (Schäfer, 1919/1974). The simple static poses of Egyptian figures were not intended to divorce the individual from the outside world, but were a typical Egyptian rendering of grandeur and solemnity. The art was not designed for the living beholder and as such did not demand naturalistic representation. It was meant instead as "a presence for the dead who 'own'" it (Frankfort, 1951, p. 38).

The timelessness, in part, created the potency of the Egyptian image; a "newly discovered eternity of art" held out a promise that the power of the lucid image could preserve life and conquer its evanescence (Gombrich, 1960, p. 125). The Egyptians, with their mummies and their funerary art's guarantee of connecting the deceased with his or her lifetime activities, struggled for the preservation of life. Egyptian art served primarily a ritual function and was part of an attempt to maintain integrity and definition in the face of the threat of death, annihilation, and disintegration. This was achieved not by our conventional sense of time stretching backward and forward to infinity, but by the ancient conception of recurrent time and the repetitive life cycle. The preoccupation with life in death in the Old Kingdom, and the monumentality in the art of the Middle Kingdom, was replaced in the New Kingdom by a concept of timeless existence. Timeless existence is achieved by an individual's status that allows one to participate in a divine order. The relationship of life and death—the basis for all Egyptian funerary art—is expressed in the concept that life is like death and that death is only a new phase of life. The eternal in life is achieved only through death (Frankfort, 1951).

There is a basic similarity in the content and function of Egyptian and Paleolithic art. Both presented ritualized images that sought to preserve life by creating a realistic image of an object. The origins of art in the Ancient period are in the action context of ritual, fetish, and cult (Gombrich, 1960), and it expressed concerns about basic needs and functions: life and death and pleasure and pain. The ritualistic function and content of Ancient art are closely tied to issues of sexuality, fertility, and the natural cycles of harvest and hunt, life and death. Themes abound of need-gratification based on safety and preservation (bodily well-being) in a dangerous and destructive universe. Likewise, Egyptian art served primarily a ritual function and was an attempt to transcend the phenomenal world and to preserve and continue life. Both Ancient and Egyptian art are primarily at a sensorimotor-preoperational level of representation.[15]

In summary, a fundamental characteristic of all pre-Greek or aspective art is the rendering of nature in two-dimensional frontal or

---

[15] Art in "primitive" tribes and societies is also often at a sensorimotor-preoperational level. It expresses preoccupations with survival, security, power, and safety; powerful spiritual forces are personified because they are believed to be essential for life, health, and fertility, or to ward off danger and death. Primitive images produce powerful illusions (Arnheim, 1954/1974), they attribute superhuman power to the body and are an attempt to conserve life. Art serves primarily a magical-ritual function. Part properties of the body are often exaggerated—such as the mouth, breasts, genitalia, and various parts of the sensory apparatus—parts most often involved in sensuous gratification or in attempts to survive in dangerous situations. This is not an abstract representation in which part properties have some symbolic relationship to the total object. Rather, bodily parts most involved in need-gratification and/or sensorimotor activity, are emphasized. The size and detailed elaboration of the various parts of the body are based on their importance in the sequences of pleasure-pain. If there are attempts to achieve proportionality in primitive art, parts of the body are usually represented in equal proportions with one-third each devoted to the head, body, and legs. There is an attempt to balance equally the three major segments of the body as opposed to contemporary western art's proportional representation. In primitive art, there is usually a distortion of the size based on the importance of the part property in sensuous gratification or a segmented representation of the body without relative proportionality for each of the segments.

profile images that depict all the essential features of an object. This was a necessary step in the history of art, in much the same way that the development of perspective in the Renaissance was essential for the art of the centuries that followed. The Egyptian representation of the human figure in both a profile and frontal image was an attempt to achieve a concrete and accurate rendering of nature (Schäfer, 1919/1974).[16] One must ask why ancient peoples, before the Greeks, represented the object as they knew it as a concrete entity and did not draw the object as it was seen. Schäfer (1919/1974) explains that the pre-Greeks must have noticed that objects in the distance appeared smaller than these same objects when they were seen from a shorter distance because they were able to calculate the trajectory of an arrow to hit an animal in the distance. Schäfer also cites a Babylonian poetic fragment in which Etana flies to heaven on an eagle and comments, as he looks down, on the decreasing size of the world below him until he notes its eventual disappearance. Further evidence supporting this fragment is found in early Chinese and Hebrew literature (Schäfer, 1919/1974), but drawings of the flight in Babylonian cylinder seals show no aerial view, only people looking upwards. Schäfer (1919/ 1974, p. 84) concludes that the basis of the pre-Greek representation of the concrete object rather than the visual image "must be a general perceptual-cognitive tendency of the human mind." "Ignorance of foreshortening in those [pre-Greek] cultures is not constitutional but is connected with a definite *Kunstwollen* (artistic aim)" (Gioseffi, 1966, p. 192). Schäfer (1919/1974) takes his cue from Plato who, many centuries after the Ancient period, objected to perspective art because it is an illusion, a distortion of the facts of reality. The same objection is voiced, says Schäfer, by the person unfamiliar with perspective drawing, who balks at having a portrait drawn from an oblique angle because it foreshortens the moustache he had taken great pains to trim evenly. Foreshortening deprives the object of some aspect of its

---

[16] There are some forms of painting in primitive art that seem to contradict the formulation that the primary emphasis is on the concrete, literal object. For example, in paintings from a variety of primitive cultures, inner organs are often represented simultaneously with external form and contour. While this could be seen as an abstraction and as a contradiction to the basic literal representation, it is important to stress how these representations are actually very concrete. They depict the object in its essential features and details, with little regard for how the object would appear to the observer. Thus, they depict simultaneously the inside and outside of an object.

objective symmetry. Accepting foreshortening and perspective, which require that the object's reality be abandoned, involves overcoming one's natural predisposition for preserving reality. When the pre-Greeks depicted an object and included not only the side from which it was viewed, but also adjacent sides and details, they were trying to assure the object's definition and identity. For this reason, the Egyptians, as well as all pre-Greek art, did not paint shadows. Shadows were incorporated into painting by the Greeks only in the last generation of the 5th century B.C. (Schäfer, 1919/1974). Schäfer (1919/1974, p. 269) concludes that a major transformation occurred with the Greeks who made the "intellectual sacrifice" of renouncing objective reality for the distortion of appearance.

Richter (1970, p. 8) considers pre-Greek art as a "convenient convention," and Schäfer (1919/1974, p. 149) comments on "the *fixed character of the forms once they have been invented*" (Schäfer's italics). Modes of representation are "characteristic signs of man's relationship with the world, with God, and with himself" (Brunner-Traut, 1974, p. 444). The Egyptians did not seek to achieve a personal viewpoint; they conceived their task as an attempt "to integrate themselves into the absolute and universal order which was laid down once and for all by God" (Brunner-Traut, 1974, p. 427). They derived their knowledge from believing acceptance, not critical perception. Thus, for the Egyptian, there was only one possible correct representation of the object—literal and absolute, everywhere, for everyone, always; that is, independent of observer and spatiotemporal context.

Even as late as 360–342 B.C., in the last pure Egyptian period (Nectanelus II) before the Ptolemy Kings, fixed, stylized, and stereotyped figures combined frontal and profile views. It was only with the Greco-Egyptian temples, such as the one at Edfu, begun by Ptolemy III (Euergetes I) in 237 B.C. and finally completed in 57 B.C., that there are the first known consistent attempts at naturalistic representations with foreshortened curved shoulders, frontal facial views, and realistic portrayal of the body in the breasts and the stomach. But even these examples of naturalistic representation during the Ptolemic period are limited and rare. An emphasis on realism, emotion, and movement in art begins only with the full Roman influence in the 1st century A.D. and is seen in portraiture in late Egyptian art with full frontal views portraying distinctive individuals (see Fig. 10).

Pre-Greek art, including Egyptian art, is based on sensorimotor-preoperational modes of representation and utilizes primarily topo-

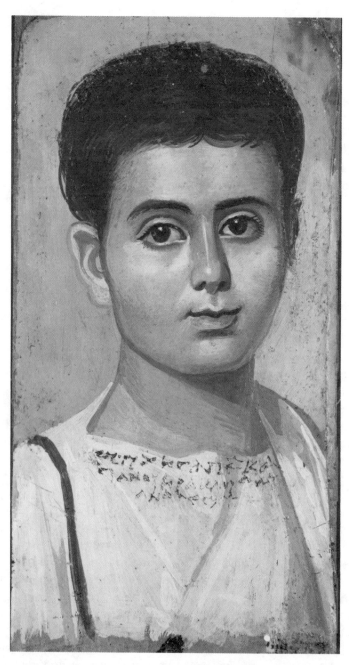

FIG. 10 *Portrait of a Boy* (c. 2nd century A.D.), Egypto-Roman, Probably from Fayum, Upper Egypt. (The Metropolitan Museum of Art, gift of Edward S. Harkness, 1918).

logical concepts of space that emphasize clearly defined boundaries and contours. Initially, in Paleolithic art, objects are depicted as static, fixed entities, as lifesize and in isolation. Individual objects are treated as a collection of separate partial elements and essential features. An object is depicted in isolation with no relationship to other objects or to a context. Subsequently, objects are represented in diminutive form and in an aggregate of objects placed in simple linear order. Space is still fragmented by the contours of each individual configuration, but individual objects are placed in coherent groups based on a theme, even though they are not really interrelated. Each object is defined in isolation by its contour and boundary and placed in simple juxtaposition or order to another object, but without a unified organization of space. Later in the Ancient period, in Egyptian art, space begins to be organized by the introduction of a baseline upon which figures are placed. Figures are flat, usually in profile and/or frontal view and not extended in space. A fixed concept of proportionality is uniformly applied to all figures. The emphasis, however, is not upon the representation of a unified object, but upon each essential feature of the object and upon the overall boundary and contour. It is only the Greeks who made the "intellectual transformation" (Schäfer, 1919/1974), away from the representation of separate, concrete, literal parts of an object, to a representation based on visual appearance. The Greeks inherited from the Egyptians a strict concept of proportionality. In addition, they developed a mode of representation based on object constancy in which they were able to assume that the identity of the object could be established and maintained from the representation of only those partial details of an object seen from a particular vantage point.

As Brunner-Traut (1974) points out, the Egyptian method of representation is most appropriate to the Egyptian's general orientation. It is not the product of philosophical, epistemological reflection and does not indicate the level of their cognitive or intellectual capacities. It is instead their attempt to express their experience of the world within the limits of the social organization and modes of representation available to them. Within these limits they achieved a rich aesthetic tradition. Certainly no one could maintain that Greek art is "superior" to Egyptian because the former achieved a more developed level of representation. The rigid conventions of Egyptian art, in fact, served as an effective representational system for nearly

3,000 years (Gombrich, 1960, 1975). But, more important, Egyptian art occurred early in man's intellectual history and served as the foundation for the development of all subsequent modes of representation.

GRECO-ROMAN ART

The Greeks accomplished a major revision in the mode of artistic representation. They moved beyond the emphasis in Ancient art on topological dimensions of boundary and contour and the utilization of art as a ritual for dealing with issues of life and death. Based on their interest in the dignity of the individual and the importance of subjective experience, Greek culture progressed to a new level of representation involving rudimentary concepts of projective space such as foreshortening and perspective, and the representation of feelings and emotions. Classical art involved a major transformation from the depiction of objects as they concretely exist in nature to a depiction of the way they are visually perceived. An initial emphasis upon ideal proportionality and symmetry in Classical Antiquity led to realistic representations of an idealized, constant object. This stabilization of the concept of the object allowed artists to go beyond a concrete, literal mode of representation to explore representing an object at a specific moment and from a particular point of view, utilizing foreshortening, shadows, and rudimentary (intuitive) concepts of perspective. According to developmental psychological concepts, intuitive or empirical perspective occurs as part of the beginning phases of projective concepts of space. Initially, perspective is partial and intuitive; subsequently, the representation of perspective becomes more extensive, elaborate, and systematic. In Classical art there is a progressive shift from sensorimotor-preoperational representations involving topological concepts of space, to an intuitive level of representation involving early forms of projective concepts of space. Because early concepts of projective space are essentially transitional, they are initially supplemented by continued reliance on topological spatial concepts such as an emphasis upon boundary and contour of an object in isolation.

The progression from topological spatial concepts to an intuitive utilization of projective concepts of space depends upon the development of object constancy—the recognition that an object can be identified from the representation of part features seen from a defined point of view. Pliny cites a Hellenistic critic who praises the painter Parrhasios for his skill in creating the illusion of roundness by the outlines of his figures: "for the outline must go round and so end, that it promises something else to lie behind and thereby shows even what it obscures" (Pliny, *Natural History*, XXXV, 67, 68, cited by Gombrich, 1960, p. 138). The viewer is expected to complete the figure even though parts of it are not seen or reproduced by the artist. The representation of the object is no longer a literal, concrete image; instead it involves an appreciation of the viewer's capacity for object constancy whereby parts of an object can be inferred and constructed, independent of their presence in the immediate perceptual field. Object constancy also enables one to know that an object represented as smaller because it is at a distance is equivalent in size to an object represented as larger because it is much closer to the viewer. Object constancy is an important milestone in cognitive development.

The development of projective concepts of space begins during the intuitive phase of object representation. The intuitive phase is a transitional one, leading to the development of operational modes of representation in which the capacity exists for coordination and transformation of different dimensions of the object. But operational coordination and transformations can occur only after the concept of the object has stability and object constancy has been established. Thus the search for symmetry and perfect proportionality of an idealized figure is an essential part of the intuitive phase of object representation and for the subsequent development of operational modes of representation.

Egyptian art dealt with concrete, objective reality, Greek art was based on "a phenomenon of appearance, not of reality" (Richter, 1970, p. 2). Ancient art represented an object of action, early Greek art depicted the visual image of an ideal object of stability and constancy, and later, more meditative Greek art depicted objects of contemplation and introspection. Progress in the mode of representation in Greek art occurred gradually over several major phases, from the Protogeometric and Geometric (1100–700 B.C.) and Early Archaic (700–530 B.C.) periods, to the Later Archaic and Classical (530–323 B.C.), Hellenistic (323–31 B.C.), and Roman (31 B.C.–313 A.D.) periods.

In the Protogeometric and Early Geometric Greek periods there was a search for order, structure, and patterns in nature to reduce the sense of vulnerability to the awesome powers of nature and the uncertainty and unpredictability of life. This search was expressed in art in the representation of repetitive patterns of basic geometric forms of the straight line, circle, rectangle, and their derivatives: the arc, triangle, diamond, and zigzag line. This was not a representation of nature in the abstract but a fascination with basic geometric forms. Later, an intricate and repetitive "key pattern" or "meander" was used with increasing frequency to achieve more complex patterns and to add a sense of rhythm and motion to the severe, fixed regularity of basic geometric forms. Angular geometric patterns were later integrated with floral and curvilinear patterns and eventually the geometric designs were separated into symmetrical panels and registers.

Late in the Geometric period (750–700 B.C.) the emphasis on strict geometric form was supplemented by attention to details of nature. Isolated figures of animals were drawn as a simple, single silhouette still utilizing basic geometric forms. Subsequently, human figures were represented, often in the context of cult and ritual action. Themes of death and burial or of battles were frequent. Art began to assume a narrative function, but the human shape was still represented only in its simplest form—a frontal torso and a profile view of the head and feet, without a uniformity of scale or proportion. As it had been in Ancient Art, the object was represented as it was known to exist, not as it was seen by an observer.

Funeral scenes on a large, mid-8th century Attic Geometric krater, *Lamentation and Procession of Chariots* (Fig. 11), illustrate figures drawn in frontal silhouette according to a rigid, fixed, geometric formula. Heads, however, are in profile, with a central dot indicating the eye. Animals are also drawn in profile according to a fixed formula, but they have somewhat greater vitality and freedom than the human form.

Interest in more detailed representation of the human form and narrative art increased in the 7th century B.C. The strict adherence to geometric form with regularity and order was replaced by a somewhat freer style as more naturalistic figures were placed in a less formal and regular manner. The frieze from the shoulder of a late Protocorinthian oinochoe from the mid-7th century (Fig. 12) illustrates the overlapping of silhouetted contours of human forms, but the forms now have greater detail. The bodies begin to have proper proportion and volume, internal details enrich the silhouette, and faces begin to have somewhat greater clarity and individual features. Depth is suggested in the complex overlapping of figures, but there are no three-quarter views; shields, for example, are presented frontally without foreshortening. Also, figures at a distance do not dimin-

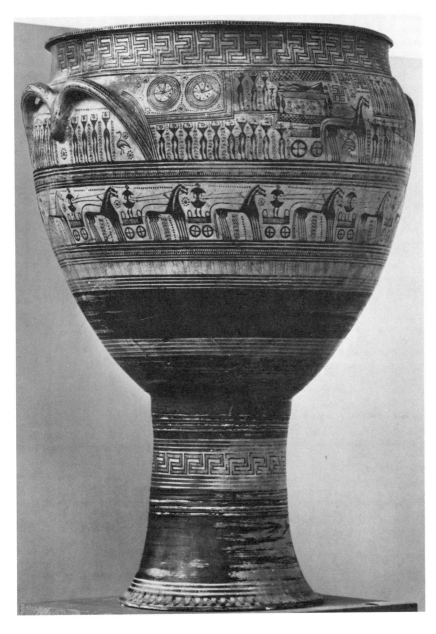

FIG. 11   Attic Geometric krater, *Lamentation and Procession of Chariots* (middle to late 8th century B.C.), National Museum, Athens (Hirmer Verlag).

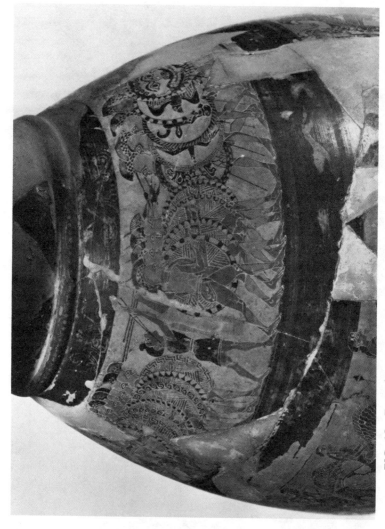

FIG. 12 From late Protocorinthian oinochoe, so-called Chigi Vase. *Hoplites Going into Battle* (c. 640 B.C.), Villa Giula Museum, Rome. (Hirmer Verlag).

ish in size and receding parallel lines do not converge. Figures are all placed on a common ground-line and each figure is confined to its space within the plane without any potential for movement outside that plane.

The Archaic period (700–530 B.C.) marked the beginning of a freer representation of humans in their actual and mythical exploits. At the beginning of the 6th century the influence of Egyptian art led to an increased awareness of proportionality. The development of the "black-figure" technique with increased details allowed representations to be less formal and fixed. As illustrated by Fig. 13, a neck-amphora attributed to Exekias entitled *Achilles Killing Penthesilea* (c. 540 B.C.), the dark figures of the black-figure technique are silhouetted against the background of the natural red clay. The figures are painted in black on the baked red clay, and other colors, such as white and purple, are painted over the black, but the inner details within the figures are added by incising through the paint to expose the red clay beneath. The use of color and greater detail contributed to a new style in which dramatic themes were represented in the silhouettes of human and animal forms, placed in a field in a more liberated manner. Human figures are still presented in the Archaic blend of frontal bodies with profile head and feet, without foreshortening, but they have greater vitality and action. Also, objects, such as shields, are now presented in the oblique, with foreshortening.

Early Greek art, like Ancient art, emphasized outlines and silhouettes. Figures were presented in their broadest aspects (Loewy, 1900/ 1907); emphasis was placed on outline and contour, without gradations in color to express light and shade. The use of marked contrast in early Greek art was part of the topological separation of figure from ground that had been established in the Ancient period. For example, the early black-figure style and its mirror image, the later red-figure style, set off the intended shape from the unintended ground (Gombrich, 1960; Noble, 1965, p. 52). Figures were detached from the background by strong contrast in brightness, which also created areas at different depths.

The development of the red-figure technique in the late 6th century (about 530 B.C.) led to further innovation in the depiction of action and emotion in narrative art. In the red-figure technique, the natural color of the red clay was reserved for the figures set against

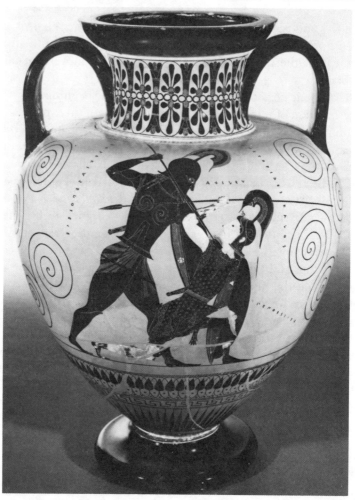

FIG. 13   Black-figured neck-amphora by Exekias, *Achilles Killing Penthesilea*
(c. 525 B.C.) (British Museum).

the painted black background. Internal details are now painted in the
dilute black glaze with a fine brush. Instead of incising details, as done
earlier in the black-figure technique, the freedom and flexibility
gained by painting led to a greater capacity to represent subtle details
and more vigorous action. Figures and background details, dramatically outlined in black, and a fuller elaboration of internal details
facilitated the representation of greater vitality and drama. Red-
figure painting increasingly replaced the black-figure style in an effort to create more powerful emotional effects by having bright

figures dramatically emerge from a darkened field. A 6th century calyx krater (c. 515 B.C.) by Euxitheos and Euphronios of *Dead Sarpedon Carried by Thanatos and Hypnos* (Fig. 14) illustrates the red-figure style. The freedom and flexibility of the red-figure style led to representations of human forms with foreshortened limbs and to three-quarter and rear views of a torso twisting in space. This imparted an organic unity, a quality of solidity and substantiality, and a sense of volume and depth to the human form. The red-figure style continued through the Late Archaic period, with increasing representation of corporeality of human and animal form, dramatic action, and powerful emotional content.

The high point of Greek art is considered by many to have occurred with the development of the Classical tradition. In the 5th century, mythological explanations of the universe and people's ac-

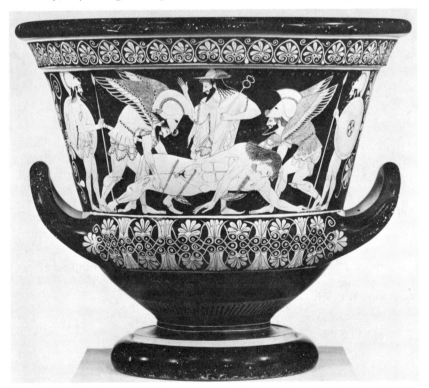

FIG. 14   Red-figured calyx krater by Euxitheos and Euphronios, *Dead Sarpedon Carried by Thanatos and Hypnos* (c. 515 B.C.) (The Metropolitan Museum of Art, Bequest of Joseph H. Durkee, Gift of Darius Ogden Mills, and Gift of C. Ruxton Love).

tions were replaced by an assertion of the individual's role in society, his capacity for exercising reason to discover truth, and the belief that people control and determine their destiny. The conception of God and man was merged and this was expressed in art in the representation of the exact proportions of an idealized human figure (Foss, 1946). The ideal figure was a universal form and image, free of individual characteristics, blemishes, or feelings. Regardless of the action or the context, figures maintained a cool, detached expression. This representation of the human form was an idealized abstraction, not an interest in a particular individual.

With the stabilization of an idealized, universal form in the Classical period, the representation of figures could become increasingly solid and volumetric and their actions more deliberate and energetic. Figures were no longer confined to the flat two-dimensional picture surface of Archaic art but could now begin to move more fully in space and be located at different positions with a variety of gestures expressing a range of emotions and thoughts. Figures began to have more individuality and were represented in interaction. Partial perspective was achieved within individual figures through foreshortening, and they were often interrelated psychologically. But each figure was confined to his own space and the total composition had only limited spatial unity.

Polygnotos, in the first half of the 5th century, broke with the Greek principle of arranging figures on a single baseline. He replaced the horizontal baseline with lines indicating irregular ascending and descending terrain and different levels within the composition. Idealized figures were placed at different ground levels throughout the composition. Unfortunately none of his work survived, but as described by Pausanias, Polygnotos also used marked foreshortening, shadows, and color to create the illusion of depth; but this illusion was thwarted somewhat by his use of a uniform size for all figures regardless of their location in the composition.

Examples of Polygnotos' style can be seen in the work of the Niobid Painter. The Circle of the Niobid Painter, influenced by Polygnotos, placed superimposed figures and groups at various locations and levels throughout the composition to create a unified epic narrative. This dramatic use of foreshortening and a rudimentary form of perspective created bold figures with a quality of monumentality. This is well illustrated by the calyx krater, *The Battle of Greeks and Amazons,* of the Circle of the Niobid Painter from the middle of the

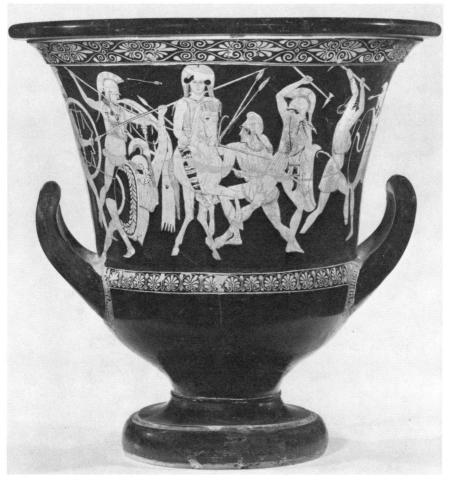

FIG. 15   Red-figured krater, attributed to painter of Berlin Hydria (Niobid Circle), *Battle of Greeks and Amazons* (460-450 B.C.) (Metropolitan Museum of Art, Rogers Fund).

5th century (Fig. 15). These attempts to create an integrated spatial context were limited, however, because each figure had its own spatial orientation and there was no diminution in the size of figures located at a greater distance.

The art of the Classical period was bold and dynamic, representing human emotions and vigorous action of full, corporeal figures in a spatial context. Representation of a somewhat broadened spatial context in which figures seem to move, think, and react was accompanied by an interest in representing an expanded range of emotional expressions. A "new confidence led the Early Classical artists to begin experimenting with the representation of conscious inner life" (Pollitt, 1972, p. 24) and the expression of affects and emotions, particularly in facial features (Pliny, 77, A.D., XXV, 98; cited by Pollitt, 1972). It is important to note that this increased interest in representing emotions coincided with the first experiments with perspective. Perspective and the representation of emotion were central factors in Classical art and essential expressions of the Periclean Humanism dominant in the second half of the 5th century (Haynes, 1981). The Periclean emphasis on the importance and dignity of the individual allowed artists to represent nature from a subjective orientation—using foreshortening, an intuitive form of perspective, and the expression of emotion.

The development of white vase painting in the High Classical period (450–400 B.C.) allowed for a greater representation of subtle emotions in uniquely defined figures. Contemplative figures replaced the representation of active and violent ones and the mood of these figures seemed eternal. Colors and gradations of light and shadow increased the capacity to represent volume and spatial depth as well as capture a wider range of affects and moods. Once object constancy and the representation of perspective were established, the Greeks could relinquish the topological emphasis on the boundary of the figure and begin to integrate gradations of color and shading within the figure without the threat of losing its basic differentiation. (See Fig. 16).

A three-tone code was used for modeling light and shade instead of simple alternations of high contrast (Gombrich, 1960). The use of gradation, shading, and variations of light and color within the object itself contribute further to the sense of fullness, roundness and depth that had already been achieved by foreshortening. Shadows were incorporated into Greek paintings in the last generation of the 5th century B.C. Although some representation of depth had been achieved in the techniques of foreshortening and perspective, the impact of the development of shadow painting was so great that the term for shadow painting *(skiagraphia)* "became a term for perspective as a whole" (Schäfer, 1919/1974, p. 73). The use of cast shadows enhanced the illusion of three-dimensionality. Color and shadow had been employed to some degree earlier, but it was only in the High Classical period that "local colour of objects and figures was subordinated to a single system of light and shade applied to the whole

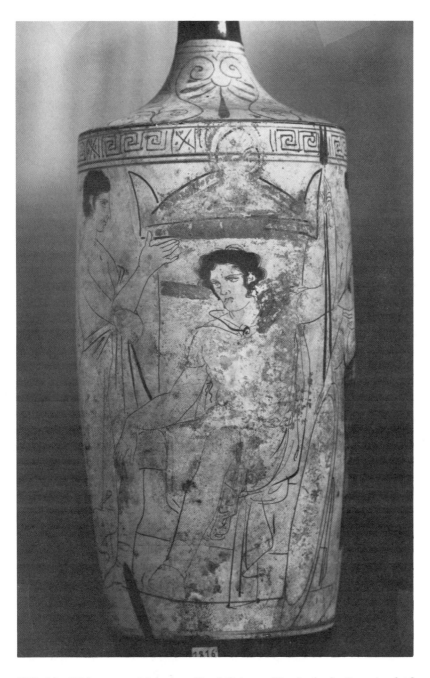

FIG. 16   White-ground lekythos, Reed Painter, *Warrior by the Grave* (end of 5th c. B.C.), National Museum, Athens (Hirmer Verlag).

picture, and when the individual forms were subjected to modelling by gradations of light and colour in accordance with this system" (Dörig, 1976, pp. 376–78).

The rich and elaborate High Classical style continued into the first quarter of the 4th century with an interest in mythic themes and scenes of love, abduction, and intimate aspects of the life of women. An increasing gracefulness and softness was expressed in the representation of elegant feminine forms and ornamental decorations (see Fig. 17). Throughout the 4th century, figures were increasingly full and corporeal, representing a wide range of emotions and communication between figures.

The struggle with perspective in 4th century vase painting is well illustrated in a red-figured hydria by Apulia of *Iphigeneia and Orestes in the Land of the Taurians* (c. 370–360 B.C.) (Fig. 18). Individual figures and objects are represented with depth and volume, but an overall spatial organization is lacking. The solidity of the altar upon which Orestes is seated is achieved through perspective recession of a series of slanted parallelograms and the use of shading. The use of perspective in the temple on the hill, however, is less successful. There is little sense of a consistent spatial orientation, no convergence of parallel lines, and the capitals of the Ionic columns are all frontal and inconsistent with the orientation of the temple. The open doors, however, contribute to a sense of depth and receding space. Despite this partial success in representing depth and volume in individual objects, there is a lack of continuity in the spatial orientation and in the size of figures and objects at different locations in the composition (Pollitt, 1972).

The expansion of Greek society in the 4th century and the wider distribution of wealth and power transformed not only Greek life and society, but its art as well. New art centers and a wide range of patrons enabled artists to break with the 5th century Classical tradition and move toward greater individuality, including the expression of specific human emotions and the representation of personal identity, leading eventually to portraiture. A greater naturalism was achieved in the integration of foreshortening, perspective, and gradations of color, light, and shade. Crowd scenes were replaced by a greater subtlety in the representation of a few figures, each with inner feelings and emotions that are shared and communicated in intimate interpersonal relationships.

The Hellenistic period (323–31 B.C.) extended the style of the early

4th century. Portraits expressed emotions and personal feelings, and scenes emphasized the sharing of emotions in interpersonal interactions. In addition, landscapes became more realistically scaled and proportional through the extensive use of color, light, and shadow as well as foreshortening and perspective. The representation of spatial depth was achieved through a more effective and extensive use of

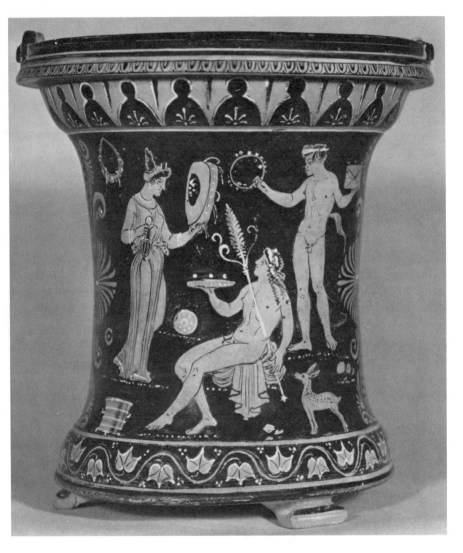

FIG. 17   Red-figured terracotta situla, Manner of the Lycurgus Painter (c. 350 B.C.), Italian (The Metropolitan Museum of Art, Fetcher Fund).

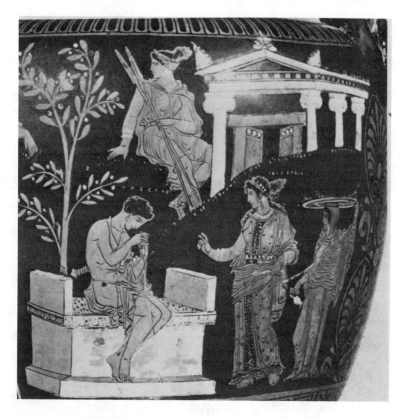

FIG. 18   Apulian krater, *Iphigeneia and Orestes in the Land of the Taurians* (4th century B.C.) National Museum Naples (Alinari).

perspective. Portraiture, naturalistic representations, and narrative art established in the Hellenistic period provided the basis for the art of Rome.

In the Hellenistic period, from the death of Alexander the Great in 323 B.C. to the battle of Actium in 31 B.C., Greek culture spread into Egypt and Asia, and Oriental and Egyptian concepts began to influence Greece itself. Also at this time, Rome emerged as a dominant political force in the Mediterranean. These widened horizons of thought were paralleled in art by a broadened conception of space (Fuchs, 1976) expressed in the representation of landscapes and action. Whereas Archaic Greek art sought to represent the object world in absolute terms, Classical art endeavored to represent the ideal, and Hellenistic art sought to capture the realism of a relative world filled with personal and subjective experiences and meaning (Pollitt, 1972).

Themes from mythology were replaced by an interest in pastoral landscapes and scenes from everyday life. The calm Classical Greek figures were given a new dynamic form in Hellenistic painting that captured emotional states and affective intensity. The Hellenistic representation of emotions and dynamic movement has been discussed as reflecting a "baroque persuasion" (Fuchs, 1976, p. 500) and as "rococo" (Klein, 1921; cited by Pollitt, 1972). The lively use of color, shadow, and contrasts of light and dark, as well as the representation of the human form in a spatial context and an interest in a fuller and more comprehensive understanding of nature are all aspects referred to as the Baroque quality of Hellenistic art (Fuchs, 1976).

These changes in modes of representation in art were not, as Plato claimed, a descent into an art of deception and illusion, but a move from representing nature concretely to a beginning recognition of the importance of subjective experience. Such changes occurred during the period when Greek philosophy was occupied with the problem of reality or non-reality of phenomena, arising out of the quest for the basic substance of the universe. Greek science, previously a collection of explanatory myths, was emerging at this time as a discipline in its own right (Schäfer, 1919/1974, p. 272) concerned with the problems of the physical process of vision (e.g., Empedocles). Schäfer (1919/1974) concludes that these simultaneous changes in philosophy, science, and modes of representation in art are not a matter of chance but an integral aspect of a basic change in Greek culture.

Beginning in the 6th century B.C., signatures began to appear on Greek works of art and artists increasingly became important and influential members of society. This recognition of the individual artist not only reflected a change in the culture's attitude toward art, but it expressed the emerging Greek humanism with its emphasis upon the dignity of the individual (Kris, 1952; Kris & Kurz, 1934/1979). Earlier, when art primarily had a magical or ritual function, there was little interest in the resemblance of art to nature and in the identity of the artist. The quest for naturalistic representation and the identification of the individual artist were both expressions of Greek humanism which began in the 6th century B.C. Prior instances of naturalistic representation, such as foreshortening, were based simply on the observation of an individual artist. Such efforts, however, were not part of a general style and, when achieved, remained isolated. Each instance tended to be confined to an individual work, without any systematic effort to develop consistent techniques for naturalistic representation. With the Greeks, this changed radically. For the first time man strove to represent pictorially what he saw visually in accordance with a theory of vision. Greek humanism expressed itself partly in an interest in the individual's visual experiences and the codification of these experiences in a theory of vision and optics.

Greek culture had a pervasive influence on all subsequent representation in art. Since so much of the evidence has been lost, it is uncertain why the Greeks originally wished to represent objects as they appeared to an observer. But there are a number of overlapping explanations to account for this important development in Greek art. In addition to simultaneous changes that were occurring in philosophy, science, and the social order, there was also the beginning of historical writing. Narrative, historical writing—an interest in the subjective eye-witness accounting of events—was another indication of an increased self-consciousness and confidence, and an appreciation of the dignity of man.

In Classical Antiquity there were major shifts in the structure, content, and function of art. Pre-Greek art, as we have seen, served primarily magical and ritual functions in portraying struggles around the basic polarities of existence, such as hunger-satiety, pleasure-pain, and life-death. Egyptian art provided a means for trying to achieve immortality, but it was the Greeks who were bold enough to emancipate artistic representation from the domination of the magical preservation of life in order to offer insight into the world and the nature of personal experience (Bernheimer, 1961). Greek art discovered both a more convincing mode of representation and the narrative function of art. The "Homeric freedom of narration," developed in the 9th or 8th century B.C., was a major factor in this revolution in the history of art (Gombrich, 1960, p. 133). Sometime during the 7th century B.C. there was a shift away from trying to control the inevitable cycles of life and death toward an interest in the historical recording of major events in the society. The rise of what has been called "craft literacy" (Havelock, 1963, p. 39) in the 6th century B.C., after the invention of the alphabet either late in the 7th or early in the 6th century, led to the keeping of records by some Greek towns that were then used in local histories. The logographers, the most important of whom was Hecataeus (500 B.C.), collected information without any clear chronological scheme. Emphasis was on consulting eyewitnesses rather than mere hearsay or folk memory. True historical writing came later with the rise of science and rationalism. Art itself also came to assume a narrative and eventually an archival function. Narration, story-telling, or what happened and how it appeared to an *eye-witness* (Gombrich's foreword to Schäfer, p.x, emphasis added) brought a systematic emphasis on the subjective point of reference for the first time in the history of art.

The move from an objective to a subjective mode of representation was a major development in art. The Greeks achieved "systematic modifications of the schemata" (Gombrich, 1960, p. 141), which involved a shift from the representation of the concrete literal object as it existed in nature to an emphasis on the object as it appeared to the viewer from a personal vantage point. Gombrich maintains that this shift should not be considered a function of the desire to imitate nature more accurately, but rather the result of "ceaseless experimentation" (1960, pp. 141–142) in a sort of avant-garde rivalry as the Greeks pursued their aesthetic interests within their cultural context. Kitto (1951, p. 61) considers the Greek emphasis on subjective experience to be a function of the change in the image of the individual, no longer "a mere nothing in the sight of the gods," but an expression of their respect for the beauty and dignity of the individual. Pollitt (1972) notes that the confidence and optimism of the Greeks arose from the fact that against overwhelming odds they won the Persian War. The Greeks considered Hellenic man as separate from the barbarians. They had an awareness of man as a uniquely endowed creature; they were preoccupied with the beauty and elegance of nature and man was considered the highest form of nature. Their appreciation of the dignity of the individual was expressed in the establishment of democracy as a political system and the artistic creation of the natural image—the representation of reality from the vantage point of a particular, individual observer. Jaeger (1937; cited by Gardner, 1975, p. 124) comments that, in contrast to a concept of a God-King and the "suppression of the great mass of the people . . . the beginning of Greek history appears to be the beginning of a new conception of the individual." The Greek sense of the dignity of the individual and the Greeks' "superb self-confidence in humanity" (Kitto, 1956, p. 61) were conducive to the shift from an objective to a subjective orientation, from an "aspective" to a "perspective" (Brunner-Traut, 1974) mode of artistic representation.

There are numerous comments about the Greeks' conception of space in the considerable philosophical, scientific, and mathematical writing on Greek architecture and optics from Greek and Roman sources as widely scattered as Plato, Aristotle, Seneca the Younger, Euclid, Lucretius, Vitruvius, and Sextus Empiricus (Pollitt, 1965, 1974). Most writings indicate that the Greeks accepted the general principle that receding parallel lines appear to converge, but they did not apply this observation to optics (Ivins, 1946). Although the exact nature of their theoretical knowledge about the perception of space (and the extent to which it influenced artists) is a subject of speculation, it is generally agreed that the Greek artist had an intuitive (perceptual) sense of perspective. Richter (1970) discusses three aspects of the development of the representation of three-dimensional space in Greek art: foreshortening or three-quarter view, the size of objects varying with their distance from the viewer, and perspective or the unity of objects in the picture plane by the projection of three-dimensional space using points of sight and converging lines. Richter's (1970) detailed figure-by-figure analysis and Bunim's (1940) discussion of cast shadows and the pictorial surface are major contributions to understanding the Greeks' development of the capacity to represent three-dimensional space.

Foreshortening was a primary technique in the Greek development of perspective. During the Geometric and Early Archaic periods, there was no foreshortening, but instead a continuation of the frontal/profile alternation inherited from earlier traditions. There were frontal eyes on profile heads and frontal shields held by profile bodies. Around the end of the Early Archaic period, attempts at a three-quarter view began. The three-quarter view was mastered, especially in drawings of the human body, presumably because a foreshortened body is more likely to indicate action (White, 1967). There were numerous examples of foreshortening by the 5th century B.C., less than a century after the first attempts to depict a three-quarter view. Once mastered, this technique remained unchanged throughout the remainder of the Greco-Roman period.

Typically, there were changes in the rendering of the eye. The eye first began to correspond with that of a frontal or profile view of the head. The early eye had a round iris in the center. As the iris was elongated and able to move from the center to an inner corner of the eye, the eye became capable of expressing a wider range of human feelings. Added lines suggested lashes or an upper lid whereby the eye could be partially closed to indicate a somber mood, or fully opened to portray hope, fear, or surprise. Changes also occurred in other details such as horns, wings, chariots, chariot wheels, and shields. Shields that would earlier have been drawn round in a frontal view were now shown in three-quarter view as elliptical (Richter, 1970).

Another major factor in the Greek development of perspective was the development of stage space. Bunim (1940) discusses the concept of stage space, that is, a sense of depth created by juxtaposing two planes at right angles so that one forms the ground and the other the rear wall. Bunim discusses this primarily in terms of changes in the treatment of the picture plane. In Paleolithic art, the picture plane is an unprepared and untreated surface. In Egyptian art, it is a constructed surface, unframed except for the baseline serving as the lower limit and support for the figures. During the Hellenistic period of Greek art, the picture plane was first transformed into stage space: the plane of the foreground was differentiated from that of the background. The term "stage space" comes from the theater, where, according to Vitruvius (Bk. VII, praef 11—see Pollitt, 1974, p. 240), perspective was first developed. "*Skenographia,*" or scene painting, is one of the Greek technical terms for perspective, "The 'funnel-shaped' stage with its floor inclined upward and its side flats inward . . . gives an illusion of much greater depth than it really possesses." For the floor to appear to be a receding rectangle, the planes of the "floor, ceiling, and two side walls [must] form four trapezoids that the audience sees as receding rectangles" (Gioseffi, 1966, p. 192).

Previously, in early Greek art, depth was indicated by the aspective method of overlapping—a series of horses' legs and heads may be seen as if on a single body. Early Greek art, like Egyptian art, used the overlapping technique for incorporating several objects within a composition. While this method lacked realism, it created an atmosphere that clearly conveyed the meaning of the scene. Richter (1970) suggests that this accounts for the long period of time that elapsed before more naturalistic means of representation were developed. In fact, this technique persisted side by side with more naturalistic ones even after they had been discovered. Alternately, Archaic Greek art used another aspective technique to indicate depth in which above means behind. The illusion of depth was developed further by Polygnotos in the mid-5th century B.C. by the introduction of irregular ground lines, such as a hill for figures to stand on, creating different levels and a contrast between the surfaces of the vertical hill and the level

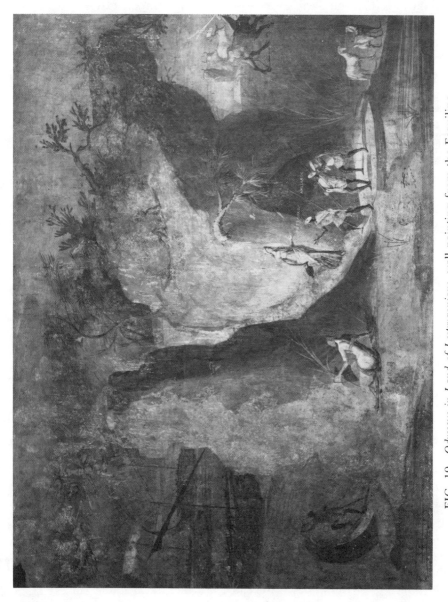

FIG. 19 *Odysseus in Land of Lestrygonians*, wall painting from the Esquiline (late 1st century B.C.), Vatican Library, Rome (Alinari).

ground. Although the effect of depth was gained, no differentiation in size was indicated for figures at different distances (Bunim, 1940; White, 1967/1972).

The diminution of objects at a distance began in the Hellenistic period. Roman landscapes of 1st century B.C. such as *Odysseus in the Land of Lestrygonians* (Fig. 19), derived from the Hellenistic interest in landscapes, showed an approximate relationship between size and distance. Background figures are smaller than foreground ones, but there was no systematic relation established between distance and size and, therefore, it is difficult to estimate actual distances among various parts of the picture.

This narrative wall mural was obviously conceived without a consistent unified sense of space or perspective. There is a generalized and vague spatial environment, and the figures seem to recede in a dissolving mist rather than stand on solid ground. The *Odysseus Mediterranean Landscapes* integrate a consistent sense of space with the use of color, light, and shade to create the experience of limitless space. The light, however, seems to come from several sources rather than a consistent one that would cast predictable and unifying shadows. Also, the relationship between figures and background is casual, not inseparable, and there is no pervasive unity, no coordinated and measurable system that includes both the figures and the picture plane (Bunim, 1940).

Another major advance toward three-dimensionality was accomplished in Greek art with the advent of shading and shadows. There were no shadows in Egyptian art and none in Greek art until the end of the 5th century; their use was developed in the Late Classical and Hellenistic periods. They were used throughout Roman painting, disappeared during the Medieval period, and then reappeared with Renaissance and Baroque *chiaroscuro*. Cast shadows greatly enhance the three-dimensionality of Greek art, creating a ground plane on which the figures stand, and from which and onto which they cast their shadows. Ground planes had been suggested in pre-Greek art by baselines, but only in Greek art did they develop into a stable horizontal platform (White, 1967) that transformed the lower part of the picture plane perpendicular to the figures, giving a greater sense of the existence of a horizontal ground plane with the rest of the plane behind the figures as a vertical rear wall. This was an important step in the development of stage space (Bunim, 1940). Thus, in the well-known Pompeian mosaic, *Alexander's Victory over Darius* (c. 100 B.C.) (Fig. 20), copied from a Hellenistic painting, a neutral picture plane

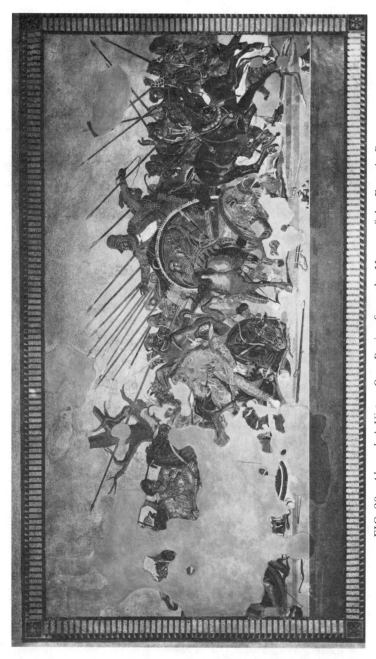

FIG. 20 *Alexander's Victory Over Darius*, from the House of the Faun in Pompeii (a first century mosaic copy of a late 4th century B.C. Greek painting), National Museum, Naples (Alinari).

becomes a three-dimensional space through the effective arrangement of the figures. The brown strip across the bottom gives the
effect of a vertical edge of a platform. The cast shadows create the
sense of a horizontal ground and vertical walls (Bunim, 1940). A
remarkable sense of depth is achieved through the extensive use of
foreshortening and perspective that creates a receding picture plane
and a coherent spatial organization. The use of shadows and a rich-
ness of color contributed further to the remarkable capacity to represent action and intense emotional experiences in the expression of the
figures.

The elaborate background and complexity of the composition increase the emotional intensity of this work. Since the picture is littered
with objects and overlapping forms, the viewer is forced to identify
with the work in order to sort out the various parts and to comprehend or complete an experience of the human figures (Gombrich,
1960). The artist relied on the viewer's capacities for object constancy
to construct a full image of the object based on the representation of
partial details. The viewer was expected to construct the presence of
the person whose face is reflected in the shield in the lower center
foreground. The spectator is brought into the picture by complex and
incomplete shapes, and by increased emotional content. The intense
foreshortening of the horse in the foreground, for example, leads the
viewer to experience a scene of urgency, panic, and slaughter. This
mosaic demonstrates effectively the subjective power of the Homeric
narrative tradition (Auerbach, 1946; Gombrich, 1960).

The development of perspective in Greek art is a topic of considerable controversy. While it is evident that the Greeks had at least
an intuitive sense of perspective, the exact nature of their theoretical
knowledge of linear perspective and its formal use in art is uncertain.
Many of the conclusions about perspective in Antiquity are based on a
consideration of artistic evidence of the 1st century B.C. Pompeian
frescoes, specifically the wall paintings from the Villa at Boscoreale,
the Villa of the Mysteries, and the House of the Labyrinth, and the
most recent and very controversial finds discovered in 1961 on the
Palatine in Rome in the Room of the Masks, and in the Villa at Uplontis (de Franciscis, 1975). In the frescoes in the Villa at Boscoreale (Fig.
21), the projecting balconies and colonnades have receding parallel
lines that often converge, but not all the lines converge to a central
vanishing point. The space of the fresco is not a unified whole—the

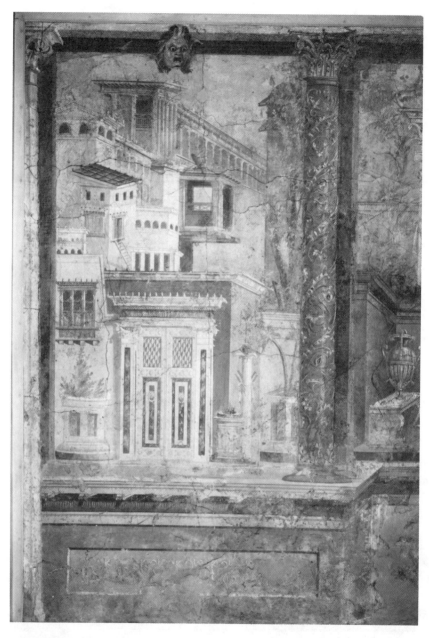

FIG. 21 *Wall painting from Villa at Boscoreale* (1st century B.C.) (The Metropolitan Museum of Art, Rogers Fund).

148

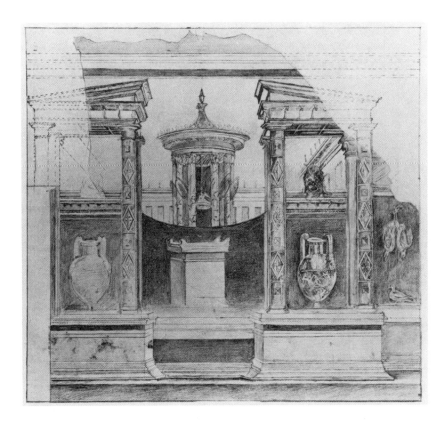

FIG. 22a   *Wall painting* from House of the Labryinth, Pompeii, (Alinari).

parts are pieced together from different points of view and are improperly interrelated. While there is a basic scheme of perspective, there are multiple vanishing points (White, 1956, 1967/1972).

In the wall paintings of the House of the Labyrinth, there are over 40 receding lines vanishing to one point in the altar located at the lower, central portion of the painting (Fig. 22a). As indicated by Beyen's perspective reconstruction of this work (Fig. 22b) six more receding lines miss this central vanishing point by an inch. This is repeated on the fragments on the opposite wall and "therefore represents a definite intention," but it still contains inconsistencies and lacks unity (White, 1967/1972, p. 259).

In the House of the Mysteries, an extensive architectural complex in a single, limited area has been unified to a single point. But the only extant painting with a single central vanishing point was found in

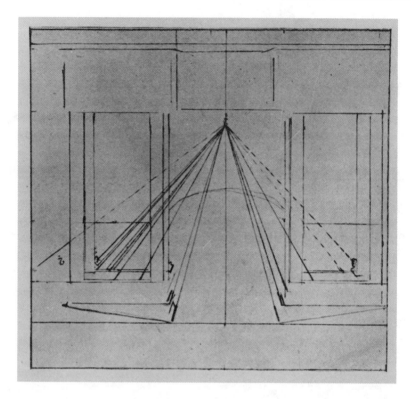

FIG. 22b   *Perspective construction of wall painting* from House of the Labry-inth, Pompeii. (*Die Pompejanische Wanddekoration,* H.G. Beyen, Hagg: Martinus Nijhoff, 1938, p. 37).

1961, in the Room of the Masks on the Palatine in Rome (Figs. 23a and b).

Richter (1970, p. 53), basing her argument on the discovery of the Room of the Masks, reaffirms her original position (1937, p. 35) that there may have been sporadic expressions of the use of a central vanishing point that "may be due to the correct observation of an individual artist." But the artist's success was based on his superior ability to draw what he saw, not on the laws of perspective. Gioseffi (1966, p. 197) comments, however, that this argument is somewhat weakened by the fact that the painting in the Room of the Masks is a Roman copy of a Greek original, probably produced "by a humble team of decorators . . . reproducing standard motifs taken at third or fourth hand from the great models of Hellenistic scenography and decoration." Even within the fresco in the Room of Masks, however, there are several other vanishing points in addition to the primary central one.

Thus, there has been considerable controversy about whether scientific, mathematical, linear perspective, with a central vanishing point, was known to the Greco-Roman world. Extensive debate has raged about the explanation of the perspective that was achieved in the recent discovery in the Room of the Masks, which appears to be the only existing Classical work where much of the painting is organized around a central vanishing point. Some consider it as coincidence, the result of intuitive skills, while others view it as an example of the deliberate execution of the mathematical formula. The issue, of course, is not an aesthetic judgment, but a consideration of the development of the concepts and techniques of perspective.

The primary written documentation on Greco-Roman perspective is provided in the work of Euclid (3rd century B.C.), and Vitruvius and Lucretius (1st century B.C.). Only Vitruvius, however, mentions art. In *De Architectura* (25–23 B.C.), Vitruvius (Bk. I, 2,2; Bk. VII, praef. 11) writes about pictorial perspective in the design of theatrical scenery in which objects in the distance appear smaller than those in the foreground. Vitruvius notices that planes in depth appear foreshortened, but does not formulate a geometrical method of organizing or unifying the receding lines in planes. The exact meaning is unclear at several points and different translations are cited as

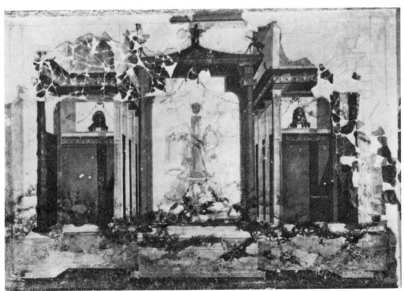

FIG. 23a   *Wall painting* from Room of Masks on the Palatine, Rome (Alinari).

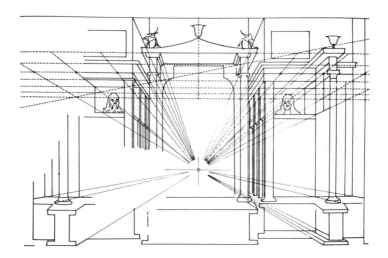

FIG. 23b   Perspective drawing of wall painting from The Room of the Masks on the Palatine, Rome (Carlo Gandini).

evidence in favor of different types of perspective. In Bk. I, 2,2 Vitruvius wrote:

> Skenographia (Perspective) is the method of sketching a front with the sides withdrawing into the background, the lines all meeting in the centre of a circle. (p. 14)

Also in Bk. VII, praef. 11 Vitruvius continues:

> In the first place Agatharcus, in Athens, when Aeschylus was bringing out a tragedy, painted a scene, and left a commentary about it. This led Democritus and Anaxagoras to write on the same subject, showing how, given a centre in a definite place, the lines should naturally correspond with due regard to the point of sight and the divergence of the visual rays, so that by this deception a faithful representation of the appearance of buildings might be given in painted scenery, and so that, though all is drawn on a vertical flat facade, some parts may seem to be withdrawing into the background, and others to be standing out in front. (Vitruvius, *The Ten Books of Architecture*, transl., M. H. Morgan, p. 198)

Panofsky (1924/25), in an interpretation that has been disputed by both art historians (e.g., Edgerton, 1975; Gombrich, 1960; White, 1967/1972) and investigators in optics and perception (e.g., Doesschate, 1964; Gibson, 1960; Pirenne, 1952), argued that perspective according to Vitruvius was based on a curved, not linear intersection of a visual cone. Panofsky, primarily relying on Vitruvius and Euclid, argued that the ancient Greeks and Romans conceived of the visual world as curved because the eye is a concave surface and we tend to view straight lines as curved. If visual rays are projected on to subtended arcs and these dimensions are transferred from the arcs or their chords onto the picture plane, the resulting perspective approximates a vertical axis construction. Panofsky attempted to demonstrate that Greek compositions based on a vanishing axis, first seen in the Apulian Greek vases of the 4th century B.C., and that persisted throughout Antiquity, the Middle Ages, and even into the Renaissance, were based on a curvature form of perspective.[17] Though Panofsky's formulation of a curvature form of perspective has been actively disputed (e.g., Edgerton, 1975), there is general agreement that the central vanishing axis dominated painting even though single-point perspective is less difficult to achieve and is more realistic. Carter (1970, p. 846), in an extensive review of the development of

---

[17] Panofsky (1924/25) relied on Euclid for much of his discussion of perspective in Antiquity. Euclid's "Optics" *(Ta Optika)* deals with the appearance of objects at a distance and expresses geometrically the relationship between the real magnitude of the object and the apparent magnitude of our visual image of the object. The apparent size, writes Euclid, is proportional to the visual angle subtended at the eye. Panofsky distinguishes between Euclid's visual angle theory and the Renaissance ray theory, which hypothesizes that the size of an object's appearance is a function of its distance from the eye. Panofsky also cites Vitruvius' definition of skenographia: "a method of sketching a front with the sides withdrawing into the background, the lines all meeting in the center of a circle" (Morgan transl., Bk. 1, 2, 2; p. 14). Panofsky hypothesized that a sphere of projection became a simplified and visually reproducible circle of projection—all lines converging on a vanishing axis rather than to a vanishing point. Based on the evidence from Euclid and Vitruvius, Panofsky concluded that perspective in Greek art would have to have been spherical, not linear. Levy (1943, p. 52) also concluded that Vitruvius appears to define spherical, not linear perspective in the comment that "the incline of the Parthenon columns by two lines drawn from the eye of the spectator, the longer reaching highest and giving the impression of a backward bend." In Greek columns, there was an awareness that in order not to appear curved, they must be slightly convex—a straight line is seen as curved, and curved as straight. Levy (1943), discussing the interaction between architectural composition and pictorial invention in Antiquity and the Renaissance, stresses the distinction between the curved perspective achieved by the Greeks, as an expression of natural law (Vitruvius, Bk. VII, praef. 11) and the linear perspective of the Renaissance.

linear perspective, concludes that there is no evidence of single-point perspective until the 15th century, "except in one brief period of Pompeian painting and then only in the upper parts of the pictures." Carter, based on Doesschate (1964), concludes that the discovery of one-point perspective was delayed because we do not perceive more than two parallels as being directed toward a common point. The more a pair of parallels is situated to the left or right, the less the degree of apparent convergence. This observation deterred artists from using a single point for the convergence of an entire group of parallels until one-point convergence was demonstrated in the Renaissance via a projection plane and a fixed eye point. Numerous authors have stressed the differences between the inconsistent perspective that the Greeks achieved on the basis of optical adjustment and the angle axiom of Euclid's visual theory, and linear perspective achieved on the basis of the Renaissance theory of representation. Some authors (e.g., Bunim, 1940) have even argued that it was essential to abandon the Greek mode for the representation of perspective based on the angle axiom and the vanishing axis in order to achieve linear perspective.

Euclid's *Optics* was concerned with the perception of isolated objects (Ivins, 1946). There was an optical adjustment in the size of an object to compensate for its placement in the vertical plane. The degree of adjustment was determined by the size of the subtended visual angle. An object higher in the vertical plane is experienced as smaller than an object lower in the plane because it subtends a smaller visual angle. The higher the object, the less the angle and therefore the smaller the visual size of the object. The size of an object is determined by its placement in the vertical plane and the size of the angle subtended on the eye of the viewer. While this formulation established a fixed reference point within the individual, it was primarily concerned about the appearance of an object in isolation. This visual angle principle of Euclidean optics precluded the possibility of discovering the inverse size-distance relationship of objects over successive planes. The visual angle principle was an adjustment for size only in reference to the placement of an isolated object in the vertical plane. Differences in the distance of objects in the lateral planes at right angles to the viewer are defined only in the linear perspective of the Renaissance by the inverse size-distance relationship established throughout the picture plane. The establishment of linear perspective in the Renaissance required abandoning the angle axiom of Euclid for the more counter-intuitive abstraction of an inverse size-distance relationship (Veltman, 1979a).

   White (1967/1972), in disputing Panofsky's curvature (or spherical) theory of perspective, points out that although a consistent system can be derived from the law of optics developed in Antiquity, its application in art would have been impossible. White rejects Panofsky's formulations about a spherical theory of perspective and instead believes that Vitruvius and Lucretius, in the 1st century B.C., asserted the existence of ideas that produced a true vanishing point and a perspective capable of unifying the whole picture plane. White (1956, 1967/1972, p. 251–254) argues effectively that the word translated as "correspondence" in Vitruvius (Bk. VII, praef. 11) can also be translated as "convergence" and that Vitruvius had in mind single vanishing point perspective. White (1967/1972) also cites Lucretius (*De Rerum Natura*, IV, 426ff), who wrote about the effect of distance on the appearance of a colonnade—how it seems to vanish into the point of a cone. White also believes that there is evidence of central perspective in the Pompeian frescoes, between the time of Lucretius' death (mid-1st century B.C.) and Vitruvius' treatise around 25–23 B.C. It is possible that Vitruvius was trying "to give ancient lineage to a relatively new invention" (White, 1967/1972, p. 258). White's thesis is that in Pompeian art, perspective derived and developed from the art of other cultural centers. So, in early (style II) Pompeian art we see the best traces of perspective, while later (styles III and IV) Pompeian art goes in other directions. In the late frescoes (Pompeian styles III and IV), there is more spatial coordination in the representation of isolated objects than in the spatial organization of the total composition. These late frescoes depart from perspective and are more oriented toward the composition, content, and texture of the surface (White, 1967/1972)—an interest that continued into the Middle Ages (Bunim, 1940). Because there is no evidence of linear perspective beyond the early Pompeian frescoes in the three houses (and the 1961 discovery of the Room of Masks), White (1967/1972, pp. 260–61) concludes that there was no development of perspective at Pompeii, and that the advances expressed in some Pompeian frescoes "were made elsewhere" and "at an earlier date." Because it was derived from a prior "parent system," there was only a brief and intermittent use of perspective in Pompeian art. But the frescoes that remain for us to consider demonstrate that the parent system "must originally have been no less than a completely unified vanishing point construction"

(White, 1967/1972, p. 261). The existence of a few exceptions of equivalent quality leads White (1967/1972) to the conclusion that there was an inclusive pattern:

> Twenty to forty lines upon a wall do not converge upon a single point by chance. Just one example of a system's use is proof of its existence, if not of its popularity. . . . Each of the three remaining complexes of first quality, early Second style decoration at Pompeii has revealed clear traces of a vanishing point perspective. (p. 261)

White (1956, p. 69) concludes that there is a good probability that there was the use of a single vanishing point in Greek art, as indicated by the evidence in the Pompeian frescoes and the writing of Lucretius and Vitruvius. With more evidence, "probability comes near to certainty."

Despite the arguments by White, most authorities seem to agree that although the Greeks had some intuitive sense of perspective, there is little consistent evidence to suggest that they were able to achieve linear perspective. Given their intense competitiveness and preoccupation with perfection, it is curious that the Greeks never culminated their pursuit of perspective and were almost satisfied with a limited representation of space. They achieved a basic use of planes, but were unable to develop a plane section of the cone of sight that would establish a consistent and systematic construction. The ancient theories of space did not reach the point of defining space as a coordinated system of relations between height, breadth, and depth, in which objects are located along three spatial coordinates in an integrated conception of three-dimensional space (Panofsky, 1924/25). Perspective was achieved in the representation of isolated objects but not as a method for unifying space (Richter, 1970). Objects were not represented as they appeared relative to each other in their respective shapes, sizes, and positions from a single point of view. Rather, each separate body and object was seen by itself in its own private space (Ivins, 1946). The Greeks lacked the basic concepts that were necessary for the development of linear perspective and the more advanced concept of space as isotropic, homogeneous and infinite (Ivins, 1946).

In summary, the Greeks began to develop foreshortening and perspective in the late 6th and early 5th centuries B.C., supplemented by variations in light and shade in the 4th century B.C. (Gombrich, 1960). Foreshortening, especially in the representation of the human body, was quickly attained. Perspective developed more slowly and, although competence was achieved, it appears to have remained, for the most part, partial. There was an interest in representing three-dimensionality, but with a limited capacity to do so. Individual objects were defined, but the three-dimensional elements were seldom integrated into a unified conception of space. Objects were placed above or behind one another, but figures and the space between them did not form a spatial whole. There was an emphasis on foreshortened orthogonal lines and their convergence, yet the lines almost never met in a single horizon, much less a single center. In general, magnitudes diminished with distance, but in neither a consistent nor proportional way. The representation of depth was limited to the three-dimensional structure of separate figures, objects, or buildings. It did not integrate the picture plane and transform it into a deep space or vista. The illusion of depth came from the optical depiction of individual objects (Bunim, 1940). In Panofsky's (1924/25) terms, Greco-Roman space remained "a spatial aggregate"; it never became "a spatial system."

While there were occasional and sporadic expressions of one-point perspective, they seemed dependent upon the particular ability of an individual artist. As Richter (1970) notes, a particularly observant artist, faithful to what he sees, will empirically draw perspective. The Greeks were very much interested in the illusion and the illusionistic images of foreshortening and perspective. Plato's dismay (Richter, 1970, and Schäfer 1919/1974) and protest against the illusion of art testifies to the prevalence of illusionistic devices. Plato objected to the deception and trickery involved in substituting appearances for reality (i.e., the moustache drawn shorter on one side; four chair legs, but two drawn shorter). We can say for certain that the Greeks were concerned with creating the illusion of perspective; there was a real sense of a quest to achieve naturalistic representation. Perspective, however, was probably grasped only intuitively and primarily with multiple vanishing points along a vertical axis.

Levy (1943) and Kitto (1951) discuss the Greek development of foreshortening and some form of perspective as an attempt to bring the spectator into the picture. Artists were interested not only in the object as viewed by an observer, but also in the organization of these objects into a single scene. The Greeks extended their conception of space beyond topological emphasis of boundaries, separations, contours, and surfaces and established a projective conception of space based on the unique vantage point of the observer. The narrative frescoes (e.g., Alexander Mosaic, Odyssey Landscapes) illustrate the combined use of topological concepts of space (e.g., boundaries and contours) established by the Egyptians and the early phases of projective concepts of space (e.g., object constancy, foreshortening, approximate coordination of distance and size in an early, intuitive form of perspective). The use of projective space, however, was not a fully elaborated and integrated system.

The contrast of the modes of representation in Egyptian and Greek art vividly expresses the important developments in modes of artistic representation that occurred during the Greco-Roman period. In Egyptian art, objects are represented as they exist in reality, not as they appear to the viewer. Colors are rendered without shadow or variation and there is little expression of emotion. In Egyptian "aspective" art (Brunner-Traut, 1974; Schäfer, 1919/1974), individual parts of an object are rendered without foreshortening, as they exist in isolation, and then are added together to form a whole. Action is presented simultaneously as several fixed, single acts occurring at the same time. In Egyptian art the literal, concrete object is central. Greek art, in contrast, attempted to represent the object as it appeared visually to the viewer. Depending on the position of the viewer, sides are foreshortened, angles distorted, and lines made finer as distance increased. Variations in color and shading added subtle distinctions which enriched the representation of depth and of emotions. In Greek art, the observer is central. In Brunner-Traut's terms (1974, p. 426), "An Egyptian artist gives himself to the object, while a perspective artist takes his distance from it." With this distance from the object, the perspective artist has a more comprehensive view of the object. This, according to Cassirer (1927), indicates greater object-subject differentiation.

Before artists could experiment with representing transformations and "distortions" of the object, it was necessary to stabilize the image. As stated by Gombrich (1960, p. 206), "It was when art withdrew from the Pygmalion phase of action that it had to cast around for means to strengthen the illusion and to create the twilight realm of suspended disbelief which the Greeks first explored." There was a shift from a sensorimotor-preoperational representation of objects of action to a beginning, intuitive representation of objects of observation and contemplation. Perspective art reflects a more differentiated and integrated observation of the world—the entire object is viewed in its context. The size of objects and the mutual relationship between objects depends on their distance from the viewer; the values and the conditions of the existence of objects are defined in relative terms. In perspective art, the individual parts of an object and the objects themselves are subordinated to the whole, and their elements are represented in a functional interdependence. In perspective art, "there is always a certain tension between the object, which exists on its own, and the 'subject' who perceives it" (Brunner-Traut, 1974, p. 426). The development of perspective was a unique event in the history of civilization. "The sudden leap to perspective is part of the general transformation of man's relationship with the world. . . . Perspective presupposes a different ranking of man in the cosmos, that he take up a different position" (Brunner-Traut, 1974, p. 427). With the development of perspective, the represented object becomes a dynamic entity standing free in its environment, encompassed by space and time. The change from the aspective to the perspective mode of representation was part of the enormous transformation of the Greek miracle (Schäfer, 1919/1974); it was a "milestone in man's journey toward self-consciousness" (Brunner-Traut, 1974, p. 444).

THE ART OF THE MIDDLE AGES

The Middle Ages, the thousand years from the 5th to the 15th century, was a period of turmoil and social instability and upheaval. Any discussion of the art of this period must include the developments in the Eastern and Western Roman Empires, the Carolingian and Ottonian Renovatio, and the Romanesque and Gothic periods. The Eastern Roman (Byzantine) Empire at Constantinople developed separately from the urban structure of the Roman Empire in the West until about the 10th century. From the 5th to the 8th century, Western Europe gradually sank into a period of confusion, turmoil, and oppression—a period often referred to as the Dark Ages. Beginning as early as the 9th century, there were a number of renascences or periods of proto-renaissance in the West (Panofsky, 1960/1972). The transition from the Medieval period to the Renaissance was thus a gradual and evolving process and the selection of any specific date to mark that transition is somewhat arbitrary. For the purpose of our analysis, we will mark the Renaissance as beginning in 1400 with Lorenzo Ghiberti's first trial panels (1401–02) for the bronze doors of the Baptistry in Florence.

Because of the profound social instability and marked undulations in artistic interests, the history of art of this period is complex and contradictory. There are two basic sets of interpretations about the art of the Middle Ages. Some consider Greek and Roman humanism and their interest in realistic representation as the zenith of figurative art. The Middle Ages is viewed as a regression from the ultimate synthesis in representation of three-dimensional space and idealized proportions of the human form achieved in the Classical period. Beginning with the decline of the Roman Empire, the Classical Greek mode of representation was replaced by arbitrary rules for the depiction of human form and of space that had powerful religious connotations. The naturalistic representation of idealized form was replaced by schematized Byzantine contours, flattened frontal view of figures, and a loss of interest in the representation of depth and space. The intuitive integration of individual forms within a spatial context (projective concepts of space) achieved in Antiquity was discarded in the Middle Ages and replaced by a rigidity and an isolation of individual objects. Interest in the representation of depth and modeling of light and shade of figures in landscapes and closed interiors began to decline and eventually was lost (Levy, 1943; Panofsky, 1924/25). The representation of objects apparently behind each other gave way once again to objects above and beside each other. The sense of components integrated within a coherent space was replaced by forms that were flattened and lined up on a plane without regard for classical compositional structure. The use of figures and cast shadows to define the perpendicularity of ground plane to picture plane was relinquished and figures were increasingly aligned in isolation along the edge of the baseline of the picture plane. The ground plane became a vertical surface. Even though vestiges of stage space were retained, the picture plane essentially became a two-dimensional surface (Bunim, 1940). The picture frame was no longer a space to be looked through, but the frame defined the boundary of a surface to be filled. The foreshortening and intuitive perspective of Hellenistic and Roman art disappeared, and the stress once again was on topological concepts of space—the outline or contour of individual figures in isolation. Space became uniform, without dimension or measure, and reduced to a flat surface, enhanced by the value of the basic element of this new flatness: the line. Depth and volume were eliminated and there was a simplification of posture, gesture, and expression in an attempt to dematerialize man and his world and to elevate the spirit and exalt the eternity of life in heaven. Color and light were viewed as emanations from God and as expressions of God's presence. Naturalistic representation began once again only when the concepts and standards of Antiquity were rediscovered in the late Middle Ages and in the Italian Renaissance.

Classical modes of representation, however, were not completely lost in the Middle Ages. Some of the classical characteristics of Antiquity were retained in Byzantine art (Weitzmann, Chatzidakis, Miatev, & Radojčić, 1966; Weitzmann, 1979). In the art of the Eastern Empire at Constantinople, as exemplified by the frescoes and icons at the Saint Catherine monastery at Mount Sinai (Fig. 24) and the mosaics at Ravenna (Fig. 25), there are vivid depictions of full, well-proportioned, realistic human forms, boldly placed against a flattened background. Although little interest was shown in the representation of space, there was intermittent but continued progress in the representation of realistic human forms in the images of biblical figures. These figures were represented in isolation as well as in aggregate but non-communicating groups. Straight, simple, substantial shapes and forms, and symmetrical compositions expressed the stability and discipline of classical modes of representation (Arnheim, 1954/1974). The apse mosaic from San Vitale in Ravenna, of *Justinian and 12 Members of His Court,* (c. 547) (Fig. 25) is an excellent example of the Byzantine style that began with the golden Justinian era in Constantinople. The figures are tall and slender with powerful expression and ceremonial grandeur. All sense of time and space has been excluded to achieve a synthesis of regal and divine, eternal qualities. Individual features are differentiated to some degree but there is a fixed, stereotyped quality to the solemn frontal images with uniformly defined bodies and faces.

Other art historians (e.g., Bunim, 1940; Panofsky, 1960/1972) reject the interpretation that the Middle Ages was a regression in the representation of space. They contend that the loss in the Middle Ages of the advances made during the Greco-Roman period in the representation of space should be considered as a necessary transition in the development of modes of representation. Bunim (1940) and Panofsky (1960/1972) argue that the Renaissance development of linear perspective could never have come about without the changes

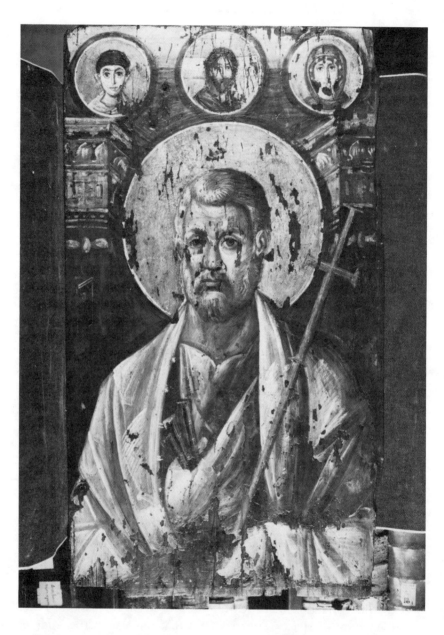

FIG. 24 *St. Peter Icon* (7th century), Monastery of St. Catherine at Mt. Sinai. (Michigan-Princeton-Alexandria Expedition to Mount Sinai).

in the picture plane that occurred during the Middle Ages including the relinquishing of the Greco-Roman vertical vanishing axis. It was necessary to transcend the "optical" or intuitive mode of representation of the Greco-Roman period in order to achieve a systematic, mathematical method for the integration of objects within their three-dimensional environment in the more pervasive unity that could be built around the consistent point of view of a spectator and the central vanishing point. In order to transform the picture plane into a consistent and homogeneous pictorial space, it was necessary to go beyond the partial and intuitive level of perspective achieved in Antiquity on the basis of Euclid's theory of vision. Greco-Roman, intuitive, optical "stage space" had to be reduced to a vertical surface to develop a fuller and more systematic theory of perspective that would apply to the spatial context as well as to the representation of figures. Although the picture plane as such disappeared in Medieval art, it was eventually rediscovered and subjected to the same visual laws that were applied to the representation of figures (Bunim, 1940).

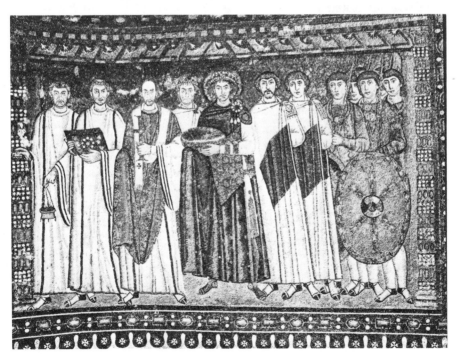

FIG. 25   San Vitale Mosaics, *Justinian and 12 Members of His Court* (6th century) Ravenna, Italy (Alinari).

The Medieval lack of interest in the representation of three-dimensional space did not begin abruptly in the Middle Ages but had already started in the late Pompeian period (stages III and IV) when an interest in the content and quality of the surface of the picture plane began to replace illusionistic methods. Roman stage space, the intersection of a horizontal ground and a vertical rear wall with cast shadows, was relinquished as figures were isolated and aligned along the baseline of the picture plane. The ground plane and the rear wall gradually became a colored vertical pictorial surface of sharply defined horizontal zones of "stratified space" (Bunim, 1940, p. 40). Figures became isolated in arrested, uniform, three-quarter, or frontal poses, staring blankly into space.

Bunim attributes much of the lack of interest in illusionistic art and the preference for a flattened and decorative quality in late Roman and early Christian art to the influence of an oriental mode of representation. Greco-Roman art had not developed a systematic procedure for the representation of three-dimensional space and Medieval art was interested in a religious, transcendental, symbolic orientation; hence the turn toward the oriental mode. During the early Middle Ages, the primary interest in man and his natural environment was replaced by an interest in the spiritual. The human image was rendered abstractly and symbolically, naturalism became irrelevant, and color, size, gesture, and position of figures assumed religious significance and meaning. Human figures in art were replaced by symbols or became symbols themselves, and the picture plane became a decorative, pictorial surface (Bunim, 1940).

Thus, there is considerable controversy about this complex period in the history of Western Civilization. Given the profound instability and social upheaval of this period, however, it is not surprising that there was some interruption in the development of art, literature, and science. But such an interruption is not necessarily inconsistent with the identification of a more extended developmental sequence in which powerful external forces can sometimes facilitate progress and at other times create a negative climate that can cause temporary disruption or even a regression (Meiss, 1951). Based on developmental psychological principles, the representation of space in the Middle Ages clearly ignored projective concepts of space and the intuitive form of perspective achieved in Antiquity. But, at the same time, the representation of the human form occasionally became increasingly realistic and substantial. The icons at Saint Catherine and the mosaics at Ravenna illustrate the lack of interest in space and perspective as well as the occasional increased emphasis placed upon the representation of substantial forms of religious figures. In fact, it may have been the lack of interest in representing depth in an embedding spatial context that contributed to the increased attention given to the representation of substantial human figures.

The thousand years of Greco-Roman art had come to an end in the 3rd century A.D. with the beginning of the new Christian world. Early Christian art, prior to the Edict of Milan in 313 A.D., was primarily funerary painting in the Catacombs and entailed simple transformation of pagan themes, motifs, and manners. Greek and Roman gods were replaced by themes from Christianity. Images of Christ's life and passion, portraits of saints, and aspects of the liturgy became the dominant content of art. Art functioned as a didactic medium to explain religious concepts—to communicate biblical stories from the Old Testament and the Gospels, the revelation of the Divine, and the nature of man's salvation. The individuality, realism, and vitality of Greco-Roman portraiture were replaced by expression of universally divine qualities of spirituality and contemplation (Weitzmann, 1979). Early Christian art de-emphasized Greco-Roman naturalism and instead returned to more Archaic Greco-Roman prototypes. The replacement of Greco-Roman naturalism and illusionism with a new religious symbolism involved utilizing body attitudes and gestures for religious significance. The naturalism of bodies in action was replaced by simplified, rigid, and stiffened gestures. For a while the continued use of Greco-Roman cast shadows and modeling gave the figures a three-dimensional substantiality. But eventually figures lost their naturalism, and landscape and architectural settings became symbolic rather than substantial and descriptive. (see Fig. 26).

At first in Christian art, the Church sought to emphasize more spiritual values and to represent the body in a dematerialized, abstract manner. The major theme was the glorification of the spiritual and the transcendental. Reality and naturalism were minimized and the major concern was the iconographic significance of figures—their religious symbolism. Hebraic, Greco-Roman, and Christian themes and styles were interwoven. Simple and crude figures appeared in hieratic compositions in which there was a denial of naturalism and three-dimensional space. Based upon biblical law, the portrayal of the human image was prohibited and art was limited primarily to symbolic renderings. Panofsky (1960/1972), citing von Schlosser, notes that at

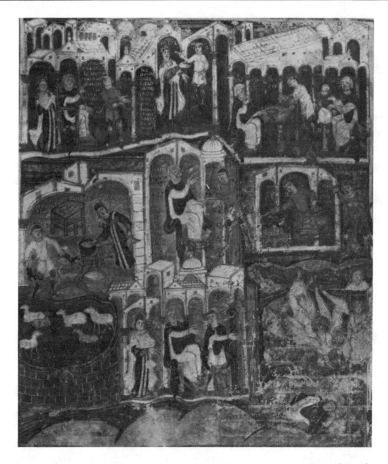

FIG. 26   Ashburnham Pentateuch, *Illuminated manuscript, Story of Jacob and Esau* (c. 7th century) (Bibliothèque Nationale, Paris).

the time of Emperor Constantine and Pope Sylvester all statues were dismembered and mutilated, and the books, treatises, and pictures that provided the rules and guidelines for naturalistic art were destroyed. As Arnheim (1974, p. 147) notes, earthly life was viewed as a interlude and preparation for life in heaven. The body represented temptation and suffering. Art avoided expressing the beauty of the body; instead, the body, in dematerialized form, was used as a symbol of the spirit. Man and his world were simplified and dematerialized. Straight, sharp, simple shapes and lines had an ascetic quality much like the asceticism of the Church. Emphasis was upon ornamentation and spiritual meaning, not upon realistic human figures in a spatial context. The decoration of the surface of the picture plane took precedence over the realism of space and proportionality. Figures became fixed, posed, frontal views with little sense of action.

There were alternations, however, in the enforcement of the biblical ban against creating graven images, and when it was abandoned there was renewed interest in the representation of the human form and Greco-Roman naturalism to communicate biblical stories from the Old Testament. The 6th century Justinian revival led to a new Byzantine style expressed in the monumental mosaics at Ravenna. The mosaics from this period in Constantinople have all been destroyed, but primary examples still remain in San Vitale and San Appollinaire Nuovo at Ravenna. The primary focus was no longer upon the spatial context but upon isolated figures that loomed large with massive solidity. Remnants of the Greco-Roman naturalism were retained in the volume of individual figures. But these substantial figures were placed in isolation and treated as symbols. They convey in vivid form the complex symbolism of Christian dogma. This veneration of the symbolic image created a sense of presence (von Simson, 1948) in which the spiritually powerful symbols and images were "like the magic of the Paleolithic caves, where the hunter-artists believed they summoned and controlled their animal quarry by the miracle of representation" (Gardner, 1975, p. 273). This hieratic Byzantine style was the basic form and content of the art of much of the Middle Ages. The emphasis is upon the figures—tall, angular, elegant, and powerful—and upon glittering light and vivid colors that create an otherworldliness, spirituality, and sense of mystery.

From the 3rd to the 7th centuries A.D., there were ascendances and declines of Classical and Christian themes and styles (Panofsky, 1960/1972). Often, these different styles would appear simultaneously, even within the same work of art. In the apse mosaic of the Saint Catherine Monastery at Mount Sinai (548–565 A.D.) (Fig. 27), for example, the Christ figure is represented abstractly, while the faces of the Prophets, Moses, and the Apostles Peter, John, and James are represented as lively, emotional, and quite corporeal and vital. Divinity was represented in abstract form, whereas human figures were expressed more naturalistically. These two modes were "used for different purposes" and were the foundation of the great variety of styles found in the art of the Middle Ages that integrated abstract-symbolic and naturalistic-classical elements (Weitzmann, 1979, p. xxvi).

Subsequent to the Justinian revival, the interest in naturalistic

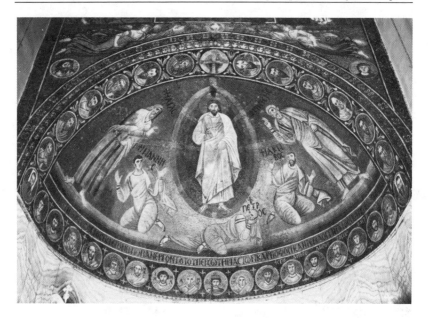

FIG. 27   Apse mosaic, *Transfiguration of Christ*, Monastery of St. Catherine at Mt. Sinai. (Michigan-Princeton-Alexandria Expedition to Mount Sinai).

figures was again lost in the frequent periods of prohibitions against creating graven images. There was a severe setback in representational art during the 8th and early 9th century violent Iconoclastic Controversy. Eighth century Iconoclast Emperors were concerned about a lapse into idolatry and they restricted religious art to abstract symbols and the forms of plants and animals throughout the Byzantine Empire for over a hundred years. When the iconoclast ban was finally lifted in 843, a new style emerged that was based on a subtle blend of Hellenistic naturalism and Byzantine abstraction and symbolism. It integrated the "simplicity, dignity and grace of classicism . . . with Byzantine piety and pathos" (Gardner, 1975, p. 280). Byzantine abstraction and the disinterest in space produced a timeless spirituality, while Hellenistic naturalism gave the figures a vitality and substantiality. With the relaxation of the biblical prohibition against graven images, the abstract, decorative, linear Byzantine devotional icon eventually became increasingly realistic.

Beginning in 843 there was a return to representation of substantial human forms in elaborate mosaics and elegant miniatures of ivory and silver. In mosaics, the human figures were placed against a solid gold background that gave them a vivid presence as they seemed to float in space. Angular and highly stylized poses also contributed to the sense of these figures as removed from the world of nature and reality. This "second golden age" of Byzantine art lasted until Constantinople was conquered by the Fourth Crusade in 1204. Although this crusade destroyed much of Constantinople's art, it also brought about the dispersion of the art treasures of the Byzantine Empire throughout Western Europe. With the return of Greek emperors in 1261, Byzantine art once again flourished until 1453, when Constantinople finally fell to the Ottoman Turks. Despite considerable pressure and turmoil, the Eastern Empire survived precariously until the middle of the 15th century. By this time, Byzantine art was well established and existed throughout Europe in manuscript illuminations and miniature art such as small ivory reliefs, embroidery, and gold and enamelwork. Though this miniature art lacked the monumental effect of fresco paintings and mosaics, the Byzantine style had a major influence on the eventual development of Italian Renaissance art.

Thus there was a complex development within Byzantine art. Early forms of Byzantine art, like early Christian art in the Western Empire, were based on the forms of Antiquity. Subsequently, naturalistic representation and classical form were repudiated and Christian spirituality and the sense of the Divine were expressed in abstract forms and a complex iconography markedly differentiated from the natural world. Figures were defined by unbroken contours of flattened silhouettes against a neutral background. Later Byzantine art became increasingly naturalistic and contained dramatic action and expressions of emotion in facial features and gestures, while still including elements of the earlier abstract, decorative, linear, Byzantine style. This late Byzantine period was a time of rediscovery of the naturalistic traditions of the classical past which were integrated with the early Byzantine emphasis of the hard, firm, well-defined line (topological concepts of space). The late Byzantine work entitled *Enthroned Madonna and Child* (Fig. 28) from very early in the 13th century clearly expresses the integration of Classic and Byzantine elements. The Madonna's graceful pose and the emotional expressiveness of her face are integrated with more schematic and abstract dimensions to create an effect that is neither flat nor fully spatial (Janson, 1969).

In the Western Empire interest in classical themes and admiration of Greco-Roman art and science waxed and waned. From the 3rd to the 6th century A.D. Christian and Classical philosophy were integrated; Greek thought was given Christian form and nature was seen

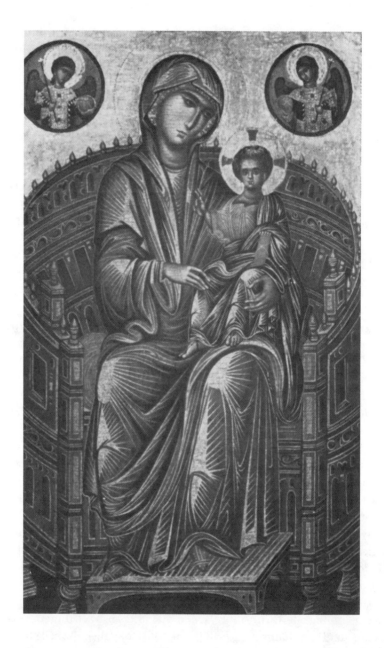

FIG. 28   Byzantine School, *Enthroned Madonna & Child* (c. 1200) (National Gallery, Washington, D.C.).

170

as revealing spiritual truth. Interest in classical naturalistic forms and themes alternated with attempts to ban the worship and the representation of pagan (Roman) gods. The concerns about idolatry led to a more hieratic and spiritual approach in art, expressed in more abstract geometric forms. Three-dimensional space was collapsed into a flat, two-dimensional representation and luminous colors and flat geometric forms emphasized the otherworldliness of the images. Spirituality emphasized a hierarchical and vertical view of the universe, expressed in church frescoes and mosaics in which the figure of the all-ruling Father was at the central dome. Below him, usually at the base of the dome, were the angels and the archangels, and closer to the common level of man in the congregation, on the wall of the church, were the figures of the saints. The Virgin Mary was often placed to the side, high in one of the alternate domes. The composition of the art reflected the organization of the universe. The figures in the mosaics and frescoes were symbolic images of the divine. Individual features were suppressed and figures were flattened. Highly stylized frontal poses and stereotyped facial expressions of isolated figures against a gold background created a remote otherworldliness.

But all this came to an end with the conquest of the Western Empire by the barbarians in the latter part of the 5th century. Rome was plundered several times in the 4th and 5th centuries and the Western Empire finally collapsed in 476 A.D. and was continually fragmented by frequent invasions and conquests. In contrast to the precarious continuity of the classic tradition in Constantinople, the Western Empire was unstable and in great turmoil. It required centuries for the West to recapture and reappropriate fragments of classical culture and incorporate them into the Western way of life. While Byzantian civilization was able to maintain a continuity for a thousand years, the Western Empire disintegrated into continually warring barbarian kingdoms beginning in the early 5th century. Despite constant strife, anarchy and warfare, Christianity was well established in the various barbarian groups and served as a unifying force. But Western Europe, from about the 5th to the 8th century gradually disintegrated into conflict and confusion. The artistic images of the migrating barbarians were replete with themes of war, monsters, and terrifying supernatural forces derived from pagan tribal experiences and rites. Art was non-naturalistic, abstract, decorative, and geometric (Gardner, 1975).

The changes from Classical to Medieval art were not restricted to the loss of naturalism in the representation of space and of human and animal form. Also involved was a change in the content and function of art. The content of art became primarily the "timeless re-enactment of the life of Christ in the liturgy of the Church" (Gombrich, 1960, p. 145) and its function once again became ritualistic. When art in the Middle Ages assumed a narrative function, it was for the teaching of religious dogma and ritual, not for representing reality. Objects were included in art, not because of the way they were organized in nature, but to emphasize a religious theme.

There was also a fundamental change in the conception of man and his role in the universe during the Medieval period. The Classical emphasis on the importance and dignity of the individual was replaced by a conception in which man relinquished his role in submission to a powerful deity. Man was considered as different from, and inferior to, God (Panofsky, 1960/1972); people were insignificant in contrast to God's divine scheme and power. Medieval art portrayed eternal, fixed, divine events with little sense of time and space. The art of this period, much like the concept of God and man, was based on a rigid and fixed formula. Ambivalent attitudes existed toward the representation of space and the human form; and once again the individual artist became anonymous. The identity of individual artists and the biographic account of their lives, which began during the Classical Greek period, was lost during the Middle Ages and reappeared once again only with the Renaissance and its rediscovery and elaboration of Greek humanism (Kris, 1952; Kris & Kurz, 1934/1979).

In terms of developmental psychological concepts, the modes of representation during the Middle Ages, both in the Eastern and Western Empire, were at a transition point between sensorimotor-preoperational and concrete operational modes. The concepts of space were also fluctuating between a primary reliance on topological concepts (an emphasis upon the boundary and contour of objects in isolation) to the beginning stages of projective concepts of space. Artistic style throughout the thousand years of the Middle Ages wavered back and forth within this transitional zone; the function of art alternated from being primarily ritual and dealing with powerful, threatening, external, mystical forces to more naturalistic representations that recognized the role of the individual in constructing an understanding of nature.

From the 10th century on, invasions were repelled in the West, stability was restored, and Western Civilization began a remarkable advance and ascent, culminating in the Renaissance. The Byzantine preservation of classical content, form and style and its eventual dispersion throughout Europe was an important factor in the eventual development of the Renaissance. A primary aspect of the long process leading to the Renaissance was the numerous attempts to recover and assimilate the form, style, and content of Antiquity. But it is important to stress, as Butterfield notes (1957, p. 191) in discussing the history of science, there was no indication "that the ancient world, before its heritage had been dispersed, was moving towards anything like the scientific revolution" that occurred in the Renaissance. No evidence shows "that the Byzantine Empire, in spite of the continuity of its classical tradition, would ever have taken hold of ancient thought and so remoulded it by a great transforming power." The scientific and artistic revolution of the Renaissance was the creative product of the dynamic quality of life that had been developing in Western Europe, beginning in the 9th and 10th century.

A pre-Renaissance around 800 A.D., the first move toward a new civilization in Western Europe after the collapse of the Roman Empire, occurred with Charlemagne in the Carolingian Renascence. Charlemagne sought to emulate the art, culture, and political ideals of Christian Rome and to revive aspects of Classical Antiquity. He was impressed with Greco-Roman naturalism that had been preserved in Byzantine illuminations and appreciated its marked contrast with the anti-naturalistic tendencies in the art of the West. The Carolingian revival was one of the first rapprochements with Classical traditions. The Carolingian masters utilized Roman and early Christian prototypes in book illuminations as well as reliefs in stone and stucco, ivory carvings, cameos, and coins (Panofsky, 1960/1972), and they attempted to represent the human body according to the laws of anatomy and physiology. Narrative art and the representation of expressive figures in action appeared in a variety of different forms. The Carolingian Renascence was the first indication of a return to some form of naturalism and realism. As noted by Holländer (1924), a skillful rendering of space in the later scripts of Charlemagne's court school went far beyond the Justinian Byzantine imitation of classical perspective. The artists in the court at Aachen related the picture space to the central figure in order to stress its importance and give it added significance. According to Panofsky (1960/1972, p. 50), "Carolingian art acquired a rich and authentic vocabulary of . . . classical 'images': figures (or groups of figures) classical not only in

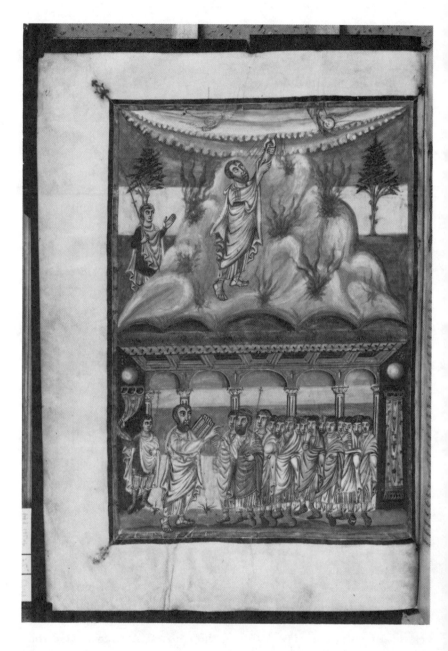

FIG. 29 *Moses Displaying the Tablets of the Law,* The Bible of Moutier-Grandval (second half of the 9th century) (The British Library).

form . . . but also in significance." The lower half of Fig. 29, *Moses Displaying the Tablets of the Law* in the Bible of Moutier–Grandval from the second half of the 9th century, illustrates the Carolingian appropriation of some of the techniques of perspective preserved from late Antiquity, such as interiors defined by walls and converging lines of coffered ceilings, canopies, or small segmented domes supported by four columns (Panofsky, 1960/1972).

The Carolingian revival ended in 877, followed by eight or nine decades "as barren as the seventh century" (Panofsky, 1960/1972, p. 52). The collapse of the Carolingian empire brought on a period of confusion and darkness. As far as art is concerned, the years between 880 and 970 were a "period of incubation," (Panofsky, 1960/1972, p. 53) prior to a general resurgence of artistic competence and discipline in the last third of the 10th century—a resurgence referred to as the Ottonian Renascence. This revival from 970 to 1020 not only preserved the Carolingian culture and tradition, but extended and enriched it. Inspiration was also drawn from early Christian and Byzantine sources. The Ottonians used a sharply defined, firm line that often partitioned off clearly modeled shapes and forms and created a strong sculptural relief and silhouette. Although Ottonian art lacked Classical realism and naturalism, it emphasized the spatial context and expressive figures.

The Carolingian interest in classical form was extensive, but it imitated only minor works of art that usually did not predate the 4th or 5th century A.D. Classical values were appropriated in the Carolingian revival, but classical forms were used only to a limited degree (Panofsky, 1960/1972). In contrast, the Ottonian revival of the 10th century, derived from the Carolingian and Byzantine sources, was less extensive and widespread, but their strongly modeled figures were new and powerful. An illumination from the *Gospel Books of Otto III*, entitled *Otto III Enthroned Receiving the Homage from Four Parts of the Empire* (997–1000 A.D.) (Fig. 30), though like the Justinian mosaics in Ravenna, indicates a powerful new expressiveness in the representation of the human form in art. Also, a renewed interest in the representation of space was indicated by the emperor enthroned under a canopy and the recession into space of the two figures on either side representing the Church and the State.

The Carolingian and Ottonian Renascences involved primarily architecture and sculpture, and painting and illuminated manuscripts only secondarily. Each period was relatively transitory, and each was

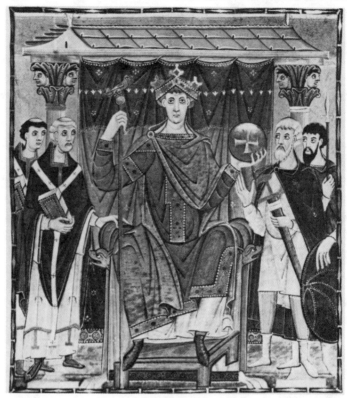

FIG. 30 *Otto 111 Enthroned Receiving the Homage from Four Parts of the Empire*
(flanked by nobility & clergy), from the Gospel Book of Otto 111 (997–1000),
Court School of Otto 111. (Bayerische Staatsbibliothek, Munich).

followed by a relative estrangement from Classical traditions. Thus,
the Middle Ages involved a succession of attempts to assimilate and
reject Antiquity. The eventual revival of Antiquity in the Renaissance,
however, was stable because it was embedded in a more basic change
in society that also involved the revival of mathematics and natural
science. The movement toward the Renaissance was the result of the
artistic revival that first began in the monasticism of the 10th century,
after Europe regained a degree of political stability. By the mid-11th
century Europe had begun to emerge from the confusion of the
barbarian movements. The further development of monastic orders
as educational centers, the growth of feudalism as an economic order,
and the expansion of economic centers of commerce and trade partly
as a consequence of the Crusades, all created a climate that brought
increased contact with and interest in Islamic texts that had retained

much of the Greek tradition in mathematics, philosophy, and science. These Islamic texts provided the basis for succeeding periods of renasence including the Romanesque and Gothic periods.

Much attention has been given to the degree to which Medieval art turned away from the principles of Antiquity. Panofsky (1960/1972) points out that the greatest transformation—the complete renunciation of perspective and naturalistic representation as developed in Antiquity—occurred in Northern Europe during the Romanesque period (1050–1150). Romanesque art was a fusion of Roman, Carolingian, Ottonian, and Byzantine elements. As part of a growing religious enthusiasm as seen in various crusades and pilgrimages, the interest in Romanesque art was on the religious content rather than on the pictorial effect. Naturalism was gradually replaced by nonrepresentative forms as the details of the environment and the spatial and temporal context became less important. The background in Romanesque painting became a closed, vertical, two-dimensional, decorative surface without depth or space. Figures were also modified and became more linear and schematized rather than organic and plastic. Poses became fixed and stereotyped, without movement or action. Both the background and the figures were limited in depth to a single plane. All pictorial effects including foreshortening, perspective, tonal values, and gradations of light and shade were replaced by nonrepresentational, abstract, symbolic, schematic forms.

The picture plane became strictly a two-dimensional surface for the representation of the contour of objects. Firmly drawn lines were the hallmark of Medieval Art (Gombrich, 1960) and they were used to bound and ornament a surface. Firmly drawn outlines and heavy, dark contours defined the figures. Figures were kept flat, without movement or emotion, and partitioned into separate molded segments that almost broke the figure into independent parts (Gardner, 1975). This segmentation flattened the human figure and interrupted its integrity and definition, and it created a continuity between the figure and the background. Romanesque painting reduced body and space to a common and homogeneous surface. The illusion of perspective was rejected and replaced by a surface in which there was an indissoluble unity between the figure and the background plane. This occurred primarily in sculpture, but also in painting. Architectural sculpture was no longer set into the architecture or applied to it, but made to conform to the architectural mass itself (Panofsky, 1924/25). In Antiquity, "bodies" were substantial and had individually determined extension, and form, but in Romanesque art they were a union of indistinguishable functions. Natural figures were transformed into religious images of severe linear design and symbolic distortion that expressed transcendental, spiritual values. These images were in marked contrast to the gentle, naturalistic forms of Antiquity and to the work that was to occur in the more humanistic Gothic age (Panofsky, 1924/25).

A comparison by Bunim (1940) of a late 11th century manuscript illustration of Philippe I and his court (Fig. 31a) and a copy of the illustration made two centuries later (Fig. 31b) serves to demonstrate the differences between Romanesque and Gothic modes of representation. In the 11th century Romanesque illustration the figures overlap each other slightly, their eyes are large and full, and the pupils are placed in the center of the eye. The trunks of the figures are frontal and the heads are also frontal or twisted slightly. The same hieratical gesture is repeated in each figure. The drapery is a series of simple lines. Philippe I is seated with legs crossed and his toes turned inward. His head is in three-quarter view, but his eyes, like those of the other figures, are frontal with the pupils in the center. His seat and footstool lack the rudiments of perspective and the rounded arch above seems to isolate him from the rest of the scene.

The figures undergo a marked change in the 13th century Gothic illustration. Intercommunicating, expressive groups replace the flat alignment of isolated figures. Figures are more naturalistic, proportional, and their gestures vary. Heads are turned to the right and left with foreshortening in the three-quarter view and only part of the eye is shown on the foreshortened side of the face. The drapery has more naturalistic folds with gradations of light and shade. Philippe I has a naturalistic foreshortened appearance as his body is turned to the right in a gesture and a glance directed toward his court. The architectural detail has become a Gothic pointed arch. And the chair of Philippe I has changed from a typical Romanesque "foldstool" with crossed legs to the more substantial, blocklike, Gothic throne. The compact and unified composition of the 13th century manuscript is characteristic of the Gothic mode of representation in which a distinctive spatial form is created in both the background and in the figures (Bunim, 1940).

Bunim (1940) and Panofsky (1960/1972) stress that the Romanesque radical renunciation of all spatial illusion and perspective was a necessary transition for the development of a modern view of space.

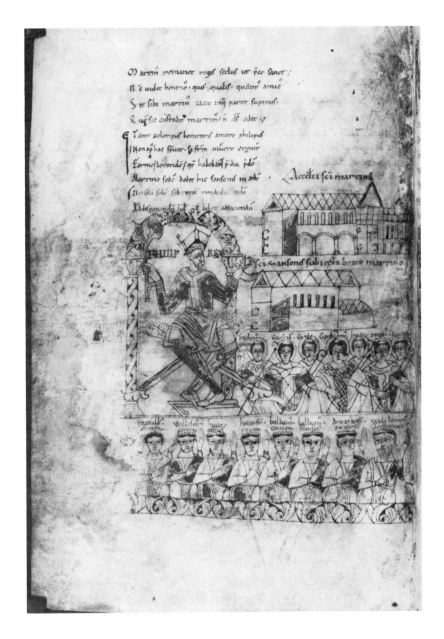

FIG. 31a *Philippe 1 and His Court, Charter of St. Martin-des-Champs* (11th century manuscript) (The British Library).

179

Romanesque mural painting of the 11th and 12th centuries contained two basic and competing trends: a commitment to iconoclasm and the iconoclastic era (Trinkaus, 1970) and an interest in creative realism and the natural world (Auerbach, 1953). An ambivalent tendency to preserve traditional forms and religious symbols competed with an interest in experimentation and a curiosity about the natural aspects

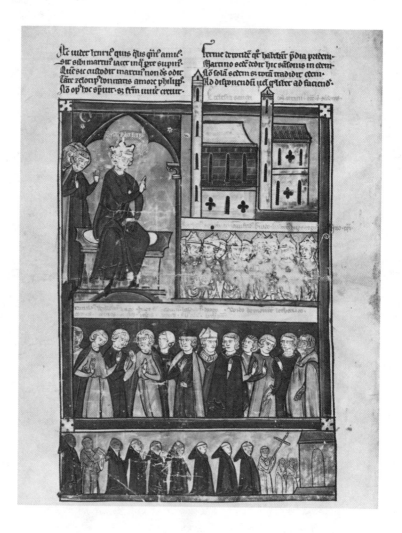

FIG. 31b *Philippe 1 and His Court, Charter of St. Martin-des-Champs* (13th century manuscript) (Bibliothèque Nationale, Paris).

of the real world. But the linear and schematized forms of the non-representational picture surface, conducive to expressing spiritual forms, did not lend themselves easily to being able to suggest nature in form or content. Romanesque painting was primarily religious in content and traditional, nonnaturalistic, and abstract in form. Early Romanesque art was non-representational and two-dimensional, the picture was more decorative than naturalistic. Figures had limited depth and volume. There was little relationship among figures and movement was avoided (Bunim, 1940).

In later Romanesque painting, portraits of a living person, other than a reigning monarch, begin to reappear. In later Romanesque painting, there is a softening of the segmentation and patterning, a renewed interest in foreshortening, three-dimensional forms, and the movement of the figures as the composition becomes more integrated. The differentiation of the body and the surrounding field (including drapery), was finally achieved in Gothic art, leading to a sense of depth that increased and deepened into a rich naturalism. Subsequently, in Gothic art, the mass of figures was differentiated into quasi-corporeal structures, the statue emerged from the wall as an independent structure, and the relief was free of its surroundings (Panofsky, 1924/25). Monumental sculpture was revived after being dormant for at least six centuries and was used in relief around the columns and massive doors of churches to express biblical history and religious doctrine. Structure, discrete form, and openness were emphasized along with a revival in a feeling for and an appreciation of the human body. The gentle, naturalistic Gothic figure was simple, clear, and substantial. In painting, as the figure was defined as separate from the picture surface, there had to be a corresponding development of space. Bodies and the sphere of space containing the bodies were simultaneously emancipated. The Gothic figure was assigned a definite place in empty space; it had a definite zone of space, a stage (Panofsky, 1924/25). In Gothic sculpture the statue stands out from the plane of the wall and is treated as a three-dimensional volume. Mask-like, fixed Romanesque features are replaced by unique features of specific individuals. Initially, these individual qualities were expressed as part of a religious image, and later as portraits of specific individuals. For the first time in a millennium, faces began to have unique features and personal expressions. Emotional expressions appeared in sacred figures to create the sense of human feelings with which an observer could identify (Gardner, 1975). And for the first time since the Classical period artists began to sign their work (Kris & Kurz, 1934/1979).

Progress in the development of new modes of representation in the West began around the 9th and 10th century when there was increased stability in society and a greater emphasis on the importance and dignity of man. Changes in modes of representation occurred at the same time as basic revisions in social order and a renewed interest in man and nature. This interest was expressed in a return to naturalistic representation, including the intuitive use of perspective and early forms of projective concepts of space. The emerging Renaissance emphasis on individual dignity (e.g., by Ficino, Pico della Mirandola) created the cultural context that facilitated the further development of representation of perspective—the representation of how the world appears from an individual vantage point.

From the fall of Rome to the reign of Charlemagne in the first half of the 9th century (800–814 A.D.) God was portrayed as a critcal, judgmental, potentially punitive figure. An oppressive relationship existed between God and man. In the porticoes of Romanesque churches (as late as 1075–1125 A.D.), for example, Christ sat in judgment at the entrance of the church. Subsequently, in the Gothic church beginning around 1150 A.D., the figure of Christ in the porticoes was complemented by the image of the more supplicating, accepting, maternal Virgin. The tone of the relationship between man and the Divine was enriched by this addition. Man was defined once again as different from both barbarians and the Divine—as unique and valued, different from animals because he controlled his instincts, and, though less than God, beloved by God and created in His image. There was a "conviction of the dignity of man, based on both the insistence on human values (rationality and freedom) and the acceptance of human limitations (fallibility and frailty)" (Panofsky, 1955b, p. 2). Heretical religious sects began to criticize ecclesiastical authority. Approved sects, such as the Franciscans and the Dominicans, began to stress the need for closer contact between people and the clergy, and the appreciation of the earthly as well as the heavenly realm. The cult of the Virgin during this age of chivalry was an expression of an increased respect and spiritual recognition of women (Bunim, 1940). This cult was part of a less dogmatic, more acceptant, compassionate religion. The severity of judgment and the threat of damnation of the Romanesque period were modulated and modified by the gentleness, compassion, and emphasis on salvation in the Gothic period. The image of Christ as Judge was changed to that of loving Saviour (Gardner, 1975).

Gothic art in the late 12th, 13th, and 14th centuries was the cumulative effect of movement begun in the 11th and 12th centuries with the Crusades and the development of a secular culture with humanistic tendencies. Gothic art was an extension of the Romanesque, but it was based on a philosophy of personal faith in God rather than on God's supremacy. Artistic style also was based more on individual aesthetic judgment than on strict aesthetic or religious formulas. This emphasis on individual judgment encouraged exploration and experimentation and facilitated a wide range of stylistic variations. The Romanesque period was dominated by archaic feudal tendencies with constant conflict and warfare. Gothic social order was also feudal, but not as disrupted and disjointed as the Romanesque. Centralized governments were established and a number of urban centers sprang up. A middle class began to be defined around craftsmen and their guilds, and the emergence of a mercantile and a professional class was part of a newly developing social and economic order. Greater openness between the monasteries and secular society led to the growth of intellectual centers as part of civil communities. Universities began to appear in urban centers and they, rather than the isolated monasteries, became the educational centers. Profound changes also began to occur in man's conception of himself. The Romanesque conception of the body was in contrast to the spirituality of the soul—the body was frail and vulnerable to temptation. This view was replaced by a conception of the body and soul as closely interrelated and the belief that an individual's soul is made manifest through his or her body. Individuality and personal uniqueness were acknowledged as important in both physical form and spiritual quality (Gardner, 1975).

By the 13th century Western Europe began to achieve a synthesis of the Greco-Roman classical heritage and aspects of the Byzantine and Islamic traditions. Islamic texts had retained much of the classic heritage in mathematics, philosophy, and science and were an important source for the eventual recovery of the classical tradition in the West. Arabic translations of the texts of Antiquity influenced scholars throughout the 12th and 13th centuries. A new curiosity about nature and systematic attempts to describe the appearance of nature were seen as an expression of God's glory. Religious views were supplemented by secular intellectual curiosity. Impressive technological advances, the development of craft guilds, and urban economies created the social context for the emergence of a period of remarkable discovery. Increase in travel, trade, and skilled crafts along with the development of municipal government were all part of an increased self-consciousness in society.

Increased interest in the natural world during this period led to the beginning of scientific inquiry and technological advances such as the construction of the compass and the lens, and books on optics by Roger Bacon and others. Lay artists began to replace monastic artists as art became more secularized, competitive, and experimental (Bunim, 1940). In both Romanesque and Gothic painting figures were still limited to a single plane, but in the Gothic there was increased communication among figures and a beginning definition of an architectural frame in the integration of a ground plane with the background surface. Figure and background were separate but coordinated, leading to a beginning sense of unification within the picture plane.

Subsequent to the Carolingian and Ottonian Renascences, Medieval art developed a procedure in which "the ground has congealed into a solid, planar working surface while the design has congealed into a system of two-dimensional areas defined by one-dimensional lines. . . . Thus for the first time in the history of European art a consubstantiality had been established between the solid objects (figures or things) and their environment" (Panofsky, 1960/ 1972, p. 131–132). Medieval art remained unalterably nonperspective and thus never abrogated the complementary principles of "mass . . . and surface consolidation" (p. 131). In Classical art the background had been a single color (usually black or white) on a neutral surface. The Medieval picture plane was two-dimensional and had an expressive function as either a symbolic color or a decorative surface. Medieval art transformed the picture plane into an independent two-dimensional surface and figures and objects were all reduced to this surface. Three-dimensionality was then reintroduced into the figures and objects as well as into the picture plane through the use of stage space. Based on Byzantine stage space the picture plane was divided into two parts: a ground plane and a vertical background. Although figures were flattened, the stage space maintained the vestiges of three-dimensionality. Eventually, the ground plane once again became perpendicular to the picture plane and figures became less stylized and began to be represented as freely moving and actively communicating in groups. This led to the development of three-dimensional space in the picture plane and to techniques for representing figures and objects naturalistically (Bunim, 1940).

The integration of this Medieval sense of solidarity and coherence with the preservation and revival of the illusionistic Greco-Roman tradition established the sense that space could be continuous and infinite. According to Panofsky (1960/1972), the Renaissance concept of space and linear perspective was the result of the unification of classical perspective with the principles of mass and surface consolidation. The figures and the architectural settings in the early Renaissance paintings of Cimabue, Cavallini, Duccio, and Giotto had a new sense of coherence and stability as well as a sense of depth, in which there was volume allocated to every solid as well as to every void. Despite technical limitations and inaccuracies, artists in the late 13th and early 14th century were able to construct a space that was "no longer discontinuous and finite," but now had the potential to become "continuous and infinite" (Panofsky, 1960/1972, p. 137). The picture plane was no longer an opaque and impervious surface, but a window on which one could construct a genuine projection plane. The evolution of the picture plane into definite, substantial, enclosing, and potentially measurable planes reintroduced the problem of the representation of perspective.

The representation of a unified composition began in the late 13th century through the use of a simplified two-dimensional stage space with a unified background and ground plane that formed architectural interiors as a frame around the figures. The Byzantine preservation of stage space and the occasional representation of substantial human form contributed to the development of Gothic naturalism with its coordination of figure and background. And this Gothic naturalism at the end of the 13th century, as seen in the work of Cimabue (Fig. 32) and Cavallini (Fig. 33), was the prelude to the remarkable changes in the representation of space in the Renaissance. The distinct and well-defined naturalistic Gothic style emerged in the mid 13th century in manuscript illuminations and panel paintings in the north and in Italian frescoes.

Gothic painting was strongly influenced by the Byzantine style, and integrated it with the development of a less harsh and more realistic style and an interest in the representation of subtle details. The discovery of light and shade to model figures contributed to advances in the representation of depth. Cavallini, Duccio and Giotto in large

murals and frescoes created figures that were able to communicate
with each other by gesture and expression. In these large-scale paintings, Byzantine style was combined with expressive narrative sequences. Well-molded figures, with expressive features and gestures,
were set in landscapes and architectural structures that convincingly
enclosed them (Bunim, 1940). Artists were interested in the depiction

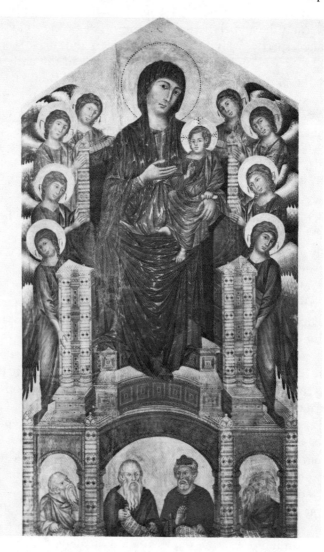

FIG. 32   Cimabue, *Madonna Enthroned* (1280–90) Uffizi Gallery, Florence
(Alinari).

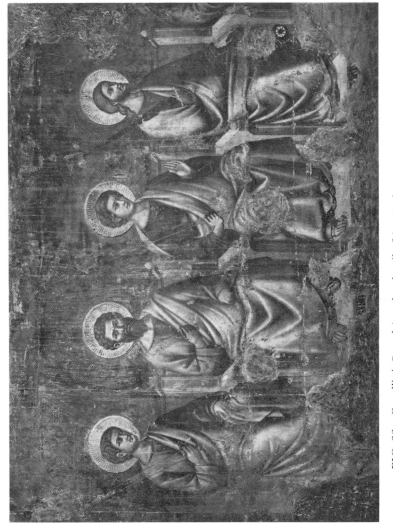

FIG. 33   Cavallini, *Seated Apostles*, detail of *Last Judgment* (c. 1290), Church of St. Cecilia, Rome (Alinari).

187

of expressive figures in large, realistic, and carefully constructed settings. With the achievement of narrative composition and the illusion of reality, more stylized and abstract Byzantine conventions were discarded. The large-scale murals and frescoes of the Gothic period provided an important opportuty for the development of perspective and the naturalistic representation of three-dimensional space.

Alberti's treatise *Della Pittura* (1435), was the foundation for the development of a geometric method for representing perspective in the Renaissance. Alberti suggested procedures for the convergence of parallel lines in a logically determined vanishing point and for diminishing the size of figures as a function of their distance from the edge of the picture plane. Alberti's techniques of central projection and projective sections provided a basis for establishing rules for a "reciprocal . . . metrical correspondence between the pictorial representation of objects and the shape of those objects as located in space" (Ivins, 1938/1973, p. 10). The solution of more complex problems of linear perspective was subsequently introduced by Piero della Francesca, Leonardo, and other Italian artists of the late 15th and early 16th century. These techniques and procedures provided a method for representing a unified perspective scene in relation to a spectator that was potentially measurable. Renaissance perspective was an integral part of the development of a theory of representation in which it was possible to establish logical relations between the forms and locations of objects within a consistent symbol system (Ivins, 1938/ 1973). While Renaissance perspective developed out of Medieval optics and Alhazen's theory of vision (1270), it constituted a major conceptual contribution that enabled artists to establish integrated compositions that were isomorphic representations of a segment of nature on a two-dimensional surface. As such, Renaissance perspective was part of the development of a new conception of space as homogeneous, infinite, and isotropic. The operational procedures developed for the construction of perspective in the 15th and 16th century eventually received independent mathematical confirmation, initially in Kepler's postulation in 1604 that parallel lines meet at a position in infinity, and in the mathematical formulations and projective geometry of Gerard Desargues and his student Blaise Pascal developed around 1635.

As discussed earlier, there is considerable debate about whether to consider the art of the Medieval period as a major setback or a necessary transition in the history of art. The Middle Ages were a period of profound social upheaval that involved the temporary relinquishing of naturalism and the partial, intuitive solution for perspective that had been achieved by the Greeks. Some consider this period as a regression in the development of science and art (e.g., Butterfield, 1957), others (e.g., Bunim, 1940; Panofsky, 1960/1972) see Medieval art as a necessary phase in the eventual unification of the intuitive perspective of Antiquity with the principles of mass and surface consolidation of the Middle Ages. Bunim and Panofsky discuss this period as a necessary transition in the development of a more systematic and comprehensive system for representing three-dimensional space on a two-dimensional surface. While it is beyond the scope of this chapter to resolve this debate, Panofsky's (1960/1972) formulations of an undulation in the development of art in the Middle Ages suggest that both interpretations may be partially correct. There was intense ambivalence in the Middle Ages about the representation of the human form. At times the human form was represented as flat and in isolation and at other times as substantial and corporeal. Residuals of Greco-Roman stage space were maintained, yet there was no interest in the representation of perspective. The flattening of the picture plane into a two-dimensional surface and the preference for religious symbols and an "otherworldliness" rather than naturalism facilitated the conveying of the religious concepts of the Medieval period. But the lack of interest in the representation of space and of perspective may have enabled artists of the Middle Ages to develop fuller and more substantial representations of the human form when there was a relaxation of the prohibition against creating graven images. In addition, the flattening of the optical stage space of Antiquity to a vertical, homogeneous surface that had a common unity with the figures facilitated the development of a new conception of space as homogeneous, isotropic, and infinite that was equally applicable to figures as well as to the embedding context.

The various renascences from the 9th to the 14th centuries were important steps in the reestablishment of a continuity with aspects of the form, style, and content of the Classical period and in the integration of the classical form with visual laws that were equally applicable to the representation of figures as well as to the space that contained the figures. The abandonment of the preoperational, intuitive form of perspective during this transitional period may thus have facilitated the eventual discovery of the central vanishing point and the concrete operations and mathematical principles that are the basis for linear perspective. This quest for scientific procedures for accurately representing nature from the perspective of an observer was an integral part of the 15th century philosophical emphasis upon the dignity of man and his capacities to understand nature.

PARALLEL DEVELOPMENT IN PRE-RENAISSANCE ART AND SCIENCE

As in art, a similar progression occurred in the development of modes of representation in Ancient and Medieval science. Ancient scientific conceptions and artistic representations were based on sensorimotor-preoperational modes of representation and were attempts to master natural forces in order to preserve life and to survive. The earliest concepts of space in cosmology and science were initially based on a set of immediate, concrete, accidental, affect-laden experiences rather than objective measures. Very early poetic expressions for universal space, for example, were highly emotional terms filled with fright and terror such as chaos, yawning, or gaping (Jammer, 1954/1969). Ancient cosmologies were based upon the study of astronomical phenomena in relation to the seasons and thus to food and survival. These conceptions, like the objects first depicted in Paleolithic and Egyptian art, reflect the preoccupation and concern with life and death and basic biological survival. Ancient artistic renderings of objects served ritualistic or shamanistic purposes as humans attempted to interact with the forces of nature and the will and personality of the gods. So too, cosmological concepts were initially animistic and later anthropomorphic—as gods sailing the heavenly oceans bearing the sun across the sky, or matter having will—as in Aristotelian doctrine of the natural place of the four basic elements.

One of the first steps toward a development of a cosmology was the Egyptian theories of the sun and moon as being carried systematically across the sea of the heavens by the gods in their boats. This conception marked a move from the animistic conceptions of natural forces and the simple prediction of the appearance of these heavenly bodies—the time and location of the daily rising and setting of the sun and the somewhat less regular change in the size, shape, and location of the moon. The cosmological conceptions of the Egyptians were no longer based upon immediate perception and sensory experience, but on astronomical phenomena, first studied in relation to the seasons, and motivated by curiosity as well as the need to produce food and to anticipate nature in order to survive. The transition from the Egyptian anthropomorphic conception of the planets as systematic wanderers across the heavens to the Greek conception of the universe as a system of orderly nested orbs was an elaboration of an essentially geocentric cosmology based upon the experience and perception of an unmoving earth around which all other celestial bodies revolve. While the rational naturalism of Classic Greece emerged from magical and mythical views, it rejected the animism and anthropomorphism of earlier cosmological conceptions and sought to develop a consistent theory of planetary and stellar movement in terms of observable natural phenomena.

The Aristotelian concept of the universe was schematically a closed, spherical, hierarchically organized system of bounded, concentric, nested orbs at the center of which was the earth—the zone of impermanence, imperfection, decay, and corruption. The earth was contained in successive spherical shells or orbs, each occupied by the moon, planets, the sun, and the fixed stars, in an increasing order of perfection and immutability. The cosmos was built around the earth as the absolute center, enclosed by an outermost absolute shell of the heavens that defined the universe as a fixed, finite sphere containing the entire universe. There was nothing beyond the boundary of the outermost shell and all the planets and stars were in fixed, concentric, crystalline spheres rotating around the earth in the center of the sphere. Space was neither uniform nor homogeneous, it was the separation between the bodies of the universe, each of which had a proper place in reference to each other and to the earth as the center of the universe (Jammer, 1954/1969). Nature for Aristotle was a wholly self-contained, closed system, except for a prime mover: God (Woodbridge, 1965).

For Aristotle, space was not boundless and infinite; but the universe, like everything else, had a "place" defined by the innermost layer of its container. The "place" of a body was the innermost layer of whatever surrounded it, a kind of metaphysical membrane around any object. The sphere of the fixed stars was bounded, as was the outermost shell of the world. The emphasis in Aristotle's concept of place, as in the representation of objects in art, was on the boundary or container and on the demarcations between individual bodies or the differentiation of body and non-body, primarily along a polarized vertical directionality. Just as the earliest artistic representations of objects are concerned with boundaries and outer contour, so Aristotle's concept of place had to do with the outermost surface of a body. Just as artists were at first primarily concerned with representing the boundary of isolated objects with adjacency, instead of with the representation of relative distances between bodies or their relative recession from the observer's position, so Aristotle's place was an attribute inherent to each body, and not a system for locating objects relative to one another or to a containing space. Artistic and scientific representations primarily utilized topological spatial concepts that emphasized the boundary, contour, or surface of objects in isolation.

"Place" for Aristotle also had a more active connotation. The universe was considered to be composed of four elements in various combinations. Earth, air, fire, and water each had a "natural place" toward which they strove. Earth moved spontaneously toward the center of the universe as did water, but not as energetically; fire strove toward the outermost heavens—the celestial sphere—as did air, but less forcefully. Bodies were reducible to the recognizable elements of earth, air, fire, and water, which were stratified in a predominant vertical directionality with earth at the bottom and air or fire at the top. Bottom and top were defined by motion toward or from earth. Each element sought its natural and proper place in relation to the other elements. Bodies could be endowed with souls, objects could have "dispositions" toward certain kinds of movements, and matter itself, like objects represented in art, could possess mystical qualities (Butterfield, 1957). But as discussed by Woodbridge (1965, p. 59), this differentiation of the four elements was based on something "more primitive . . . the oppositions between the wet and the dry, the hot and the cold, . . . the heavy and the light." The binary opposition (Levi-Strauss, 1963) of heavy and light defined polarized vertical directions of up and down relative to the boundaries in which the motion of elements takes place (Woodbridge, 1965).

This Aristotelian view was a sensorimotor-preoperational conception of the universe, a universe driven by spirits. Aristotle's conception of nature was based on giving motion a central position—his "theory of nature is a theory of motion" (Woodbridge, 1965, p. 55). Motion is what bodies do, not what makes them move. Bodies, by moving, make other bodies move; motion is never anything apart from bodies. Motion requires a constant cause—as long as a body is in motion, Aristotle assumed that a force must be acting on that body to produce the motion. Movement occurs because of a disturbance created in a homogeneous medium or substance by the initial movement of an object. This movement pushes and compresses the air in front of the object, which then rushes behind the object to force its movement. In this "antiperistasis" theory, the motion of the body through a resisting medium was seen as proportional to the force producing the motion and inversely proportional to the resistance of the medium. Aristotle argued against the concept of a void because then resistance would be zero and the relationship of force to movement would not exist.

The change from rest to motion involves a mover which itself is in motion so that it can initiate action by direct contact with other bodies. The prime mover of the universe is God, "an unmoved mover" (Woodbridge, 1965, p. 74). For Aristotle "everything that happens on the earth is a consequence of movements that happen in the sky" and what is intelligible in nature is seen as largely dependent upon the sun's going around the earth, making available things for visual examination (Woodbridge, 1965, p. 61). Thus motion in Aristotle's conception of space, was accomplished by a prime mover which, according to Butterfield (1957), is consistent with a concept of the universe in which unseen hands constantly influence the movement of planetary spheres.

Based on sensorimotor-preoperational modes and topological concepts of space, Aristotle was able to account for the gross structure of his geocentric universe—the relative dispositions of earth, planets, and stars, located in successively larger orbs, as well as everyday observations such as rocks (and apples) falling, smoke rising, clay eventually falling to the bottom of a once turbid mixture. Space was not an indifferent and passive container, having no impact on the way bodies behave in it; rather, for Aristotle, space had a polarized vertical directionality, and its qualities existed in relation to the qualities and components of all bodies. There was no independent frame of space, time, and infinity in which events took place. Space and time and the void did not exist independent of bodies; space was "only the fixation of the boundaries of bodies" (Woodbridge, 1965, p. 57). Aristotle conceived of the universe itself as an object, a full and bounded entity, not a void containing matter. This was not a unified concept of space; the world was an entity somehow bounded, contained, and thereby existent in contrast with an undefined chaos or void beyond.

Pre-perspective art lacked unification of objects in the composition and a consistent relationship with the position of the observer; likewise, in pre-Copernican astronomy, each of the orbs was considered independently, and indeed, a unified system would have been impossible for Aristotle's conception of nested crystalline spheres because of the requirements for individual epicycles for each planet. The Aristotelian world view, like the predominant modes of artistic representation, was essentially qualitative and descriptive and lacked a quantitative metric system (Burtt, 1931/1954). As we shall discuss in a consideration of Renaissance art and cosmology at the end of the next chapter, it was only with Kepler, after Copernicus, that there was an attempt to consider quantitative relations among all planets in the solar system in its entirety. And likewise, it was only with the introduction of concepts of linear perspective in the Renaissance that art began to utilize quantitative concepts.

Just as Greek art reveals the rudiments of projective concepts of space, so early Greek atomists held a notion of infinite Euclidean space. Techniques of foreshortening and a rudimentary form of perspective were used in Greek art to create the illusion of depth and the relative size of objects. Likewise, Greek geometers, particularly Euclid, developed mathematical techniques which assumed an infinite three-dimensional space. When applied to the physical world, such assumptions yielded the related atomistic/Platonic tradition which gave space a projective dimension by viewing it as geometric, hence infinite rather than bounded or homogeneous. In cosmology as well as in geometry, a concrete literalness allowed for the development of the beginning forms of projective concepts of space but it did not foster linear perspective. As Van Hoorn points out (1972)

> The basic postulates of Greek geometry are the tactile-muscular ones of congruence and parallelism; i.e., essentially two-dimensional conceptions of space. Mainly for this reason the Greeks had only a vague idea of central projection and thus were not able to grasp the geometrical basis of central perspective. (p. 66; cf. also p. 99)

The atomist tradition never prevailed in the mainstream of Greek philosophical thought. Dominant instead was Aristotle's concept of space with its emphasis on the opposition between body and non-body, inseparable from its emphasis on place as the containing layer with which each body is surrounded.

In Greek art each separate body, each separate object, is seen as a thing in its own private space without an expression of emotional or psychological relationships (Ivins, 1946). Space in Greek art separates objects rather than serving as an all-containing entity. It is a "negative" definition of space; it is what happens between solids (Gardner, 1975, p. 211). Likewise, Greek geometry, beginning about 500 B.C., was concerned with the measured segments of lines, angles, areas, and volumes rather than with the relations between measurement, spatial organization, and movement (Ivins, 1946). Thus, in many ways there is a correspondence of ancient Greek theoretical, mathematical, and aesthetic representations of space.

The Platonic and Atomists' view of space as an infinite void remained at most an underground intellectual current in Europe even until the late Middle Ages. Studies of perspective—a mathematical treatment of bodies in space, especially, in optics, in relation to the visual cone—were revived in the late Medieval period as the Euclidean heritage was reclaimed via Islam (Lindberg, 1978). But mathematics was not applied to natural philosophy until the Renaissance. Even then the increasing use of mathematics had little consequence in science until Copernicus, and its full effect occurred only with Descartes and Newton.

Throughout the 13th and 14th centuries there was increasing debate about a number of Aristotle's assumptions. Eventually, the question was raised about what constituted the ultimate boundary of the universe and Medieval debates on this philosophical dilemma dissipated only with the development of a new concept of space—not as a place that defines an entity's location, but as "space" that has no "place" or location since it is itself all locations. Philosophers and scientists began to think of bodies of the universe as *in* space, rather than conceive of the universe itself as a bounded object. These challenges to Aristotelian doctrine in the 13th and 14th centuries marked the first stages of the scientific revolution that was to begin in the Renaissance (Butterfield, 1957).

In both art and science during the Middle Ages there was a relinquishing of interest in the embedding context of objects. The rudimentary form of projective concepts of space that had been achieved by the Greeks was relinquished in the art of the Middle Ages for the flat surface of the picture plane. Bunim (1940) and Panofsky (1924/25) argue that this change should not be viewed as a regression, but as an essential step in the development of linear perspective and the more extensive Euclidean-Cartesian concept of space. While issues of mathematical perspective were of interest in Greek and

Medieval studies of optics, this did not lead to the development of a concept of infinite space. Likewise, in cosmology, the Middle Ages was a period of consolidation, elaboration, and eventual relinquishing of Aristotelian philosophy, concepts, and method (Grant, 1978).

The level of artistic representation and scientific and cosmological conceptions of space during the Ancient pre-Greek period dealt with objects in essential isolation. The basic mathematical structure for these conceptions was a nominal classification or scale in which mutually exclusive objects were designated to discrete groups or categories without qualitative or quantitative order. The relation among objects was reflexive, transitive, and symmetrical. During the Greco-Roman and Medieval periods, the concepts of space in art and science were also based on objects considered in relative isolation without a unified conception of space, but objects were now placed in comparison and contrast to one another. The basic structure of measurement became increasingly complex and based on an ordinal scale in which objects were considered in relation one to the other in a comparative, qualitative order. Objects were closer or further away, larger or smaller, but there was still no unified, quantitative system of measurement. There was only a qualitative, comparative, monotonic order in which the relation between objects is irreflexive and asymmetrical, and based on transitive ordering. A unified, quantified system of measurement with equal intervals—an interval rather than an ordinal scale (Stevens, 1951)—appeared as the basis for artistic representation and scientific conception only in the mid- to late Renaissance.

4
The Discovery and Development of Linear Perspective: The Renaissance, Mannerism, and the Baroque

THE RENAISSANCE

Beginning in 15th century Florence a revolutionary change in art occurred with the discovery of linear perspective. The Renaissance was the dawn of a new era in the representation of space that would maintain preeminence for at least the next 500 years. Panofsky (1924/25), based partly on concepts from Cassirer (1910/1923) and Riegl (1901/1927), contrasted the "aggregate" concepts of space of Antiquity with the "mathematical" and systematic concepts of the Renaissance. The basic emphasis in Antiquity was on the substance and definition of objects in isolation; the emphasis in the Renaissance was on the relations among objects in space. Space for the ancients had been finite, nonhomogeneous, and discontinuous whereas in the Renaissance, space was infinite, homogeneous, and isotropic. These emerging fundamental differences in world view resulted in a profound and fundamental change in the modes of representation in art (Edgerton, 1975; Veltman, 1979a).

The ability to represent a setting realistically and to arrange figures in a balanced and harmonious order within that setting was a major change in artistic style. This change coincided with important parallel developments in science, philosophy, and social order. The reemergence of the Greek self-confidence in humanity created a new sense of the individual's place in the universe, and an increased belief that people had control over their destinies (Burckhardt, 1860/1950). The development of perspective in the Renaissance was an integral part of this new conception of man (Hartt, 1964). The Renaissance brought a renewed insistence on human values, an acceptance of human limitations that gave individuals both responsibility and dignity (Panofsky, 1955b).

> So far was the Greek from thinking that Man was a mere nothing in the sight of the gods that he had always to be reminding himself that Man is not God, and that it is impious to think it. Never again, until the Greek spirit intoxicated Italy at the Renaissance, do we find such superb self-confidence in humanity—a self-confidence which, in Renaissance Italy, was not restrained by the modesty imposed on the Greek by his instinctive religious outlook. (Kitto, 1951, p. 61)

As early as the 11th century, city states and an urban culture began to develop with the increasing breakdown of feudal systems and their transfer of power by divine inheritance. Cities were ruled by merchants and bankers; power was determined by talent and ambition. The 13th and 14th centuries were also a time of turning away from a preoccupation with the supernatural and the life hereafter to an interest in the natural world and the activities of man. Medieval religious dogmas were replaced by a worldy humanism and an interest in God's creation of natural beauty and order. Scientific inquiry burgeoned as individuals studied nature with an emphasis on the importance of personal experience in knowing natural beauty and God's order of the universe. Medieval logic and Aristotelian natural philosophy and metaphysics were replaced by interests in practical, artistic, and religious matters. The Medieval preoccupation with the salvation of the soul was replaced by a secular concern for relations among people. The Renaissance stressed the importance of individuals, especially those of talent and merit. People were no longer viewed as helpless and acting only as agents of God's will, but individuals were now real and substantial, with responsibility for their actions. God was now seen as giving individuals permission to make of themselves what they would with this new found potential (Alberti, 1435/1956). People began to experiment, invent, explore, and make remarkable contributions to science and art. The increased respect for individual talent and ambition maintained continuity with the individualism of classical Antiquity and its emphasis on the need to establish a life of reason, intelligence, and nobility. Renaissance humanism "was a great stimulus to individualism" (Artz, 1966, p. 89); it stressed human capacities and dignity as well as the study of classical authors, history and moral philosophy, and the ideal of literary elegance in spoken and written prose and verse (Cassirer, Kristeller & Randall, 1948).

In Medieval philosophy, man was considered insignificant in contrast to the divine scheme and power of God. Man was viewed as fallen and had to struggle to overcome his nature to find salvation. This harsh, critical judgmental aspect of the Church was supplemented in the Renaissance, by the image of the accepting maternal Virgin. Major steps in the development of linear perspective, for example, often occurred in paintings of the Annunciation (e.g., Giotto, T. Gaddi, D. Veneziano, Lippi, Piero della Francesca) (Veltman, 1979b). People began to feel more comfortable in their relationships with God. "Mediaeval architecture preaches Christian humility; classical and Renaissance architecture proclaims the dignity of man" (Panofsky, 1960/1972, p. 29). Throughout early Renaissance literature, a frequent theme was the glorification of man (Kristeller and Randall, 1948). This change in religious philosophy and doctrine encouraged exploration and experimentation.

The implications of the creative realism (Auerbach, 1953) that the Church had introduced was gradually realized. A respect for humanity and the role of the individual and an idealization of nature began to pervade the entire intellectual and cultural climate. Numerous examples of this emerging self-awareness and confidence appeared in the Renaissance, including books in the mid to late 15th century by Ficino (1476), Pico della Mirandola (1486) and Gianozzo Manetti (1452) about the dignity and excellence of man. Clark (1969) considers the Renaissance to have begun with Brunelleschi's Pazzi Chapel because it marked a change from the immense Gothic structures to a small, light, airy chapel adjusted to the size of the individual. Clark (p. 94) views this change as yet another "assertion of the dignity of man." And in painting, for the first time in a millennium, individual works of art were consistently signed by the artist and there was interest in the lives of artists (Kris, 1952; Kris & Kurz, 1934/1979).

A humanistic conception had played a major role in the development of perspective in Antiquity; the position of the observer was central to the Greek's intuitive expression of perspective. Now, a thousand years later in the Italian Renaissance, a conception of the dignity of man was expressed once again in a renewed interest in portraying nature as viewed by an individual from a particular point in space. The development of linear perspective brought individuals back into art and gave them a role in the representation of nature. In both Greco-Roman intuitive perspective and Renaissance scientific-mathematical linear perspective (a "rational sense" of space; Panofsky, 1924/25), the subjective point of view is paramount. The development of perspective occurred in both epochs when there was a basic philosophical admiration and respect for the individual. But the role of the individual spectator was much more limited in the art of Antiquity than it was in the Renaissance.

The relationship of humanism to naturalistic representation has been discussed extensively (Kleinbauer, 1971). Worringer (1907/ 1953), for example, noted a distinction between "abstract geometrical" styles that occur primarily in societies oppressed by nature and involved with spirituality, and "organic" styles in societies that have an affinity for finding satisfaction in nature. Seltman (1953, p. 98; cited by Kleinbauer, 1971) also discussed this distinction:

> In those ages when men have subjected their minds and souls to Authority and have allowed others to tell them what to think, unrealistic or abstract art has been the rule. But when there has existed a high degree of liberty of thought—whence comes Humanism—then corporeal art has prevailed.

A free society enables individuals to establish and maintain their own perspective.

Greco-Roman perspective was primarily based upon a theory of vision, on postulates of Euclid's *Optics*. The object's size was not defined in terms of its position relative to other objects or to the observer, but rather only in terms of the visual angle the object subtended at the eye of the observer. This resulted in an intuitive, somewhat imprecise and inconsistent representation of perspective. This "angle perspectival" method had to be relinquished in order to discover the fundamental inverse relationship of size and distance that was an essential tenet of linear perspective (Bunim, 1940; Panofsky, 1960/1972). The conception of a definite proportion between the distance of objects in space and their size in the cross-section of a visual pyramid was initially suggested early in the 15th century by Brunelleschi and Alberti, and more fully explored and elaborated by

Piero della Francesca and Leonardo da Vinci toward the end of that century (Wittkower, 1953). The development of linear perspective in the Renaissance was also a consequence of an interest in "a mathematical theory of artistic representation" (Panofsky, 1940/1971, p. 97) in which the laws of geometry were used to establish a precise, isomorphic correspondence between a representation and the natural world such that there could be full reversibility between the construction and the actual experience of nature. The discovery of the principles of linear perspective was an integral part of an emerging new conception of space as infinite, homogeneous, and isotropic (Jammer, 1954/1969; Panofsky, 1924/25).

This remarkable change in art was only one aspect of the reawakening in the Renaissance. Similar changes were taking place in other disciplines including mathematics, science, natural history, and literature. There was, for example, an increasing sense of the pervasive importance of time (Quinones, 1972)—and a heightened awareness of time's destructive power. People became more interested in extending their presence through time by achieving immortality by progeny and fame. One of the major transformations from the Middle Ages to the Renaissance was the change from the religious use of time up until the 14th century to a more secular use of time in the Renaissance. Quinones (1972) considers this change an inherent part of the vitality and diversity of any renascence and an affirmation of the differentiation between the Middle Ages and the Renaissance. Italy was at the forefront of much of the development of the Renaissance until the 16th century, when it "seemed to lose that position when humanism itself was superseded" (Quinones, 1972, p. 500).

The art of the Renaissance, partly based on the Romanesque and Gothic proto-renaissance in Italy and France and the Carolingian and Ottonian renascences 500 to 600 years earlier (Artz, 1959, 1966; Haskins, 1927), was an extension of innovations in art begun by Cavallini, Cimabue, Giotto, and Duccio in the late 13th and early 14th centuries. They had achieved a synthesis of the northern Gothic feeling for space, expressed in architecture and particularly sculpture, with the fragmentary architecutral and landscape forms preserved in Byzantine paintings. Giotto and Duccio began to paint closed interiors that were pictorial projections of the northern Gothic "stage space." It was the Gothic sense of space that brought together the scattered elements into a unity. Giotto's and Duccio's representations of a closed interior as a distinctly defined containing space gave a sense of solidity to objects and led to the mode of spatial representation achieved in the Renaissance (Panofsky, 1924/25).

The remarkable reawakened interest in the representation of space in the art of the Renaissance was a function of the movement to revive classical Antiquity and to gain an appreciation of nature. These two forces were expressed by different artists early in the Renaissance. Panofsky (1960/1972) notes that Giotto was praised as a naturalist while Donatello was lauded for his revival of Antiquity. Vasari (1550/ 1965, p. 124) commented on the rediscovery of the measurement and proportions of Antiquity in the architecture of Brunelleschi and the sculpture of Donatello, as well as on how Masaccio "gave a beginning to beautiful attitudes, movements, liveliness, and vivacity . . . in a way that was characteristic and natural".

Vasari described the Renaissance return to classical Antiquity as consisting of three phases. In the first phase during the 14th century, artists, such as Giotto, became aware of the basic principles of rule, order, measure, design, and manner, and made some progress in lifelikeness, color, and composition. There were also major advances in the second phase, but Vasari felt these artists failed to attain the integration of precision, grace, and freedom that captured the perfection of classical standards. This second phase lasted until the second half of the 15th century and included artists such as Piero della Francesca, Castagno, Verrocchio, Perugino, Botticelli, Mantegna, Uccello, and Signorelli. Artists of the third phase finally achieved the grace and perfection of classical Antiquity. Leonardo da Vinci mastered the integration of order, measure, design, and gracefulness that gave life and vitality to classical forms. Giorgione, Raphael, and Correggio made important contributions to this third phase, which reached its apex in the early 16th century work of Michelangelo. Panofsky (1960/1972) describes the development of Renaissance art in a similar way. He considers that the first radical break with Medieval principles of representation occurred with Cimabue and Giotto at the very end of the 13th century. The second phase, at the beginning of the 15th century, was an intense involvement with classical Antiquity, primarily beginning with architecture and sculpture, rather than painting. In the climactic third phase, beginning at the start of the 16th century, architecture, sculpture, and painting expressed a synthesis of the naturalistic and classical points of view.

At the end of the 13th century, two major artists, Cavallini and Cimabue, attempted to represent three-dimensional structures.

Cavallini indicated depth by having the receding lines of a ceiling converge in parallel pairs and by a convergence of parallel lines from upper and lower parts of the picture plane. This representation of depth had been seen earlier in the Middle Ages. What was significant about Cavallini's work, however, was his treatment of the entire structure as a unified three-dimensional object. He attempted to transform the background into an interior that could enclose figures (Bunim, 1940). Cavallini's, Cimabue's, Duccio's, and Giotto's interests in three-dimensional structures provided the basis for the transition from Medieval concepts of space to the eventual mathematical systematization of linear perspective in the 15th century. These four artists attempted to integrate the implicit three-dimensional stage space of Byzantine art with Gothic naturalism and to coordinate figure and background. They represented figures with mass and volume and in communication with each other. Objects were coordinated with their environment in a unified composition.

Duccio and Giotto transformed the background from a facade to a three-dimensional interior structure that enclosed figures. The planes defined by the floor, walls, and ceiling of a one-room interior space made the need for coordination more apparent than when figures were placed in exterior space. As illustrated by Fig. 34, Duccio attempted to coordinate the different parts of interior space according to an intuitive, uniform perspective plan. Lines in depth were organized to a limited, general vanishing area, but there still was no single vanishing point, no geometric system, and objects were not drawn from a single point of view. Despite these spatial inconsistencies, rudiments of systematic perspective were expressed within a unified enclosing space. The primary sense of depth was in the boxed interior, but each plane tended to have its own convergence point. While there was no unified perspective, there was a convincing illusion of depth. Although Duccio was the great master of the Byzantine style (Berenson, 1956), he began to replace abstract Byzantine symbols with figures who had unique postures, gestures, and facial expressions. Duccio portrayed figures as reacting to a major, central event and as participating in a religious drama with human reactions and emotions. He began to secularize and humanize religious subject matter.

Giotto created three-dimensional space primarily within figures that were monumental—solid, full, and substantial. He used foreshortening, figures in communication, and often a back-view that demanded the viewer to extend and complete the form of the figure.

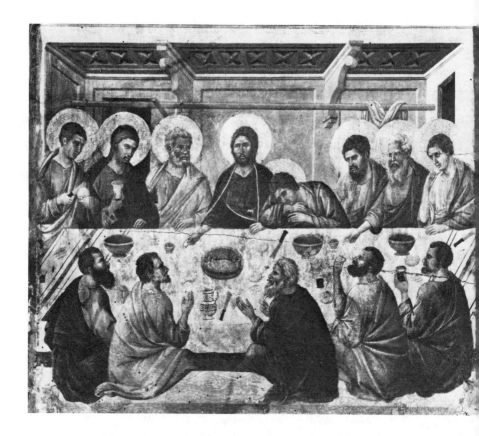

FIG. 34   Duccio, *Last Supper* (c. 1310), Opera del Duomo, Siena (Alinari).

Perspective in the stage space was rudimentary and inconsistent, but it was sufficient to contain the figures. Giotto required the observer to stand on the same ground level as the figures in the painting and thereby emphasized the spatial relationship between the observer and the painting. He not only brought the observer into the experience of the picture space, but he made the foreground figures large, simple, and tangible. Giotto's work had a sense of depth, but objects were not fully organized from a single viewpoint. Different sides and perspectives of architectural structures were presented simultaneously. But a general relationship was established between distance and the relative size of objects.

Giotto, following Cimabue, sought to replace Byzantine style with naturalism. He tried to observe nature and to appreciate its order. He represented figures with solidity, substance, and dimensionality, and was able to create the illusion of solid bodies moving through a space that contained them (see Fig. 35). His figures were simple, direct, and they participated in a human drama. As Artz (1959) notes, Giotto's goal was not to create a medieval contemplative picture that was removed from the natural world into an otherworldliness, but to create the sense that the viewer was actually observing a sacred scene.

Duccio and Giotto were among the first to create a "picture space" since the loss of interest in perspective centuries earlier. Duccio used powerful lines and surfaces to give his figures vitality. Giotto created a sense of volume as an inherent quality of objects. His figures were unique individuals reacting to one another. He presented buildings obliquely so they would take up more space in depth. Both Duccio and Giotto extended the two-dimensional painting surface. They made the painting surface a window, through which one could ob-

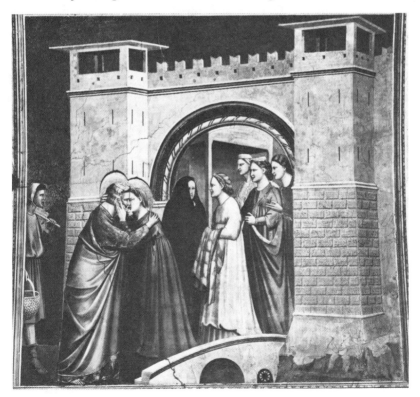

FIG. 35   Giotto, *Meeting of Joachim and Anna* (c. 1305) Arena Chapel, Padua (Alinari).

serve a segment of reality, rather than an opaque, impervious working surface. Objects were no longer simply placed on a panel or a wall, but rather the picture plane became a surface through which one looked into space, even though it was bounded on every side. Objects were defined as separate from the containing space and as substantial in their own right. The freedom of the object from its confining space allowed space to be defined in new ways and allowed the object to be appreciated as something solid and substantial. The architectural settings of Duccio and Giotto emanated a sense of coherence and solidity. Their interiors were extended in depth beyond the pictorial surface, and a definite amount of volume was allocated to every solid and every void. The use of space—though limited in extent and inaccurate in construction—had the potential for becoming homogeneous, continuous, and infinite. In Duccio and Giotto, space was enlarged from a flat surface to a transparent screen or a picture plane, to a defining space that allowed objects in the space to be unique and real. But the organization of space was still inconsistent. Some sections of the paintings converged to a common vanishing point, whereas other adjacent parts diverged sharply away from the vanishing point. While Giotto and Duccio presented the possibilities for the unification of the entire picture plane, they did not achieve the full integration that was to become possible with the development of linear perspective. But the early Renaissance paintings of Cavallini, Cimabue, Duccio, and Giotto introduced and extended the three-dimensional concepts that had been preserved in the vestiges of stage space in Byzantine art. These four artists were the primary figures marking the turn from Medieval to Renaissance art and thus are considered the "fathers of modern painting" (Panofsky, 1960/1972, p. 120).

The next generation of artists in the 14th century began to recognize the need to systematize Duccio's and Giotto's intuitive expression of perspective. They approached the problem of perspective in several different ways. Taddeo Gaddi, a student of Giotto, and Simone Martini and the Lorenzetti brothers, students of Duccio, continued to explore the representation of three-dimensional space. T. Gaddi and Martini presented large, substantial figures and attempted to express depth by the non-frontal, oblique presentation of architectural settings (see Fig. 36, 37). Ambrogio and Pietro Lorenzetti developed the checkered pavement as a ground plan to enhance the three-dimensional appearance. It gave the impression that space could be

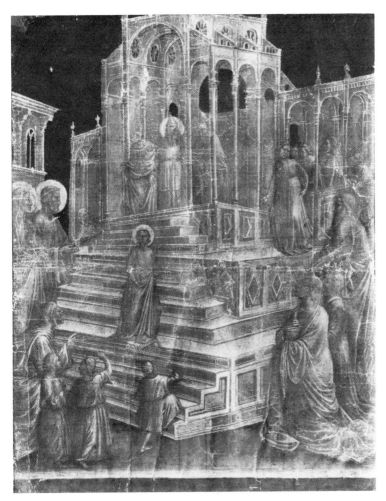

FIG. 36 T. Gaddi, *Presentation of the Virgin* (1332–38) Louvre, Paris (Giraudon).

measured with the ground square as the basic metric. The Lorenzetti brothers, however, did not use measurement but achieved a unified composition more intuitively. Portions of a floor were represented with great accuracy and orthogonals converged to a single vanishing point that created a convincing extension deep into space. The checkered floor plan, however, and later, the use of the coffered ceiling, provided the basis for systematically measuring the interval between objects (Bunim, 1940; Panofsky, 1924/25). The work *Presentation in the Temple* by the Lorenzetti brothers in 1342 (Fig. 38), had for the

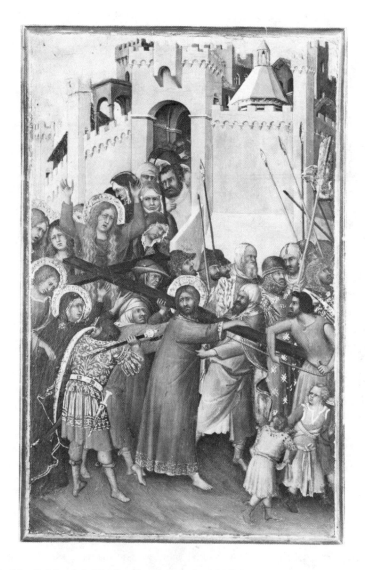

FIG. 37   S. Martini, *The Road to Calvary* (c. 1340) Louvre, Paris. (Giraudon).

first time, visible orthogonal lines of a ground plan directed toward a
single vanishing point that served to define the size and distance
between objects. The entire painting was not organized around one-
point perspective, yet it played a decisive role in the subsequent development of perspective.

The ability to create the illusion of depth on a two-dimensional surface had been achieved intuitively as early as the 5th century B.C. Numerous Greco-Roman works contain examples of foreshortening and the creation of an apparent three-dimensional expanse. Through the use of a vanishing vertical axis, Greco-Roman artists were able to create the convergence of parallel lines. Distant objects diminished in size and were blurred to give the illusion of depth. But, generally,

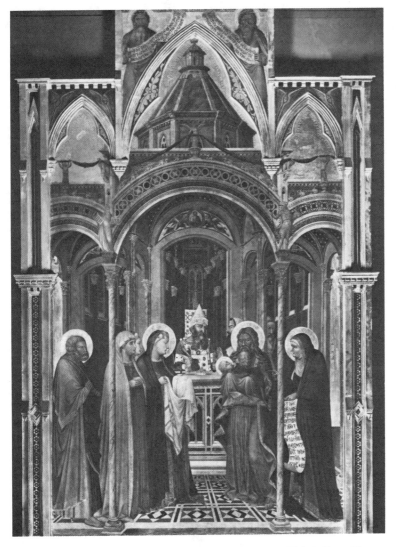

FIG. 38   Lorenzetti, *Presentation in the Temple* (1342), Uffizi Gallery, Florence (Alinari).

space in Greco-Roman paintings was a finite aggregate of solids and voids, rather than a homogeneous system. Greco-Roman art intuitively ("optically") expressed depth by convergence, diminution, and atmospheric vagueness. But the composition was not unified and attention was given primarily to the visual appearance of isolated objects or groups of objects. Greco-Roman perspective lacked a comprehensive mathematical procedure for the construction of the picture plane in which there was a systematic diminution in size directly proportional to the distance of the object from the fixed point of a spectator. Space was not organized systematically around the fixed point of a spectator; instead, space was an undefined medium between objects. Greco-Roman art utilized a generalized and unmeasured representation of space. Perspective was inconsistent and achieved only intuitively and through visual adjustment. Greek artists represented nature as they saw it in a careful observation of the world, but not through a reasoned theory of composition.

In Renaissance perspective, the size and shape of figures and objects were defined consistently by a measurable relationship to a single fixed point. Every point in space was determined by three perpendicular coordinates that extended infinitely from a single point of origin. A unified composition and perspective provided a constant structure for determining the relative location and size of all elements. Panofsky (1960/1972) describes Greco-Roman perspective as "aggregate-space" and Renaissance perspective as "systematized space." The vanishing axis with multiple vanishing points, the Greco-Roman method of perspective, was replaced in the Renaissance by the use of the single, central vanishing point that organized the entire composition.

Renaissance artists sought methods that would enable them to represent nature directly and accurately. At first it was possible to achieve a convincing illusion of perspective by copying the contours of objects on a glass plate or a mirror and then tracing them onto a panel (Edgerton, 1975). Artists also used grids of small squares that divided the picture into small units, and aspects of a scene could be entered in the sections. But these practical procedures were insufficient as Renaissance theorists sought precise rules to represent depth on a planar surface. The discovery of the scientific, geometric principles for representing perspective enabled artists to translate natural phenomena into lines and surfaces to achieve a "representational correctness" (Panofsky, 1940/1971, p. 91).

Sometime between 1401 and 1425 (Edgerton, 1975; Gioseffi, 1965, 1966), Filippo Brunelleschi developed a procedure that, according to Edgerton (1975, p. 3), "marked an event which ultimately was to change the modes, if not the course, of Western History." Brunelleschi, in preparing two panels (one of the Florentine Baptistry in the Piazza del Duomo and the other of the Palazzo Vecchio in the Piazza Signori) utilized the reflections of a mirror and a peephole procedure as an effective method to create a remarkable illusion of depth (Edgerton, 1975). These methods enabled Brunelleschi to create the first paintings that correctly utilized the principles of linear perspective. Unfortunately, these panels have been lost, but around 1480 Antonio Manetti, Brunelleschi's biographer, described the compositional features of these panels in considerable detail. It is clear that Brunelleschi used these panels to demonstrate his theories for an integrated system of perspective in which there is a mathematically defined, regular diminution of the size of objects as they proceed toward a fixed vanishing point. The Brunelleschi panels heralded the invention of a precise system for perspective that was a culmination of an attempt to define the relationship between the observer and the depiction of nature that had been developing since the beginning of the 14th century (White, 1967).

Masaccio, in frescoes completed around 1425, gave monumental expression to Brunelleschi's concepts of perspective. Several frescoes in the Brancacci Chapel of St. Maria del Carmine and the monumental fresco, *The Holy Trinity with the Virgin and St. John* in St. Maria Novella in Florence, are among the earliest existent paintings with a central vanishing point that creates a unified and systematic conception of space. The frescoes in the Brancacci Chapel are based on a central vanishing point and as a series they create a context that emphasizes the importance of the position of the observer in the experience of linear perspective. Masaccio's monumental fresco *The Holy Trinity* (1425) (Fig. 39a) is the earliest existent work utilizing linear perspective. Architecture and perspective play a dominant role in this fresco. There is a massive barrelled vault with Ionic and Corinthian columns. "The foreshortening of the architecture, in accordance with the principles of artificial perspective, is accurate both in the diminution of the coffering and in the single vanishing point which lies slightly below the plane on which the donors kneel" (White, 1967, p. 139). What is particularly impressive in Masaccio's *Trinity* is the representation of space in the vaulted ceiling. Masaccio created a full sense of receding space in which the various elements of the context and the figures are in proper proportion to each other. The ceiling provided the units of measurement for a coherent organization of space—it is as if space had suddenly become, to use Panofsky's term, "rational." As indicated in a perspective reconstruction (Fig. 39b), Masaccio's *Trinity* at St. Maria Novella in Florence utilized the basic

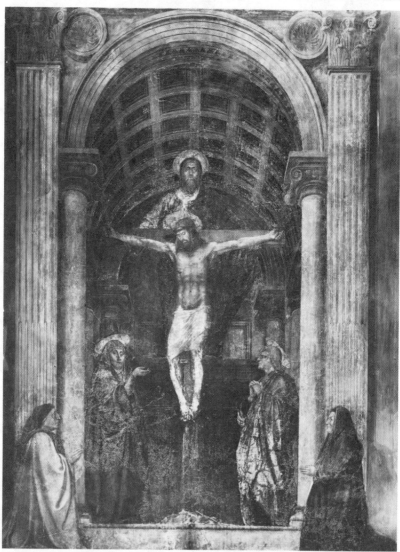

FIG. 39a   Masaccio, *The Holy Trinity* (c. 1425) Santa Maria Novella, Florence (Alinari).

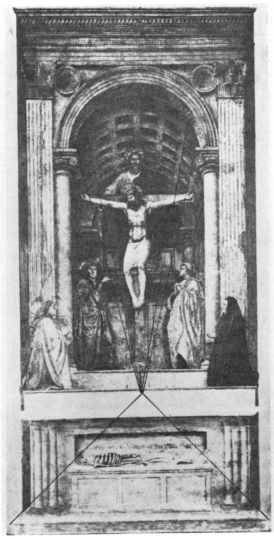

FIG. 39b *Perspective reconstruction:* Masaccio, *The Holy Trinity,* Uffizi Gallery, Florence (Alinari).

laws of perspective. It expressed this revolutionary concept in its organization of space and its representation of a majestic architectural structure as well as massive and tangible figures. The entire composition is encircled by a majestic barrel vault. The viewpoint of the observer is from below so that the vault is portrayed in all its grandeur.

The first codification of the mathematical principles of linear perspective appeared in the treatise of Leon Battista Alberti written in 1435 entitled *Della Pittura*. Perspective in its fullest sense means a transformation of the entire picture so that the surface of the painting becomes a cross-sectional plane on which the whole of space beyond the picture plane is projected, and this space encloses and contains all the separate elements (Panofsky, 1924/25). The discovery of linear perspective in the Renaissance involved the construction of a pyramid of sight in which the picture became a plane section, a window, through which we look out into a section of the visual world (Alberti, 1435). Figure 40, a diagram by Vignola (1611, from Gadol, 1969, p. 27) illustrates the optical theory of "visual rays" and the "pyramid of sight" that Alberti was to develop into a theory of perspective in *Della Pittura*.

The geometric construction of the visual pyramid depends upon the development of a ground plan that coordinates width and height. Alberti defined the picture plane as a cross section of a visual pyramid or cone with its apex in the eye of the spectator and its base in the object. The pyramid's base defines the picture's perimeter. The picture is the intersecting plane on which is projected everything within the visual pyramid extending to infinity. The representation of this cross-sectional plane requires the construction of an elevation and a ground plan. Elevation is expressed on a vertical diagram and the ground plan is expressed on a horizontal one. In each diagram the visual pyramid is represented by triangles with a common apex at the eye of the observer. The intersection of the picture plane with the visual pyramid is represented by a vertical plane. The points of intersection of the connecting lines and the vertical plane determine the vertical and transverse values of the perspective image. All orthogonal lines (lines in depth) meet in a "sight point," parallels go to a common, infinite, vanishing point that, on the horizontal plane, is the horizon. Recession into the picture plane is established in a fixed ratio, creating a fully rational, infinite, homogeneous space. Points in that space are the determinants that define the position of objects in relationship to one another. The homogeneity of geometric space is based on the reciprocal, isotropic relationships between every point in space so that constructions can be made in any direction and to any distance. There is an equivalence in the three basic dimensions of space: front–behind, above–below, and right–left (Panofsky, 1924/25). When the painting is viewed from the apex of the triangle, from

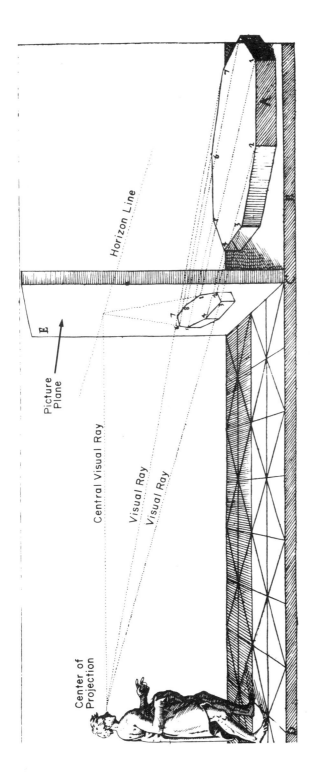

FIG. 40 Perspective projection with picture plane between the center of projection and the object. Illustration from G. B. Vignola, *Le due regole della prospectiva practica*, Rome, 1611. (From Gadol, J. 1969, p. 27).

215

the point of projection, the painting looks compellingly three-dimensional.[18]

Alberti's recognition of the importance of the spectator in defining the procedures for the representation of nature is yet another expression of Renaissance humanism. Alberti stressed that appearances are relative and that the individual has a unique role as the observer of nature. Alberti even proposed that the human figure be used as the basic metric in art. He sought to develop a procedure for the representation of nature that is organized in harmony with God's law and master plan for the universe. The fascination with perspective in the Renaissance, according to Pirenne (1952, p. 185; 1970), was "the fascination of truth." Alberti created an independent sense of space. Space was no longer defined as an extension of objects, but as containing objects arranged according to the rules of space. An earlier intuitive, quantitative concept of foreshortening and depth as a successive reduction of distances by a third was replaced by a more precise concept of diminution of size in direct proportion to the intervening distance between points in space. Qualitative conceptions of space as an aggregate of separate places and objects were replaced by quantitative concepts in which intervals of receding spatial depth diminish in systematic proportion to the fixed location of the spectator. Foreshortening was no longer defined around individual objects but was now in exact proportion to the distance from the observer. All distances became measurable in infinite, mathematically defined, homogeneous space. Orthogonal lines converge to a single vanishing point defined in reference to the eye of the observer. What Brunelleschi had achieved in practice, Alberti articulated as conceptual, mathematical principles. Alberti developed a three-dimensional coordinate system that defined the relative size, shape, and magnitude of all objects in space.[19]

---

[18] Excellent and extensive discussions of the development of the techniques of linear perspective are available in a number of sources, including Edgerton (1975), Gadol (1969), Gioseffi (1966), Gombrich (1960), Ivins (1938), Pirenne (1970), and White (1967).

[19] This new quantitative, operational mode of representation of the Renaissance is also well illustrated in the development of cartography. Medieval maps, navigational charts, and city plans depict isolated, heterogeneous places without a unified, integrated, representational scheme and without scalar quantitative dimensions. Medieval cartography depicted important, individual objects in isolation, or in a qualitative spatial comparison of the location of a pair of objects (closer or further). According to Gadol (1969),

Later statements about perspective included Ghiberti's *Third Commentary* and *De Perspectiva Pingendi* by Piero della Francesca. These works stressed the continuity between Medieval optical theory and the new representational system developed by Alberti. But the discoveries of Brunelleschi and Alberti were truly revolutionary for they provided the geometric basis for constructing space and placing figures in a consistent and precisely defined way such that there is a complete integration of space and the objects within it.

An excellent early example of the spatial harmony achieved through perspective is the Ghiberti doors, *The Gates of Paradise,* of the Baptistry in Florence—particularly the *Jacob and Esau Panel* (Fig. 41a). As indicated by Krautheimer's reconstruction of perspective in this panel (Fig. 41b), the single building in the background serves as the central vanishing point to which all lines recede, the picture base is divided in several equal sections, the height of the figures is in proportion of 3:1 in relation to these sections, the tile floor provides a

---

maps did not have planimetric views or geometrically inspired plans before the mid-15th century. No attempt was made to develop quantitative methods in which the map or chart was a scaled picture representing actual measurements and relationships. Well into the 15th century, survey diagrams of land plots, for example, often contained precise notations about numerical details, but were never drawn to scale. Maps without measure or any type of quantitative scaling persisted until the 1470s. Leon Battista Alberti, whose treatise, *Della Pittura* (1435), was the first codification of the basic principles of linear perspective, was among the first to develop methods for representing relative distances among points in a map based on a quantitative scale (Gadol, 1969). But only in the late 15th and early 16th centuries were methods developed for a true geometric representation of actual spatial geographic arrangement. The development of cartography, like the development of linear perspective, involved the introduction of a scientific, quantitative, mathematical, operational representational mode. Classical and Medieval principles of cartography were transformed by the Renaissance quest for mathematical modes of representation. "The conquest of the principle of proportional mapping in the quattrocento made possible a transformation in science as well as a transformation in art" (Gadol, 1969, p. 157). The simultaneous development of cartography and linear perspective in art was an integral part of an emerging conception of space as continuous, homogeneous, and infinite. Preoperational, intuitive modes of representation in art and science were increasingly replaced by operational modes of representation. Qualitative, comparative, ordinal organization of relative placements were replaced by coordinated, quantitative representations based on interval scaling (Stevens, 1951).

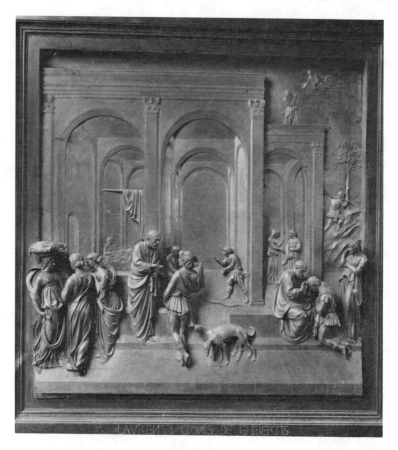

FIG. 41a   Ghiberti, *Gates of Paradise, Jacob & Esau Panel* (c.1435) Baptistry
doors, Florence (Alinari).

coordinate system for the placement of each object, and the architectural setting supplies an enclosing space that creates a sense of rational space, measurable in depth and height (Krautheimer &
Krautheimer-Hess, 1970). Ghiberti, in these doors, was able to create
an almost endless vista behind the foreground figures, but at other
times, such as in the buildings of the *Solomon* and *Sheba* panel of the
Baptistry doors, Ghiberti failed to achieve full perspective.

    At about the time of the contributions of Brunelleschi, Masaccio,
Ghiberti, Donatello, and Alberti, perspective was being introduced in
the north by the Flemish artist, Jan Van Eyck. Flemish artists such as
Van Eyck and van der Weyden achieved a sense of perspective intuitively, based on artistic practice and experimentation, but did not

develop geometric rules for the precise expression of linear perspective. Thus, there was often a disproportion between objects in the foreground and those in the distance. As indicated in Fig. 42, these Flemish artists, however, paid great attention to detail and even objects at a great distance were as sharply defined, distinct, and vivid as those in the foreground. A uniform clarity and sharpness were present throughout the picture. With the development of oil paint, these artists were able to vary the degree of reflectivity of surfaces giving objects and figures great volume and mass. Oil paint enabled Van Eyck and others to alternate opaque and translucent layers of light to create refraction, reflection, and diffusion that emphasized the surface texture and the form of objects. Objects stood out in space as solid and round, having volume and depth. These 15th century Flemish artists also developed the use of atmospheric perspective in which

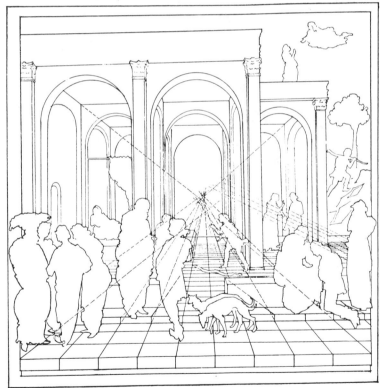

FIG. 41b   Perspective Construction of Ghiberti's *Gates of Paradise, Jacob & Esau Panel* (*Ghiberti*, Richard Krautheimer, Princeton University Press, Princeton, N.J. 1970, Diagram 7, p. 250).

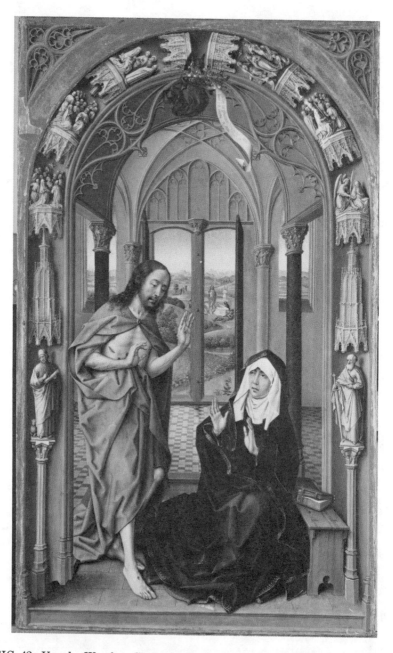

FIG. 42   Van der Weyden, *Christ Appearing to His Mother* (15th century) (The Metropolitan Museum of Art, Bequest of Michael Dreicer, 1921).

the haze of the atmosphere at a distance contributed to the representation of deep space in impressive vistas and landscapes. But the Flemish constructed perspective only intuitively. While some orthogonal lines converged, the entire composition did not converge to a single vanishing point (Panofsky, 1953). Linear perspective did not appear in Flemish art until the mid or late portion of the 15th century (e.g., Dirk Bouts, 1440); even when it did occur it was not used with consistency (Gadol, 1969). Perspective was introduced in France by Jean Viator (Pélerin) in 1505 in a volume entitled *De Artificiali Perspectiva* that contained an extensive repertory of forms presented in perspective (Descargues, 1976). This volume was translated into German and published in Nuremberg in 1509 and, along with Dürer's book on perspective, published in 1525, introduced perspective to Germany. Dürer had studied the "secrets of perspective" some twenty years earlier in Bologna (Panofsky, 1943, 1953), but, according to Ivins (1938/1973), even he continued to have difficulty with the representation of perspective.

Alberti, in addition to specifying the geometric rules for linear perspective, also discussed the role of atmospheric or aerial perspective. Objects at a distance should have a diminished intensity of color as well as blurred outlines and contours. Alberti also noted the difference in the shading of highlights and shadows in spherical, as compared to flat, surfaces. These observations led to the initial expressions of *chiaroscuro* and *sfumato* in the late Renaissance (Gadol, 1969).

In the middle Renaissance (1445–1480), artists such as Uccello, Domenico Veneziano, Castagno, and Piero della Francesca (as well as Fra Angelico and Fra Filippo Lippi somewhat earlier) elaborated the basic concepts of perspective as articulated by Alberti. A preoccupation with perspective dominated the Renaissance. Uccello was obsessed with the concept and is reported (Panofsky, 1924/25) to have commented repeatedly "how sweet is perspective." Uccello experimented extensively with perspective as indicated in his drawing of a chalice (Fig. 43) and he achieved a remarkable sense of perspective in his painting of a battle scene, but it was limited to only the bottom portion of the picture and was not integrated with the upper part (Fig. 44).

Piero della Francesca was also intrigued by the principles of perspective. His understanding and appreciation of Alberti's principles were expressed in many of his paintings such as the *Invention and*

Discovery of the True Cross (1455), *Flagellation* (c. 1450), and *Madonna and Child with Saints* (1472) (Fig. 45). After his last major work in 1472, Piero gave up painting to study mathematics and perspective. He wrote three theoretical works in which he considered the principles of perspective as Euclidean propositions and issues in mathematics and geometry (Davis, 1977; Hartt, 1969).

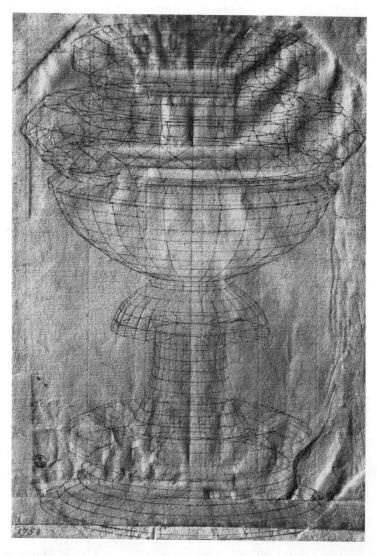

FIG. 43   Uccello, *Perspective Study of a Chalice* (c. 1451–1457), Uffizi Gallery, Florence (Alinari).

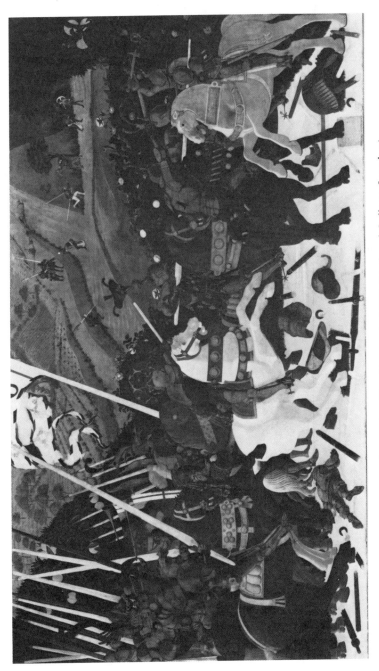

FIG. 44   Ucello, *Battle of San Romano* (c.1455) (National Gallery, London).

223

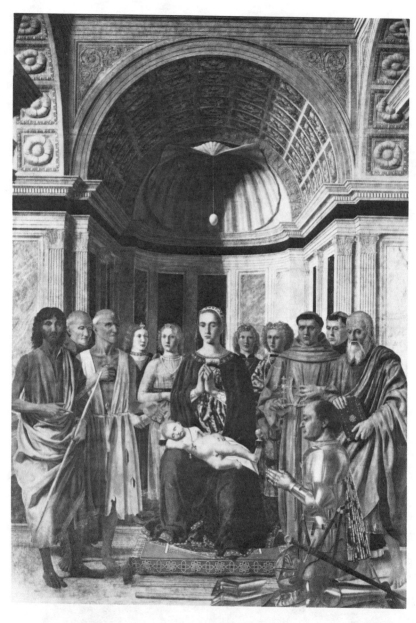

FIG. 45 Piero della Francesca, *Madonna & Child with Saints* (after 1472) Brera Gallery, Milan (Alinari).

Art became an important part of science, as artists such as Leonardo da Vinci became concerned with physics, optics, anatomy, botany and mathematics, as well as art. Leonardo, for example, was interested in proportionality not only in art, but also in mathematics, time intervals, weights and measures, and harmonic ratios in music and sound (Brachert, 1971). Natural science and art in the Renaissance both sought to represent the universe in images based on observation and mathematical laws. Artists learned the scientific procedures for representing three-dimensional space on a two-dimensional surface.

The preoccupation with perspective continued to dominate the latter half of the 15th century. Leonardo spoke of perspective as "the bridle and rudder of painting" (Richter, 1939, p. 40). But there were relatively few paintings throughout the 15th century that were totally based on concepts of linear perspective. In part this was due to difficulty with the concepts of the system but often it was the result of extensive experimentation with the principles of perspective. An example of incomplete perspective can be seen in Leonardo's *Adoration of the Magi* (1481) (Fig. 46) in which the foreground and the landscape each has a different perspective. Another exciting example of experimentation with perspective is Mantegna's *Dead Christ* (c. 1466) (Fig. 47) in which the perspective is incorrect according to mathematical rules and the painting lacks a single vanishing point. Yet there is a remarkable sense of perspective and foreshortening in which the figure of Christ becomes more supine and extends further back into the depth of the picture plane as the spectator moves away from the canvas. Mantegna was an acknowledged master of perspective and his unusual use of foreshortening and perspective in this picture creates a powerful effect.

Leonardo da Vinci's *Last Supper* (1495–1498) (Fig. 48) is one of the earliest examples of a fully integrated perspective work with a common vanishing point for both the figures and the background. The development of perspective reached its culmination in the works of Leonardo da Vinci, Michelangelo, and Raphael. In their works, generally there is a full integration of linear perspective around a central vanishing point in a unified and coherent composition. Raphael's *School of Athens* (1510–1511) (Fig. 49) is a culmination of the Renaissance development of linear perspective. The painting is constructed on the basis of a central vanishing point with a receding geometrical grid floor, a beautifully barrel-vaulted ceiling, and figures propor-

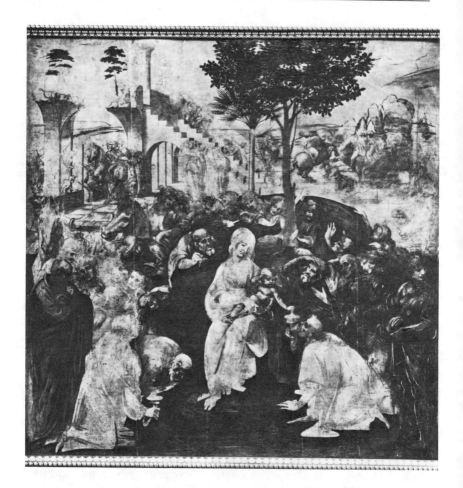

FIG. 46   Leonardo da Vinci, *Adoration of the Magi* (c.1481) Uffizi Gallery, Florence (Alinari).

tionally represented and fully integrated into the architectural field. The vanishing point is perfectly placed between Aristotle and Plato. Both in its structure and content, the *School of Athens* idealizes Greco-Roman classical Antiquity and epitomizes Renaissance tradition. Another full expression of this remarkable achievement of linear perspective includes works by Perugino such as the *Delivery of the Keys to the Kingdom* (1482) (Fig. 50).

Exciting examples of linear perspective can be found in the late 15th and early 16th centuries. But the representation of perspective and a coherent and unified sense of space did not require an adherence to strict geometric laws. Artists were able to represent perspective in a convincing fashion with only abbreviated and somewhat imprecise constructions. Interest in perspective continued into the late 16th and 17th centuries but primarily in mathematical treatises and particularly in the work of geometers. Gerard Desargues, the father of modern geometry, in 1636, one year before the publication of Descartes' *Discours de la Methode*, invented a mathematically precise method for projecting three-dimensional objects in their spatial positions on a two-dimensional surface. The geometric theory of Desargues for representing universal space was introduced into art by Abraham Bosse, but it met with considerable resistance. Heated debates took place within the French Academie Royale and Bosse was eventually expelled from membership. Mathematicians continued to explore perspective through the 19th century but debate continued within art about the importance and need for utilizing precise mathematical laws of perspective (Descargues, 1976).

As we will discuss in the section on Mannerism, in the mid and late 16th century considerable experimentation with various ways to utilize the concepts of linear perspective was taking place. Artists

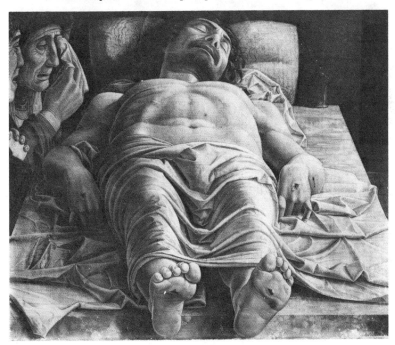

FIG. 47   Mantegna, *Dead Christ* (c.1501) Brera Gallery, Milan (Alinari).

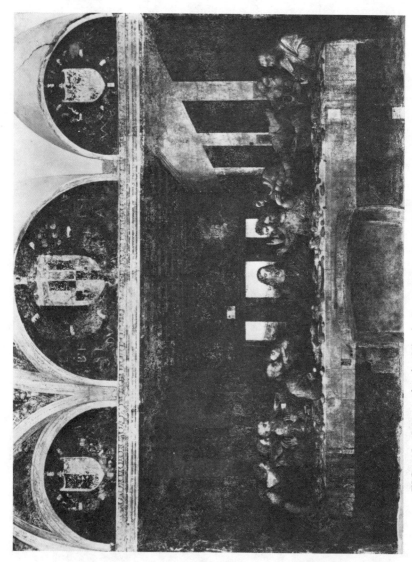

FIG. 48 Leonardo da Vinci, *Last Supper* (c.1495–98), Santa Maria delle Grazie, Milan (Alinari).

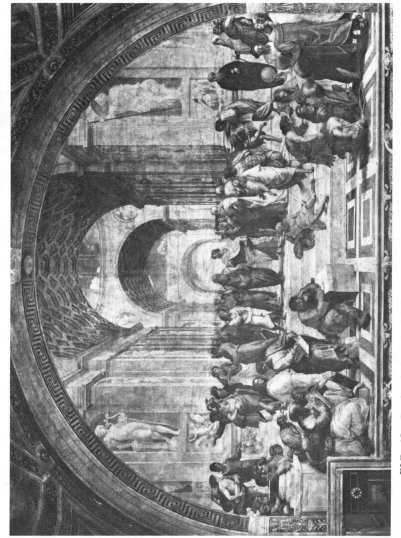

FIG. 49 Raphael, *School of Athens* (1509–11) Vatican Museum, Rome (Alinari).

229

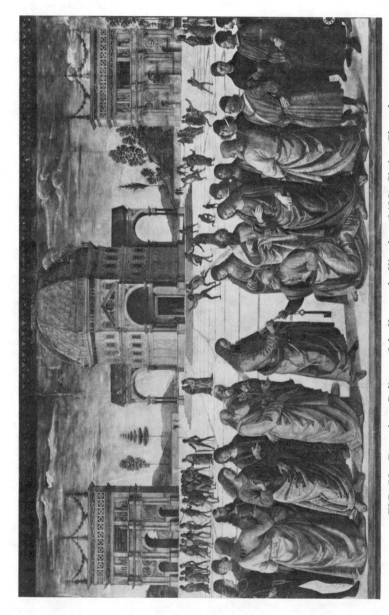

FIG. 50 Perugino, *Delivery of the Keys to the Kingdom* (1482), Sistine Chapel, Vatican, Rome (Alinari).

230

searched for alternative ways of utilizing the concepts of perspective without strictly adhering to the geometrical rules of linear perspective. Artists became concerned that paintings based on linear perspective had to be viewed "correctly"—that the viewer had to be at the one precise point defined by the artist. Despite the delight with the results of perspective, it continued to be controversial and some considered it too technical and mechanical. There were concerns that the preoccupation with perspective would result in a loss of artistic individuality. Artists sought ways to free themselves from these restrictions without destroying what had been accomplished in the discovery of linear perspective.

Linear perspective was used during the Renaissance to create highly regular, well-organized, symmetrical compositions around a central vanishing point. There was absolute order, balance, and predictability in idealized compositions of eternal perfection. In the early phase of Renaissance art, in the work of Cavallini, Cimabue, Duccio, and Giotto, perspective was represented intuitively (perceptually), utilizing early forms of projective concepts of space. Early Renaissance art, like Greek art, sought to portray realistically an idealized universal, natural image. Nature was studied and represented, not as an expression of the Divine, but for its own sake and in its own right. This interest in the ideal natural form was expressed in an interest in the nude human form, particularly in sculpture, as a subject for monumental representation. The idealized classical forms of Antiquity were a perfect vehicle for this search for universal truth. Sketch or drawing books as early as the 13th and 14th centuries (e.g., Villard de Honnecourt) indicated the ideal way to portray bodies and bodily parts. These sketch books, which emphasized projective concepts of space, formed "a reservoir of formulas or schemata which spread through Europe" (Gombrich, 1960, p. 165). Throughout the Renaissance the conviction was prevalent that artists should represent the universal and the ideal rather than the particular. This emphasis on the generalized ideal encouraged Renaissance artists to use highly stable and constant forms. And it was the attainment of the representation of these idealized constant forms that enabled artists to begin experimenting with transformations of these forms in linear perspective.

Linear perspective, as an illusionistic representation of reality, provided a particularly vivid, realistic, and veridical representation of nature. But there is considerable debate about the role of perspective in the history of art. Because of its representational effectiveness, Gombrich (1950, 1960) and others (e.g., Doesschate, 1964; Gioseffi, 1966; Pirenne, 1952, 1970) consider linear perspective as the most natural rendering of reality. Perspective was initially constructed intuitively, but the full development of linear perspective occurred only later in a geometric construction that was a unique mathematical solution based on an identity of structure and reciprocal relationships between all points, directions, and distances. Linear perspective was part of a conception of space as infinite, homogeneous, and isotropic that was emerging during the 15th to 17th centuries.

There was a long and complicated evolution in the development of linear perspective, which is the most natural and effective representational system for providing the best approximation of our visual experiences in the world around us (Pirenne, 1959). A picture drawn in perspective is "simply a device to send into the eye the same light distribution as would be sent by the object itself" (Pirenne, 1952, p. 183). Gombrich (1960, 1972, p. 148), like Pirenne, stresses that perspective is "uniquely successful" in mapping what we see from a given viewpoint, that is, it creates a compelling "genuine illusion" and is a standard with which other forms of representation must always be compared. Gibson (1960, p. 227), based on perceptual theory, states that "it does not seem reasonable to assert that the use of perspective in paintings is merely a convention, to be used or discarded by the painter as he chooses. . . . When the artist transcribes what he sees upon a two-dimensional surface, he uses perspective geometry, of necessity."

Gablik (1976, pp. 69–70), however, believes that these views of linear perspective as a set of "universal mathematical principles" reflect a conception of nature as "stable and unchanging," "permanent and fixed," "based on concepts of absolute time and space . . . in which chance and indeterminacy play no part," a world "ordered and rationally explicable" and reducible to "mathematical order by the principles of perspective and solid geometry." Gablik and others (e.g., Arnheim, 1974; Bunim, 1940; Edgerton, 1975; Goodman, 1968; Panofsky, 1924/25; White, 1967) prefer to consider linear perspective an important procedure, but only one of a number of possible ways of representing reality with fidelity. Panofsky (1924/25), in a seminal article, discussed perspective as a "symbolic form." Panofsky did not discount the importance of linear perspective, but he pointed out that it is a convention—a "symbolic form" particularly effective for representing accurately three-dimensional reality on a two-dimensional surface. For Panofsky, linear perspective is a particularly effective construction for representing space, a discovery especially congruent with the culture of the Italian Renaissance. Some art historians (e.g., Gombrich, 1960, 1972) and some investigators in optics (e.g., Pirenne, 1952) have criticized Panofsky's view that linear perspective is not the ultimate form of pictorial realism. As Edgerton (1975) states, the real thrust of (Panofsky's) argument was not to prove

> that Renaissance perspective was a mere artistic convention, but that *each historical period in Western civilization had its own special "perspective,"* a particular symbolic form reflecting a particular *Weltanschauung.* Thus linear perspective was the peculiar answer of the Renaissance period to the problem of representing space . . . (p. 157–158).
>
> Finally in the fifteenth century, there emerged mathematically ordered "systematic space," infinite, homogeneous, and isotropic, making possible the advent of linear perspective. . . . Linear perspective, whether "truth" or not, thus became the symbolic form of the Italian Renaissance because it reflected the general world view of the Italian people at this particular moment in history. (p. 161)

For Panofsky, the most important issue was not whether perspective is the ultimate method for representing nature, but why and how it was discovered during the Renaissance.

The difference in opinion about whether linear perspective is the ultimate mathematical solution or a particularly effective symbolic convention has led to considerable debate among art historians. What is most important to note, however, is Panofsky's (1924/25) emphasis that one should consider linear perspective as only one of a number of "symbolic forms" or representational constructions. Panofsky (1924/25) agrees that linear perspective is a unique and most effective form of representation and that it elevated art to science, but he stresses that it is only one phase in the development of symbolic forms or modes of representation in the history of art. Further development of symbolic forms of representation occurred subsequently in art, all built on the important contribution of linear perspective in the Renaissance. Linear perspective is a specific symbolic form, but only one of a number of symbolic forms of representational construction that have evolved through a long and complex developmental process in the history of art. While linear perspective is a mathematically unique solution for representing three dimensions on a two-dimensional surface, it is nevertheless a mathematical invention or solution—a symbolic form that expresses the general conceptual mode of its epoch. The development of the mathematical basis for perspective was an expression of the Renaissance emphasis on human dignity, the importance of man's capacity for reason, and the development of science and mathematics. Linear perspective provided the foundation for the representation of individual subjective experience: "the objectification of the subjective" (Panofsky, 1924/25).

Arnheim (1974) also discusses linear or central perspective as:

> The final result of prolonged exploration and in response to very particular cultural needs . . . as one aspect of the search for objectively correct descriptions of physical nature—a search that sprang during the Renaissance from a new interest in the wonders of the sensory world, and led to the great voyages of explorations as well as to the development of experimental research and the scientific standards. . . . The desire to find an objective basis for the depiction of visual objects, a method independent of the idiosyncrasies of the draftsman's eye and hand (p. 283).

But Arnheim (1974) also considers the discovery of central perspective as indicating a

> dangerous development in Western thought . . . a scientifically oriented preference for mechanical reproduction and geometrical constructs in place of creative imagery. . . . The lure of mechanical faithfulness has ever since the Renaissance tempted European art, especially in the mediocre standard output for mass consumption (pp. 284–285).

While Arnheim (1974, p. 294) agrees that linear perspective raised pictorial representation to a new level of differentiation, he notes that it "is at the same time a violent imposition upon the world represented in the picture" and on the viewer by requiring him or her to stand at a particular point to have the experience of convergence. Despite Arnheim's concerns about linear perspective as a dangerous development in Western thought, Arnheim (1954/1974, p. 297) considers linear perspective, as Panofsky does, as a symbolic form that was consonant with the major conceptualizations of its epoch. It was a major invention of the early 15th century, which expressed new concepts of space that had not been articulated in the Medieval period. It had a revolutionary impact on art. But there were also various forms of experimentation with the concepts of perspective. Linear perspective, as a complex convention and symbolic form, was utilized and modified in different ways in succeeding periods after its discovery during the Italian Renaissance.

In terms of developmental psychological principles, early Renaissance art was at an intuitive, preoperational, perceptual level. The representation of perspective was accomplished intuitively (empirically) without an organized, unified conceptual system. The focus was primarily on individual objects in space without a unifying conception of space. There was an interest in idealized universal forms with great stability and constancy. Developmentally, it was essential to achieve a stability (or constancy) in the representation of objects in order to enter into the operational levels in which there are transformations of dimensions of objects. Prior to the development of operational modes, object representation is consolidated around concrete, manifest, idealized forms that have stability and permanence. The emphasis in Antiquity and in the early Renaissance on the perceptual totality of the manifest features of idealized universal forms provided the stability and constancy necessary for considering objects as variable and dynamic. The interest in beauty and idealized proportionality in Antiquity and the early Renaissance provided the basis for the eventual operational transformations that are an integral part of the principles of linear perspective. Distortions in the representation of the external form of the object and of space could now be tolerated without jeopardizing the object's basic identity and definition. Early in the Renaissance, transformations and distortions were partial and intuitive (perceptual); later, mathematical operations allowed for systematic and more extensive transformations of the manifest form of objects and of space.

In the second phase of the Renaissance, in the 15th century, Brunelleschi, Alberti, Piero della Francesca, Leonardo and others discovered the mathematical basis for perspective. The representation of space moved from the intuitive to the level of concrete operations. Perspective was no longer achieved intuitively, based on perceptual experience, but was now determined operationally and conceptually, based on mathematical formulae. Operational thought involving the coordination of several dimensions allowed for transformations and reversibility as well as conservation. The same object could be represented in different ways and at different points in space while still maintaining its basic identity and constancy.

The development of linear perspective marked the advent of operational modes of representation in the history of art. The formulation of the mathematical basis for linear perspective indicated a change from preoperational to operational modes of representation. Linear perspective involves the transformation of external manifest features of well-defined, universal figures and forms in a highly structured, symmetrically balanced composition. In this sense, linear perspective in the Renaissance is an early stage of operational modes—the level of concrete operations. The beginning of operational thought, according to developmental psychological theory, is the beginning of symbolic thought. The interpretation of linear perspective as an early stage of operational modes of representation and of symbolic thinking is consistent with Panofsky's (1924/25) formulation of perspective as a symbolic form. Later forms of operational thought involve the coordination and integration of more abstract and less manifest and concrete dimensions. Thus, according to developmental psychological principles, the cognitive operations of linear perspective would be an early phase in the complex development of operational or symbolic modes of representation.

The development of linear perspective during the Renaissance was the foundation for the objective construction of subjective visual experience. It provided room for the "plastic expansion" (Panofsky, 1924/25) of bodies in space, the representation of expressive movement, and the diffusion of light throughout the space of the picture plane. These dimensions were added subsequently in Mannerism and the Baroque, and they enriched and extended the representation of subjective experiences of linear perspective by including affective and emotional dimensions. As discussed by Panofsky, the perspective view of space enriches and extends both the subjective and the objective dimensions in art. Linear perspective is subjective in that it distorts the true configuration of objects and presents the object as a function of the experience of the observer. But it is also objective because it provides a conceptual, mathematical structure for organizing elements in a coherent and integrated pictorial space based on an ordering of visual experiences. Linear perspective actually provides a basis for the synthesis of the subjective and the objective since it locates the representation of nature within the unique psychological experiences of the observer. The development of this "subjective objectivism" (Frankl, 1960) was a critical moment in the history of art. Panofsky (1924/25) questions whether the great works of the Baroque period, particularly the late paintings of Rembrandt, would have been possible without its development. The development of perspective was the

Renaissance's monumental contribution. It established and defined a precise schema for the representation of nature that, once articulated, dominated art for centuries. But, most important, it also created the basis for the representation of subjective experiences in art. Linear perspective was the introduction of the subjective dimension into art, which was to be developed more fully in subsequent centuries and integrated in increasingly effective ways with the objective dimension. The distinction of object and subject was effective for the first time in the Renaissance (Cassirer, 1927/1963) and there was an increasing synthesis of the subjective and the objective dimensions in subsequent epochs.

Linear perspective in Renaissance art was expressed primarily in highly organized, well balanced, symmetrical, pyramidal compositions. The emphasis on symmetrically balanced compositions of idealized forms persisted into the beginning of the 16th century. Subsequently, during Mannerism and the Baroque, principles of linear perspective began to be utilized in asymmetrical compositions. Paintings were still organized around a central vanishing point, but they lacked the fixed quality of absolute balance and order. Asymmetrical compositions created a sense of viewing an arbitrarily selected segment of a natural scene. Objects were no longer idealized forms but particular and unique objects viewed at a specific moment in time. In contrast to Renaissance paintings of idealized, timeless figures and places, Baroque paintings created the experience of being a participant in a segment of everyday life.

Initially, perspective was achieved intuitively, without specification of the operations involved and with little capacity for transformation and conservation. Thus there could be little variation, ambiguity, or vagueness in the representation of objects. All figures, whether in the foreground or background, were clear, precise, and well delineated. Without the mathematical operations that provide a conceptual system for integrating the entire picture plane, idealized universal figures had to have a high degree of articulation and clarity. Modes of representation in the Renaissance involved a blend of both topological and early forms of projective concepts of space. Alberti's formulations of the principles of linear perspective, for example, were based on projective concepts of space, but he still retained an emphasis on topological concepts as well. As noted by Gadol (1969, pp. 28–29), in Alberti's visual geometry "the surface or 'outer skin' of an object is the key element." Topological concepts of boundary and contour of objects were relinquished only late in the Renaissance and in Mannerism and the Baroque. Topological concepts of space (e.g., boundaries and surfaces) could be relinquished only with the consolidation of projective concepts. In the later phase of the Renaissance, when the concrete operations of projective concepts of space had been well established, figures could be represented as less articulated and vague, with increased subtlety throughout the picture plane. Variations in shading, light, and color could now enhance the sense of depth. Pliny *(Natural History)* notes a similar pattern in Antiquity— artists were free to use shading and color to enhance their art only after the achievement of intuitive perspective (Levy, 1943; Richter, 1970). And, in the Renaissance, it was only after the discovery of the mathematical, operational basis for linear perspective that Leonardo da Vinci formulated concepts of color and aerial perspective and developed the technique of *sfumato*. He wrote about the perspective of color as follows:

> In order to put into practice this perspective of the variation and loss or diminution of the essential character of colours, observe at every hundred braccia some objects standing in the landscape, such as trees, houses, men, and particular places. Then in front of the first tree have a very steady plate of glass and keep your eye very steady, and then, on this plate of glass, draw a tree, tracing it over the form of that tree. Then move it on one side so far as that the real tree is close by the side of the tree you have drawn; then colour your drawing in such a way that colour and form may match one another, and that both, if you close one eye, seem to be painted on the glass and at the same distance. Then, by the same method, represent a second tree, and a third, with a distance of a hundred braccia between each. And these will serve as a standard and guide whenever you work on your own pictures, wherever they may apply, and will enable you to give due distance in those works. But I have found that as a rule the second is $\frac{1}{5}$ of the first when it is 20 braccia beyond it.

And Leonardo wrote about aerial perspective in part, as follows:

> There is another kind of perspective which I call Aerial Perspective, because by the atmosphere we are able to distinguish the variations in distance of different buildings, which appear placed on a single line; as, for instance when we see several buildings beyond a wall, all of which, as they appear above the top of the wall, look of the same size, while you wish to represent them in a picture as more remote one than another and to give the effect of a somewhat dense atmosphere. You know that in an atmosphere of equal density the remotest objects seen through it,

as mountains, in consequence of the great quantity of atmosphere between your eye and them—appear blue and almost of the same hue as
the atmosphere itself when the sun is in the East. Hence, you must make
the nearest building above the wall of its real colour, but make the more
distant ones less defined and bluer. Those you wish to look farther away
you must make proportionately bluer; thus if one is to be five times as
distant, make it five times bluer. And by this rule the buildings which
above a (given) line appear of the same size will plainly be distinguished
as to which are the more remote and which larger than the others. (The
Literary Works of Leonardo da Vinci, Vol., I, 1939, J. P. Richter (Ed).
pp. 235–236)

In summary, the representation of space in the Renaissance was
achieved through three major techniques: linear, atmospheric, and
color perspective. In linear perspective, parallel lines recede into
space to a common vanishing point on the horizon. Objects portrayed
at a distance are made smaller by means of a scale based on the
coordination of horizontal and vertical dimensions. The coordinate
scale allowed objects to be represented in relation to each other both
in terms of size and distance. In atmospheric perspective, variations
of shading and light are also used to create the illusion of depth. Near
forms are distinct and clearly presented, while objects at a distance are
vague and less well articulated. Individual parts tended to merge in
color and form, creating the effect of an object at a distance. The
representation of depth and volume in linear perspective was supplemented by techniques of atmospheric perspective.

For the most part, early Renaissance paintings had uniform lighting throughout and objects were sharply delineated. Late in the Renaissance, Leonardo da Vinci developed the technique of *sfumato,* in
which the sharp boundaries between the figure and its surrounding
context were made blurred and indistinct. Leonardo's use of *sfumato* is
well illustrated in his *Virgin and Child with St. Anne and John the Baptist*
(Fig. 51).

It is important to stress that this relinquishing of the sharp and well-
defined boundary (topological concepts of space) occurred only after
projective concepts of space were well established in the specification
of the mathematical operations of linear perspective. From Paleolithic
art, through the early Renaissance (except for a later Greco-Roman
period), boundaries were always sharply articulated. Sfumato, the
blurring of boundaries, followed the change from an intuitive to an
operational specification of perspective and the stabilization of projective concepts of space. At the more advanced levels there was no

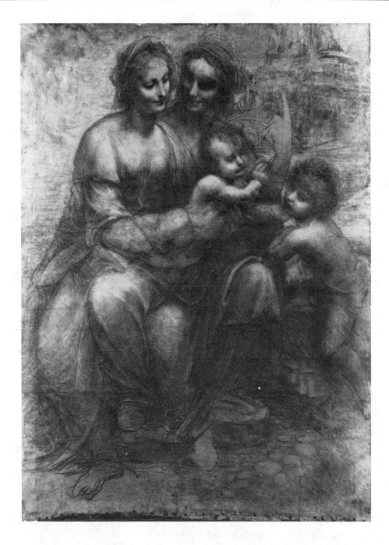

FIG. 51   Leonardo da Vinci, Cartoon, *The Virgin and Child with St. Anne and John the Baptist* (1498) (National Gallery, London).

longer a need to support the projective concepts of space with the developmentally earlier topological concepts of space with its emphasis on surfaces and boundaries. The shift from the utilization of topological to projective concepts of space is consistent with the formulations of Wölfflin (1915) of a change from a linear to a painterly style. It is also consistent with Riegl's (1901/1927) description of the move from a "haptic" (tactile) orientation, in which objects are concrete, tangible, self-contained, isolated entities, to an "optic" (or painterly or impressionistic) orientation in which objects and parts of objects are integrated with the surrounding void by a conscious, self-reflective viewer who organizes the perceptual field.

Experiments with linear perspective begun in the late Renaissance were extended in Mannerism and the Baroque and were carried on by the Impressionists in the late 19th century. Succeeding generations of artists experimented with variations and adaptations of linear perspective as they struggled to find modes of representation that went beyond the concrete operational modes of linear perspective. Leonardo's blurring of boundaries in sfumato, with its minimization of the differentiation between an object and its surroundings, was the beginning of the development of *chiaroscuro* and the increased use of modeling of light and color in the Baroque period. Baroque art utilized these techniques to extend the representation of subjective experiences first introduced with linear perspective. These new dimensions allowed artists to represent more subtle aspects of the subjective experience—mood, affect, and emotional tone. It was only with the consolidation of concrete operational modes of representation in the development of linear perspective that artists could begin to go beyond the subjective representation of external manifest form and attempt to represent more subtle, internal, subjective experiences. Objects were no longer represented as universal ideals, but were portrayed in the particular, initially with specific and unique external physical features and later with more internal, intrinsic properties such as mood and emotion.

MANNERISM

Mannerism is usually dated as beginning in Florence around 1520 and continuing through the 16th century. Mannerism, according to Friedlaender (1958), began in Florence as a conscious revolt against the ideals of the high Renaissance epitomized in the highly rational works of Leonardo, Raphael, Andrea del Sarto, and early Michelangelo. It was a 16th century aesthetic revolution against the harmonic beauty and naturalism of the high Renaissance. One of the primary factors in Mannerism was a reaction to the precise organization of space in Renaissance compositions. Some of the earliest "anti-classical" works of the Mannerist period include the paintings of

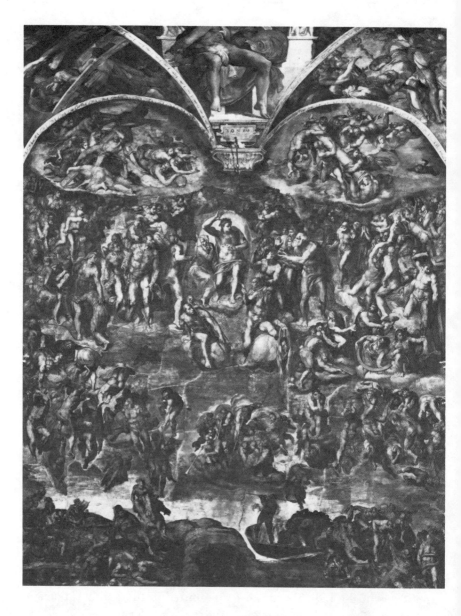

FIG. 52 Michelangelo, *Last Judgment* (1536–41), Sistine Chapel, Vatican, Rome (Alinari).

artists such as Pontormo, Rosso Fiorentino, and Parmigianino and the later works of Michelangelo, especially his *Last Judgment* in the Sistine Chapel (1535–1541). The use of space in Michelangelo's *Last Judgment* (Fig. 52) is completely different from Renaissance space. According to Hauser (1965, p. 174), the sense of space in the *Last Judgment* stands in "contrast to the homogeneous, uniformly organised, and precisely delimited spatial areas of Renaissance painting." Space in the *Last Judgment* is

> broken up into unreal, discontinuous, isolated patches, which are neither seen from one particular angle nor measured by any single standard. The discontinuity and unreality of the pictorial space is chiefly the consequence of the abandonment of the principle of creating illusion by perspective which was fundamental to the Renaissance. This is most strikingly evident in the undiminished proportions of the uppermost figures in the composition which are farthest from the observer, and consequently seem too big. However, the spatial discontinuity is perceptible everywhere; the various parts of the picture form completely independent perspective units, each with its own optics and vanishing point, with the result that the whole is a conglomeration of distinct visual systems. Thus a number of superimposed, parallel spatial areas can be distinguished. (Hauser, 1965, p. 174)

The ceiling of the Sistine Chapel is an early expression of Michelangelo's Mannerist style. The marked restriction and compression of gigantic figures of the prophets and sibyls in the narrow space of the ceiling are in marked contrast to the "powerful expansiveness" of these figures in "transcendental and divine space" (Friedlaender, 1958, p. 15). The renunciation of natural space is even more marked in the spandrels of the Sistine ceiling where gigantic figures are compressed into narrow triangular space in order to emphasize their monumentality. Michelangelo continued in his Mannerist tradition in his last two great frescoes, *The Conversion of St. Paul* and *The Crucifixion of St. Peter,* (Fig. 53) in the Pauline Chapel. In these Mannerist paintings, Michelangelo challenged the canons of linear perspective and the representation of idealized form and structure that characterized the High Renaissance. In his experimentation with the Renaissance principles of perfect harmony and balance, Michelangelo was attempting to redefine man and his place in the universe. Hauser (1965) comments on Michelangelo's Mannerist works as follows:

> Empty spaces alternate with uncannily overcrowded areas, desolate wastes with tightly packed throngs. . . . But here the emphasis is less on

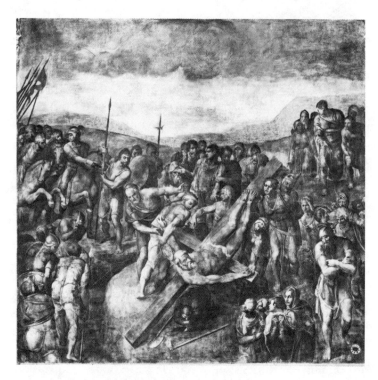

FIG. 53   Michelangelo, *The Crucifixion of St. Peter* (1545–50), Pauline Chapel, Vatican, Rome (Alinari).

the optical discontinuity of space, as it was in *Last Judgment*, than on the completely different valuation of individual spatial areas and the abrupt juxtaposition of differently occupied spaces. Spatial depth is not built up gradually, but is torn up. Diagonals break through the different levels and bore yawning holes into the background. (p. 174)

There is considerable debate and controversy about Mannerism, the 80-year period subsequent to the Renaissance and prior to the development of the Baroque style. Weitz (1970) provides an excellent summary of some of the major positions in this debate. There are art historians who focus on a new spiritualism in Mannerism, where the artist seeks an autonomous, subjective mode, rather than adhering to an objective canon (Friedlaender, 1958) or attempting to embody in art an immediate emotional certainty and mystical knowledge about the presence of God in the world (Dvořák, 1918/1967). Some (e.g., Venturi, 1956) consider Mannerism as an anti-classical revolt against the ideal form of nature and the restrictive canons of the Renaissance.

Venturi (1956) stresses the wish to cultivate abstract forms in Mannerism, and cites the "antinatural treatment of figure and space . . . sensitive handling of light . . . dexterous use of lights and darks" (Weitz, 1970, p. 198). Instead of viewing Mannerism as a revolt, Smyth (1962), Friedlaender (1958), and Gombrich (1960) consider it as a period of experimentation with the classical form of the high Renaissance. Shearman (1967) stresses content rather than form and is impressed with a pervasive interest in poise, grace, and sophisticated beauty instead of strength, brutality, violence, and overt passion. Despite these differences in interpretation, most authorities agree, however, that though there was a sense of grace and finesse in Mannerism, it was a period of dysfunction and ambivalence that attempted to alter the unity of form and content achieved in the high Renaissance (Weitz, 1970). There is considerable agreement (e.g., Friedlaender, 1958; Gombrich, 1960; Hauser, 1951/1960, 1965) that one of the primary features of Mannerism was an ambivalent reaction to the uniformity and coherence of the organization of space in the Renaissance. While the paintings of the early Middle Ages were essentially spaceless, the representation of space was a preoccupation in Renaissance art. In contrast, the spatial effects in Mannerism are sometimes exaggerated, and other times ignored. Mannerism is characterized by both a tendency to exaggerate depth and a tendency to be planimetric and emphasize surface patterns (Hauser, 1965).

Hauser (1965) and Friedlaender (1958) consider the experimentation with space a primary aspect of Mannerism. Hauser (1965, p. 278) comments that the spatial harmony of the Renaissance, the easy and comfortable relationship between objects and environment, was relinquished in Mannerism. "Figures were packed together in a corner or lost in a vast, vague, unlimited area, as if to express the sense of rootlessness and being astray." Hauser speculates that Renaissance space, like the geocentric universe in astronomy, had become too confining. Artists reacted to the narrow confines of classical art, and figures in Mannerist paintings became unreal, unnatural, and elongated. Also, there was often an ambiguous sense of space and a lack of depth in Mannerism. In Renaissance painting space behind the figure usually recedes, but in Mannerism the figure is often brought to the foreground and the receding space is lost. Figures in Mannerism retain Renaissance volume and the illusion of three-dimensionality, but the sense of perspective in the receding picture plane is markedly diminished. Mannerism, however, also distorted the volume of

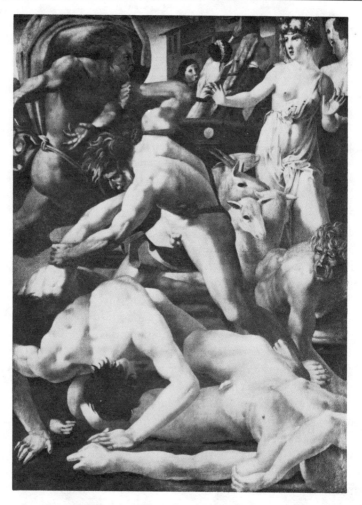

FIG. 54   Rosso Fiorentino, *Moses and Daughters of Jethro* (1523), Uffizi Gallery, Florence (Alinari).

figures by emphasizing their length and size, making figures huge, out of proportion, elongated, and unnatural. This distortion of figures is illustrated in Rosso Fiorentino's *Moses and the Daughters of Jethro* (1523) (Fig. 54) and Parmigianino's *Madonna of the Long Neck* (1535–1540) (Fig. 55).

In Rosso's *Moses and the Daughters of Jethro* (Fig. 54), monumental figures with boldly defined volume are compressed together in multiple layers, filling the entire surface of the painting. Space and a sense of depth is achieved through the layers of bodies set behind and above each other. A sense of depth is achieved, not through Renaissance perspective, but through the Mannerist layers of figures. Rosso's remarkable painting is an extreme expression of Mannerist spatial organization.

Parmigianino's elegantly charming *Madonna of the Long Neck* (Fig. 55), expresses a consciously anticlassical distortion of the relationship of figure to space. Elongated, graceful figures create an elegance of form; the unrealistic proportions of the figures are emphasized even further by their unnatural juxtaposition to the column and the prophet holding a scroll in deeper space.

In Renaissance art, unambiguous figures had a role in unambigu-

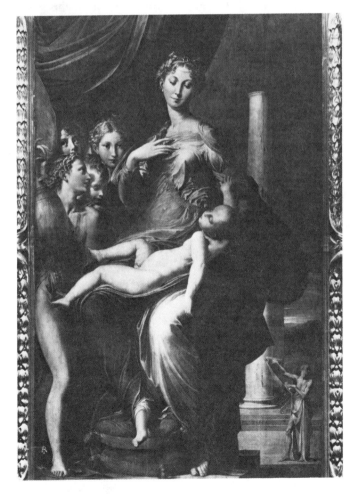

FIG. 55 Parmigianino, *Madonna of the Long Neck* (c.1535), Uffizi Gallery, Florence (Alinari).

ously constructed space. In Mannerism a basic alteration occurs in the representation of space. Some (e.g., Hauser, 1965) argue that there is a fundamental ambivalence about space; others (e.g., Friedlaender, 1958) are most impressed with the diminished sense of space in Mannerism. The illusion of space, if it exists in the picture plane, is created in some Mannerist paintings primarily by the volumes of bodies and by adding up layers or volumes of figures. Often the stress is on surfaces, on planes set behind one another. Although the paintings are more than purely flat surfaces, they have a limited sense of three-dimensional volume. Space is unnatural and unadapted to the figures; an instability exists between the figure and the surrounding space or field. The primary emphasis in Mannerism is on body volume, often at the expense of spatial context. Figures are distorted, primarily elongated, and little attention is given to background and perspective.

Friedlaender (1958) does not consider Mannerism a decay of the Renaissance, but rather a transitional phase from the High Renaissance to the Baroque. He views it as a spiritually subjective style directed primarily against the canonical art of the High Renaissance. Renaissance art, at its inception, was an expression of individuality and subjectivity, but as it became more systematized and defined by mathematics and prescribed canons and procedures, it began to limit and thwart individuality (Arnheim, 1954/1974). Artists experimented with the formal schematization of linear perspective in their continual search for creativity and innovation. Thus, Mannerism was a time of experimentation in which artists attempted to break through the constraints imposed by the canonical structure established by the Renaissance. The experimentation with space through the representation of distortions is well illustrated by Parmigianino's unnatural *Self Portrait* (1524) (Fig. 56), painted as a reflection in a convex mirror, in which the hand closest to the mirror appears elongated and overstated.

Mannerism was a period of experimentation with the precise balance and organization of space and the ideal, universal form of the Renaissance. Another indication of this interest in experimentation with the rules and procedures of linear perspective was the interest in anamorphosis—a device first developed in the mid-16th century for experimenting with the principles of linear perspective. As illustrated by Holbein's *Ambassadors* (1533), anamorphosis involved the introduction of an unrecognizable object in the painting, which becomes recognizable only when viewed from a particular position markedly different from the conventional view for the total picture. Anamorphosis is accomplished by projecting forms outside themselves in a way in which they become highly distorted except when viewed from a particular and unusual direction. Anamorphosis was a device for experimenting with the concepts of linear perspective by carrying these principles to their extreme, but without destroying them. Since

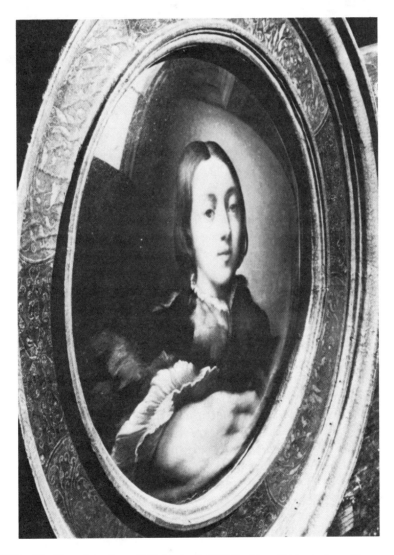

FIG. 56 Parmigianino, *Self Portrait* (1524), Kunsthistorisches Museum, Vienna (Yale University, Estate of Charles Seymour, Jr.).

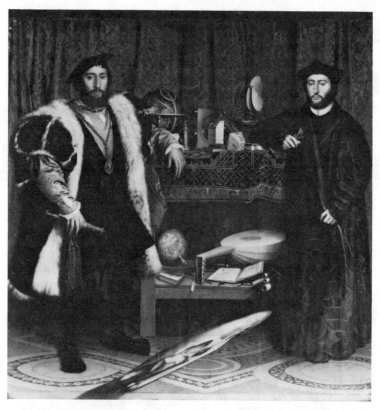

FIG. 57a Holbein, the Younger, *Ambassadors* (1533), (National Gallery, London).

these experiments were still based on the principles of perspective, anamorphosis was a system that could also be defined mathematically (Baltrusaitis, 1977). Anamorphosis began around 1531, and throughout the remainder of the 16th century several treatises discussed the rules for this procedure. In fact there is suggestion that Leonardo presented an early example of anamorphosis in his *Treatise on Painting* and in the *Codex Atlanticus* (1483–1518). "It is . . . virtually certain that those centres which developed perspective in general . . . also invented its paradoxes" (Baltrušaitis, 1977, pp. 33–34).

Holbein's *Ambassadors* (Fig. 57a) has a strange and distorted object in the lower foreground that becomes clearly defined as a skull if viewed from one particular vantage point (Fig. 57b).

Mannerism is understood by Hauser (1965, p. 111) "as an expression of the unrest, anxiety, and bewilderment generated by the process of alienation of the individual from society and the reification of the whole cultural process." The "self-conscious dissenting frustrated style" (Pevsner, 1969, p. 143) of Mannerism occurred during an age of iconoclasm, protest, and reformation. The Reformation was not only a moral and doctrinal revolt against Rome, but it also involved a rebellion against scholastic philosophy and its distorted Aristotelian structure. Aristotelian structure had continued throughout the Renaissance, despite the attacks of the Humanists on the Aristotelian structure and on the Roman Church. Their efforts prepared the way, beginning in the early 16th century, for reformers such as Luther, Calvin, Erasmus, Zwingli, and Knox (Artz, 1966). The intellectual revolt and the self-reflective, assertive quality of Mannerist art was similar to the ethic of the Protestant Reformation in which God's will was no longer to be interpreted by the established, formal hierarchy

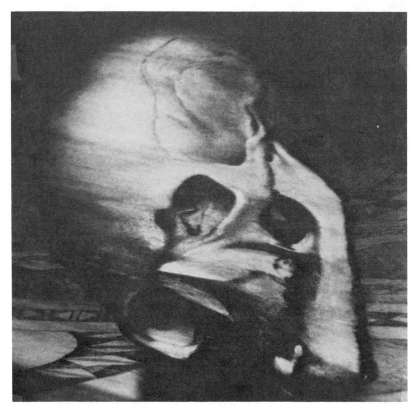

FIG. 57b Holbein, the Younger, detail from *Ambassadors* (1533), (National Gallery, London).

of the clergy but rather by each individual in his or her relationship with God. God's Grace was to be found in one's success in worldly achievements and, therefore, one was enjoined to strive and work in order to have proof of that Grace (Weber, 1958).

The Reformation was followed by a powerful Counter-Reformation that reestablished the power of the Church. The Council of Trent, which began in 1542, led to a repressive social context, a rigidity in dogma and doctrine, and an austerity in social conduct. The Inquisition was reintroduced in 1542 and the censorship of books began in 1543. There was a suppression of debate in natural philosophy and of experimentation in art. Mannerist artists were censured by the Counter-Reformation for seeking to demonstrate their own artistic skill rather than trying to achieve the most effective way to portray a religious story. Only with the new philosophical, mathematical, and scientific concepts of the early 17th century was the Aristotelian structure finally successfully challenged. Rigid and closed systems of scholastic thought were replaced by critical attitudes of observation, experimentation, and mathematical formulation. Pevsner (1969) believes that the genuine Baroque ideas, first conceived in the days of the Renaissance, were kept alive and grew during Mannerism despite its return to Medieval mentality. He characterizes Mannerism as austere, cheerless, and aloof with "no faith in mankind" (p. 146). Mannerism occurred during a complex period in which initially there was experimentation, reform, and revolt, and followed by a period of "tormenting doubt" (p. 146) and of rigidly enforced dogma and doctrine. Thus, it seems consistent that Mannerist art should be full of contradictions and experimentation with the established order. There were deliberate disruptions as well as adherence to rigid formality. Despite the contradiction and turmoil in society and in art, Pevsner calls attention to artists such as Veronese, Titian, and Tintoretto and the architect, Palladio, who remained relatively uninvolved in the contradictions of Mannerism.

Opinions about Mannerism vary widely, from seeing it as a constructive transitional phase from Renaissance to Baroque (Friedlaender, 1958), to regarding it as a conflicted, bleak, rigid, austere period whose art was a function of religious suppression and loss of individuality (Pevsner, 1969). It is quite clear, however, that the latter three quarters of the 16th century (1520–1600) were contradictory times filled with much ambivalence. In terms of the representation of space, artists during this era were struggling with the monumental discovery of linear perspective in the Renaissance. They were experimenting and struggling to transcend the precise mathematical canons for the organization of the picture plane. They seemed to be searching for ways to go beyond the monumental accomplishments of the Renaissance, to find new expressions of volume and depth. But this conscious and deliberate experimentation with space could only have occurred after the stabilization of perspective and the specification of the mathematical operations that provided a concrete operational basis for the representation of perspective. Only after the discovery of the mathematical principles and the achievement of operational concepts could experiments with transformations begin.

In terms of the level of spatial concepts, the achievement of linear perspective in the Renaissance involved basic concepts of projective space. Perspective was expressed primarily in symmetrical or pyramidal compositions in much of Renaissance art, in which the central vanishing point on the horizon was usually located in the center of the canvas. In Mannerism, this highly balanced composition was replaced by experiments with the alteration of space including the use of diagonal compositions. The diagonal appears as early as the 14th century (Panofsky, 1924/25) but its use as a systematic organizational principle began in Mannerism and was fully developed only in the Baroque. As indicated by developmental psychological research and theory, the more advanced levels of projective concepts of space involve the use of the diagonal (Dolle, Bataillard, & Guyon, 1973–1974; Dolle, Bataillard, & Lacroix, 1974–1975; Dolle, Vinter, & Germain, 1974–1975; Olson, 1970). This capacity for using the diagonal systematically is an important developmental phase because it indicates a consolidation of projective concepts of space and the capacity to represent fully volume, depth and perspective. The ability to go beyond the invariant dimensions of horizontal and vertical is based on the establishment of the concept of the self as an object unique among all other objects. The development of projective concepts of space and the utilization of the unstable structure of the diagonal requires the consolidation of the self as a highly unique and stable reference point.

While there is often a loss of depth in the receding picture plane in Mannerism, there are occasional expressions of a diagonal structure that attempt to "transform a broad canvas into a tunnel boring deeply into the background" and "break through the different levels and bore yawning holes into the background" (Hauser, 1965, pp. 158, 174). An excellent example of the diagonal structure in Mannerism is

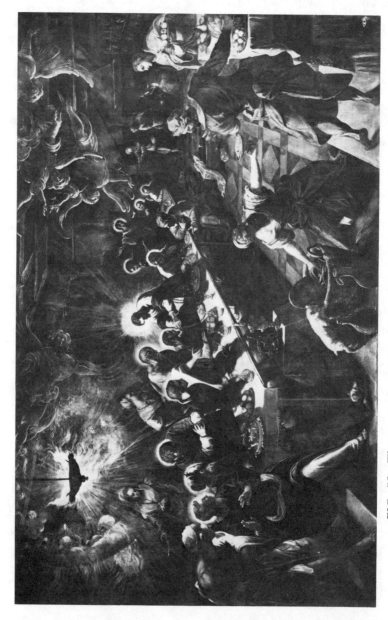

FIG. 58 Tintoretto, *Last Supper* (1592–94), S. Giorgio Maggiore, Venice (Alinari).

Tintoretto's *Last Supper* (Fig. 58). A comparison of the *Last Supper* by Tintoretto with that of Leonardo highlights a number of features of Mannerism. In Leonardo's *Last Supper* (see Fig. 48, page 228), linear perspective occurs in a symmetrical composition with Christ at the vanishing point. There is a horizontal, frontally oriented table and a background wall that supports the centrality of the Christ figure. All shapes and edges of the room lead to this central vanishing point in a symmetrical, balanced, and harmonious composition. Typical of Renaissance art, the light is from a single source, bright and uniform throughout the entire foreground. Tintoretto's *Last Supper,* in contrast, is full of depth and tension. The vanishing point has been shifted from the center to the side. After the first horizontal grouping, the diagonal composition is used dramatically. A dynamic sense of depth and excitement is enhanced by a differentiated and focused use of lighting and deep contrasts of light and dark. There are multiple sources of light. One ray coming from the front of the picture penetrates the scene and powerfully emphasizes the diagonal. Another bursts in from the side and creates deep recesses of light and shadow. A third source of light emanates from haloes that serve to highlight dramatically Christ and the Apostles. This dramatic use of light opened space to create a new sense of infinite depth and passion that was to be developed more fully in the Baroque.

In many ways, Mannerism was an extension of the representation of subjectivity begun in linear perspective during the Renaissance. Linear perspective, in its representation of how a scene appears to a spectator, was attempting an "objectification of the subjective" (Panofsky, 1924/25). This subjectivity was elaborated further in Mannerism by the introduction of the diagonal composition and by the dramatic use of lighting for emotional expression. The emphasis on the diagonal first appeared at a time when artists were seeking new and different ways to express volume and depth after having established the operational basis for linear perspective in the Renaissance. Diagonal compositions create an even greater sense of the representation of subjective experience. And the attempt to represent emotional expression through the dramatic use of light and shading is yet another example of the increased representation of subjective experiences in Mannerism. Friedlaender (1958, p. 8), in fact, considers the entire orientation of Mannerism to be toward the representation of "an inner artistic reworking on the basis of harmonic or rhythmical requirements," rather than mathematical attempts to establish idealized forms of beauty. Mannerism aimed to reconstruct the subjective experience from inside out; things are not represented as they are seen from an ideal perspective, but as they are experienced at a particular moment and under specific conditions. Canonical form is relinquished in favor of a new subjective creativity. The abstract and the internal are emphasized rather than the manifest and the external.

The use of variations of light, shadow, and color to express subjective experiences beginning in the Renaissance and Mannerism and culminating in the Baroque is similar to sequences noted earlier in the development of Greco-Roman art. In both epochs the representation of universal, idealized, eternal human form is followed by an interest in naturalistic representation based on the perceptual experience of the viewer. This interest in naturalism and perspective led to an interest in representing unique figures with specific physical characteristics, emotions, and actions. The representation of subjective experience in both these epochs was coincident with a basic emphasis on humanism that pervaded the societies. This fundamental interest and respect for the individual was not only expressed in the form and content of art, but in the recognition of individual artists. It was during these two epochs that artists first began to sign their works and there was an interest in the biographies of artists (Kris, 1952; Kris & Kurz, 1934/1979).

THE BAROQUE

After the High Renaissance and the transitional period of Mannerism, a dramatic development in style appeared, conceptualized as the Baroque. Wölfflin (1888/1964) in his seminal contribution to the concept of style in the history of art, contrasts Renaissance with Baroque art along several basic dimensions. Renaissance art is characterized by a "linear" style with sharp, unbroken, well-delineated boundaries and contours that made individual objects and figures appear substantial, solid, and tangible. Baroque art, in contrast, has a "painterly" style of broad, great masses presented with tentative lines, minimal contour, and an emphasis on shadings of light and dark, enriching the sense of depth in the picture plane. Because of the vaguely defined boundaries, individual figures blend into a composite whole. The closed, tectonic structure of the Renaissance, based on linear perspective with sharply articulated forms and definite horizontals and verticals, became a more open, atectonic composition that de-emphasized sharply articulated forms and the invariant structures of horizontals and verticals (Goldmeier, 1972). The symmetrical, pyramidal, balanced composition of the Renaissance was replaced by asymmetrical compositions in which the more variable structure of the oblique or the diagonal created a dynamic tension among different parts of the painting. The painterly style and the diagonal composition of Baroque art created a sense of infinite depth.

Wölfflin (1898/1928, 1888/1964) and Riegl (1901) discussed classical Renaissance composition as a harmony of highly articulated separate and independent parts; Baroque painting, in contrast, has an organic unity in which all elements are subordinated to a single dominant theme. The continuity of the total composition is emphasized rather than the clarity and definition of separate parts. Renaissance art achieved depth and dimensionality with the use of linear perspective and an emphasis on the sharp articulation of the relative shape, size, and position of objects in a series of planes. Baroque art achieved an even greater sense of depth and dimensionality by integrating foreshortening and the linear and atmospheric perspective of the Italian Renaissance with the use of asymmetrical unifying diagonals, and variations in light and dark that enriched and enhanced spatial recession. Colors had been sharply differentiated in Renaissance art, but now in the Baroque they began to merge and complement each other, and there was an emphasis on chiaroscuro, the subtle variations of shading. The use of shading was a major aspect of the Baroque and it created emotional highlighting, a sense of tension and excitement, deep, intimate, emotional tones, and an enriched representation of volume and depth. The Baroque was a major step in the development of "subjective objectivism" (Frankl, 1960; Panofsky 1924/25) that began in the Renaissance and culminated in Impressionism. Baroque "oblique" space (Panofsky, 1960/1972) and the representation of inner psychological states such as affects, moods, and emotions, each contributed in an interrelated way to the creation of this subjective objectivism. The Baroque was an extension of trends begun in the Renaissance and continued through Mannerism. This was true not only in art but also in general attitudes and philosophy. Preoccupation with divine authority was increasingly replaced by scientific inquiry, curiosity, exploration, and a respect for and an emphasis on the dignity and individuality of man. After long strife and civil wars,

political stability was finally achieved throughout Europe. The economically flourishing city-states, initiated at the beginning of the Renaissance, were replaced in the 16th century by nation-states that
provided an even broader base for economic growth and the development of an urban middle class. The Baroque, though an international style, had its primary impetus in Holland in the middle of the
17th century. Holland was essentially a burgher society, economically
and politically stable, and a center of intellectual activity. Protes-
tantism, prevalent in Holland and Germany, placed increased emphasis upon the individual. Responsibility for personal grace and
salvation shifted from the church and clergy to the individual, resulting in increased self-awareness and a sense of personal significance
(Weber, 1958). The 17th century was also a period of remarkable
progress in mathematics and science. Important scientific developments and discoveries included the invention of the telescope
and microscope, and the theoretical formulations of Kepler, Galileo,
Descartes, and Newton. Throughout this Age of Reason, concepts of
God, nature, man, and reason were interrelated; reason and knowledge were the vehicles for achieving freedom and happiness.

An early major figure in the development of Baroque art was
Caravaggio, who first made dramatic use of light to emphasize a portion of the picture plane. Caravaggio had a shaft of light coming into
the picture at an angle highlighting a particular figure or feature in
the painting. The shaft of light coming into the picture from an
external source was one of the first forms in which the diagonal structure was introduced into Baroque art. Caravaggio, like Tintoretto,
used diagonal lighting to give paintings an intense emotionality and a
heightened tension (Friedlaender, 1955). This dramatic use of lighting to spotlight a figure established the picture as taking place at a
precise moment in time, in contrast to the timelessness of Renaissance
painting.[20] Thus the function of art changed once again. Initially art
served as a ritualistic preservation of life, later it was a presentation of
a sacred narrative, and now it served as a dramatic evocation of a
particular event and moment in time (Gombrich, 1977).

Caravaggio and his followers used light in strong and intense con-

---

[20] The same distinction occurs in sculpture. Michelangelo's Renaissance
David, for example, is rigid, unmoving and eternal, whereas Bernini's Baroque *David* is captured at a particular moment in an action sequence, as the
sling is about to unfold and hurl the rock.

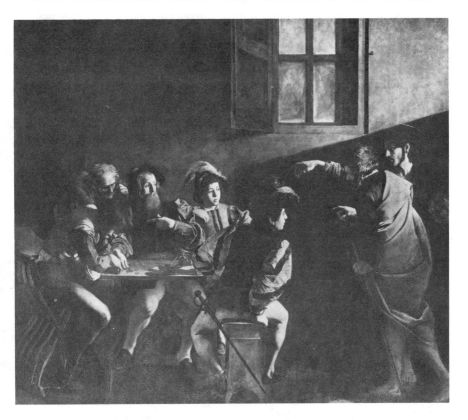

FIG. 59 Caravaggio, *Calling of St. Matthew* (1597–1600), Contarelli Chapel, S. Luigi dei Francesi, Rome (Alinari).

trast with little transition. Sharp boundaries between the illuminated figures and the parts in the shadow created clear contours in which objects stood as separate, well-sculptured figures against a dark and rather spaceless background (Friedlaender, 1955). In the Renaissance, light was generally uniform throughout the composition, with shadows used primarily to convey roundness and volume. Caravaggio (Fig. 59) used light in an intense form, as a spotlight to create deep contrasts of light and dark and a sense of depth and excitement. Shading and shadows also added to the representation of volume and depth. Shading, however, had to be integrated with color as a modification of hue. Wölfflin points out that while Leonardo was the father of chiaroscuro, he had difficulty integrating it with his sensitivity to color. The integration of shading and color began in Mannerism and the Baroque with Titian. Titian separated planes in space by

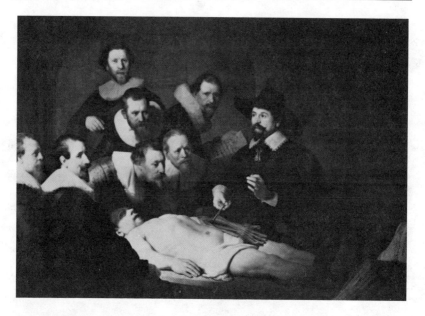

FIG. 60   Rembrandt, *The Anatomy Lesson of Dr. Tulp* (1632) (Mauritshuis, The Hague).

gradual lighting and darkening, and he used these differences to create gradients (Arnheim, 1954/1974). Although chiaroscuro had been used earlier by Leonardo and the 16th century Venetians (e.g., Titian), Caravaggio was the first to create a style based on chiaroscuro as a predominant feature (Rosenberg, Slive, & ter Kuile, 1966/1972).

Caravaggio had a strong impact on Rembrandt. Initially, Rembrandt used light very much like Caravaggio, as a way of highlighting a particular aspect. In one of Rembrandt's early paintings, *The Anatomy Lesson of Dr. Tulp,* (Fig. 60) chiaroscuro was used as a sharp external spotlight for dramatic effect. It gave the painting intensity and excitement and signaled the appearance of an event of extraordinary importance. Rembrandt went on to use chiaroscuro in increasingly subtle ways. As his work matured, Rembrandt's use of chiaroscuro became more powerful and intense. Light with deep shadows was interwoven into a rich harmony of subtle and strong tones. Nuances of light and shadow, independent of an external source, began to capture internal affective states and emotional tone. Faces and figures "appear to glow from within wherever their significance requires special attraction. A general atmosphere is created in which we become aware of the most subtle inner emotions"

(Rosenberg et al., 1966/1972, p. 115). Chiaroscuro became a powerful tool for the representation of emotional expression; it enabled Rembrandt to create an atmosphere in which there was an intimate and inseparable sharing between the figure and the surrounding space in an atmosphere of emotional and spiritual meaning. Chiaroscuro dominated Rembrandt's art from the very beginning. Throughout his work, Rembrandt made increasing commitment to chiaroscuro as a guiding stylistic principle. It enabled him to express the emotional and spiritual values that stood in marked contrast to the posed attitudes, rigid abstraction, and isolation of the idealized and universal classical figures of the Renaissance (Rosenberg, et al., 1966/1972). Rembrandt's use of chiaroscuro enabled him to portray inner psychological states that are knowable only through intuition, identification, and empathy (Kohut, 1959). Rembrandt's figures are unclear; their boundaries are vague, broken, poorly defined, and only partially visible. The use of light and shadow is suggestive and provocative, creating imperceptible transitions from the finite to the infinite, and an air of mystery. Nothing is isolated or overly distinct in the cohesive interdependence of parts. A sense of unity is achieved through a subordination of individual forms and figures to the more comprehensive elements of space, atmosphere, and chiaroscuro (Rosenberg et al., 1966/1972). The discovery and consolidation of the principles of linear perspective enabled Rembrandt to relinquish an emphasis on boundaries and contours and to replace the representation of clearly articulated figures with the representation of subtle nuances. In developmental psychological terms, the consolidation of projective concepts of space diminished the necessity for relying on topological concepts of space. This provided greater freedom for artistic representation.

In addition to chiaroscuro, Rembrandt integrated coloristic variations that enriched the deep emotional tones achieved with chiaroscuro. A radical change then took place in the mature Rembrandt. As Rosenberg et al. (1966/1977) state, Rembrandt's use of color

> not only acquires increasing warmth and intensity; it becomes a living, moving, substance which ebbs and flows through space. . . . It produces the impression of a dynamic inner connexion between all substances, and links the subjects with their mysterious dark background and even with infinite space. . . . Thus, it is chiefly in his colour and chiaroscuro that the Baroque dynamism lives on in his paintings, but it is restrained by a classical simplicity and dignity of setting (pp. 117–118).

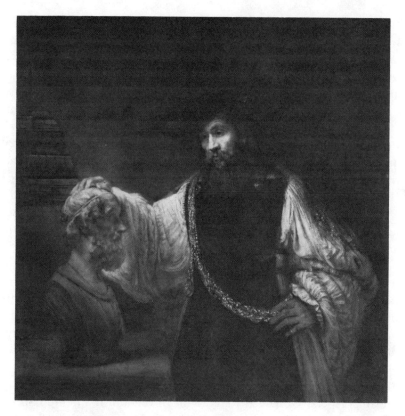

FIG. 61   Rembrandt, *Aristotle with a Bust of Homer* (1653) (The Metropolitan Museum of Art, purchased with special funds and gifts of friends of the Museum, 1961).

Expressive lighting and subtle variation in shading and color helped to create an air of excitement and to communicate nuances of emotion and meaning.

Rembrandt flourished at the height of the Baroque period in Holland. He often painted common people and was interested in capturing the expression of their spirituality and psychological states. Psychological insight, spiritual awareness, emotion, sensitivity, and compassion toward human experiences enriched Rembrandt's realism. For Rembrandt, the essence of man was the essence of nature. Rembrandt's *Aristotle with a Bust of Homer* (Fig. 61) expresses his deep sensitivity and his appreciation of spirituality, contemplation, emotionality, and the importance of cultural continuity.

Another major development of Baroque art was the elaboration of "near" space as well as the representation of space as unified, vast, and unlimited. Panofsky (1924/25) distinguished the "near" and "oblique" space of the Baroque from the symmetrical organization of space in the Renaissance. Rubens (e.g., *Fall of the Damned*, c. 1620) (Fig. 62) portrayed near space that recedes into shadow and mystery. Rubens integrated his figures into the landscape and, like Rembrandt, used chiaroscuro and coloristic variations to represent subtle psychological states.

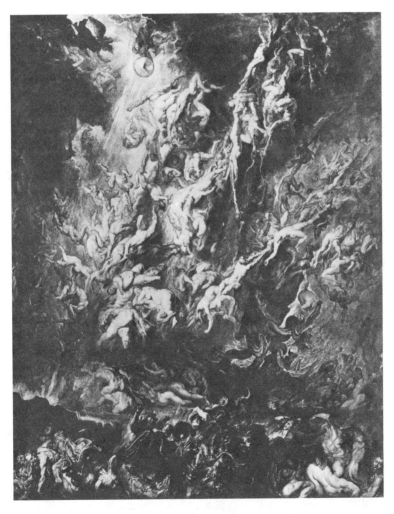

FIG. 62 Rubens, *Fall of the Damned* (c.1620), alte Pinakothek, Munich (Giraudon).

Other major figures in the Baroque, such as the Dutch artists Vermeer, De Hooch, and Steen, were particularly effective in establishing perspective in near space. Vermeer (Fig. 63) was concerned about the relationship between figures and space and was able to achieve an impressive balance between the two. Spatial recession was greatly enhanced by the rich gradations of color and the subtle variations of light, particularly with intense light in the distance in contrast to a darkened foreground. Light became more muted and subtle. The sun's rays in Vermeer and De Hooch paintings sparkle in the environment, cast shadows, give illumination and radiance, and provide vitality and a sense of time. The specific patterns of light and shade make it clear that the scene is occurring at a particular moment in a sequence of everyday events. In these later Dutch masters, the figures and the contexts are usually commonplace and often involve trivial

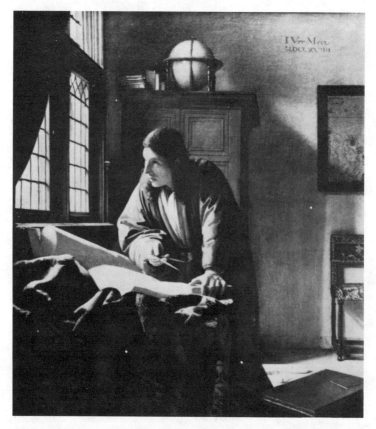

FIG. 63   Vermeer, *Geographer* (Frankfurt Studelsches Kunstinstitut).

occasions. The paintings are of real people involved in daily life with whom the spectator can readily identify. Figures are no longer universal, ideal, or generalized as they were in the Renaissance, but are real people expressing a wide range of emotions, especially those of peace and harmony (Held & Posner, 1971).

Baroque paintings created a new relationship of figure to embedding space. Objects moved about freely in intermediate space. Pieter De Hooch, a contemporary of Vermeer, explored extensively the relationship of figure to space. His elaborate spatial constructions, with open doors and windows, permitted recessions into near space. De Hooch (Fig. 64) relied heavily on rectilinear forms such as doors or windows to frame his figures and to allow the viewer to look across space into the next room or courtyard. De Hooch's colors were warm and intense, and his light from multiple sources created deep contrasts and shadows that dramatically enrich and expand the representation of space. Vermeer, De Hooch, Steen, and others often moved figures from the foreground to the background or placed them in *repoussier,* so that a dark figure appeared with light behind it to give an added sense of depth. Tiled floors, open windows and doors, as well as figures in the background, all increased the sense of depth in the near space of relatively small rooms (Wheelock, 1977).

In Baroque painting, near and remote space were unified, and the spectator's space was also integrated with the space in the picture (Held & Posner, 1971). The integration of picture space with that of the space of the spectator is well illustrated in Velasquez' *The Maids of Honor* (1656) (Fig. 65). The presence of the king and queen is indicated at the border between the spectator and the picture plane by their reflection in the mirror on the far wall of the painting. The spectator must identify with the apparent position of the king and queen since it is identical with the spectator's position. The integration of the spectator's space with the space of the picture began in Baroque art and continued in Impressionism (e.g., Manet's *A Bar at the Folies Bergère*) (Fig. 66).

Another aspect of the preoccupation with space in Baroque art was the representation of space as vast and unlimited. Numerous Baroque artists, such as Claude Lorraine and Nicolas Poussin, utilized principles of foreshortening, linear and atmospheric perspective, asymmetrical oblique compositions, and the subtle gradations of chiaroscuro and color, to achieve a remarkable sense of spatial depth in remote as well as near space. Claude Lorraine used vaporous haze to

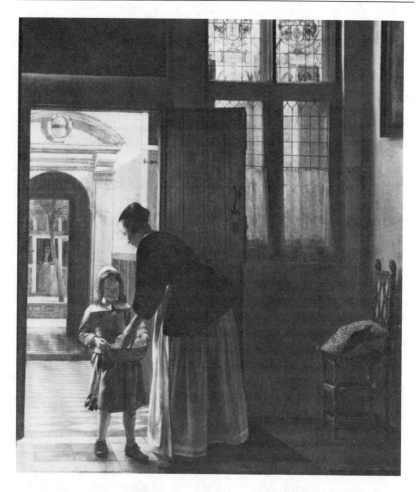

FIG. 64   De Hooch, *A Boy Bringing Pomegranates* (1660–1663), (The Wallace Collection).

represent distant and majestic horizons, and Poussin represented unlimited spatial expanse. A majestic landscape by Koninck (Fig. 67) illustrates distant space in a limitless landscape. Subsequently, landscapes included large foreground features that obscured elements of this distant space and created a striking juxtaposition of elements of near and distant space. Claude Lorrain's *The Judgment of Paris* (Fig. 68) illustrates how space could become fragmented and discontinuous in a composition still integrated according to principles of linear perspective. Asymmetrical organization along with this spatial fragmentation created landscapes that were no longer precisely coherent and integrated but became arbitrarily selected segments of natural settings (Galassi, 1981).

Numerous other examples of Baroque artists creating a sense of infinite space include ceiling paintings "of a frankly open world that goes on forever" (Arnheim, 1954/1974, p. 298), elaborate interiors of vast inner spaces in churches (see Fig. 69) and landscapes, such as those by Jacob van Ruysdael and Jan van Goyen, that used diagonal compositions along with tonal contrasts of dark foreground accented against luminous background openings in the sky to create a sense of great volume. Ruysdael (Fig. 70) integrated tectonic and atectonic forms, static horizontals and verticals, dynamic diagonals, vivid colors, and atmospheric accents to create "a mighty spaciousness" and a rich

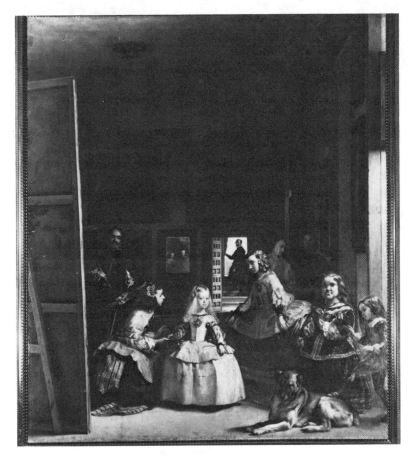

FIG. 65 Velasquez, *The Maids of Honor* (1656), Prado, Madrid (Giraudon).

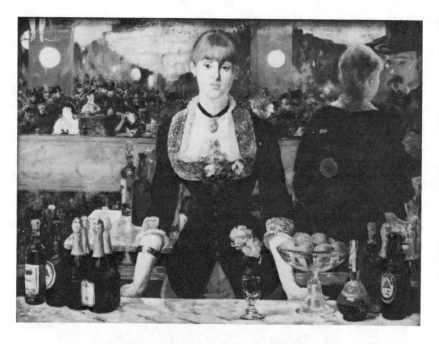

FIG. 66   Manet, *A Bar at the Folies Bergère* (1882), Courtauld Institute Gallery (Courtauld Institute, London).

three-dimensionality (Rosenberg et al., 1966/1972, pp. 262–264). Formal compositional factors, such as asymmetry, diagonals, and atectonic structure, and atmospheric factors, such as chiaroscuro and color, contributed to the capacity to represent effectively spatial recession in both near and far space. The Baroque emphasis on chiaroscuro and coloristic atmospheric dimensions provided the basis for the subsequent work of Turner and Constable, which in turn eventually provided the basis for Impressionism, late in the 19th century.

The preoccupation of Baroque artists with the representation of depth was also indicated by their continued experimentation with the distortions of perspective, including the anamorphosis that had started during the Mannerist period and the construction of "peep shows" inside boxes, which created a compelling *trompe l'oeil* when viewed from a tiny hole in the box. There was a remarkable elaboration of the representation of space in Baroque art with the development of open, atectonic, asymmetrical compositions organized around the dynamic structure of the oblique. This expanded sense of space was enriched further by the development of a painterly style in which figures were presented with tentative lines, minimal contours,

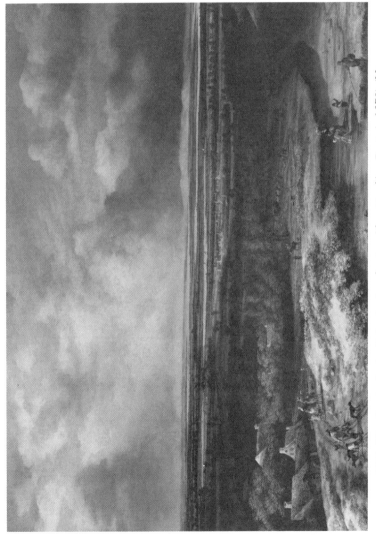

FIG. 67 Koninck, *An Extensive Landscape with a Hawking Party* (c.1670) (National Gallery, London).

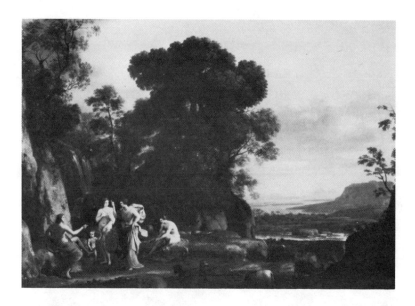

FIG. 68   Claude Lorraine, *The Judgment of Paris* (1645–46) (National Gallery, Washington, D.C.).

and an emphasis and preoccupation with chiaroscuro. Linear perspective was elaborated in the representation of complex interlocking of near space with the endless expanse of vast landscapes.

Mannerism and the Baroque were periods of experimentation with the procedures of linear perspective. Artists attempted to integrate the principles of the perspective system with new dimensions. The regular, balanced, symmetrical structure that initially characterized linear perspective in the Renaissance was extended in Mannerism and the Baroque to asymmetrical compositions constructed on the diagonal or the oblique. Baroque artists then added chiaroscuro to extend recession into space and to capture the emotional tones of an immediate event. Painting became a depiction of a segment of the continuous flow of everyday life rather than a static and fixed image of an ideal, eternal scene.

According to developmental psychological theory, the advances in representation in Baroque art are an elaboration and progression of concrete operations. Early in the Renaissance, representations were organized intuitively without the specification of the operations of linear perspective. Later in the Renaissance, artists discovered the mathematical operations for linear perspective, and for the systematic

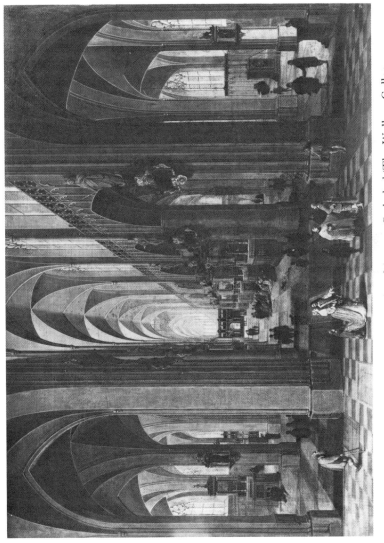

FIG. 69 Neefs, The Elder, *Interior of Antwerp Cathedral* (The Wallace Collection, London).

271

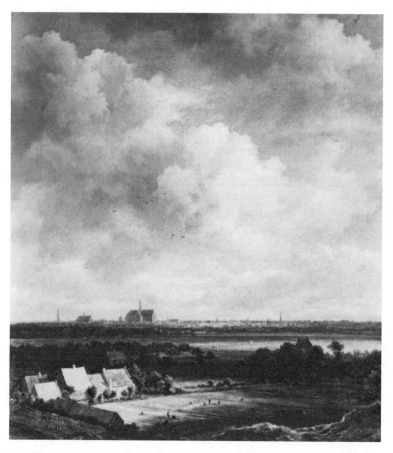

FIG. 70   J. van Ruysdael, *View of Haarlem* (c.1670) (Rijksmuseum, Amsterdam).

and integrated representation of manifest forms and features of objects. Perspective in the Renaissance, however, was expressed primarily in symmetrical compositions based on the stable and invariant dimensions of horizontal and vertical. Objects, though coordinated within the setting, were still well-defined and sharply delineated. Figures were drawn with firm, unbroken boundaries and contours and clearly differentiated from their surroundings. The sharp boundaries of figures indicated a continued reliance on topological concepts of space with the vestiges of a conception of space as discontinuous and nonhomogeneous.

Advances in the mode of representing space in Baroque art are indicated by the relinquishing of the emphasis upon the topological spatial concepts of boundary and contour. Baroque figures were represented with tentative lines and minimal contour, boundaries were vague and individual figures began to blend into the composition. With the further development of projective concepts of space, perspective could be used without the support of spatial constructs from the earlier topological stage. The development and consolidation of the techniques and theory of linear perspective enabled Baroque artists to relinquish an emphasis on contours and boundaries. Space was now homogeneous, based on subtle gradations and blendings, rather than containing discontinuities.

In Baroque art, there was also a shift to asymmetrical compositions based on the utilization of the diagonal. In individual psychological development, the representation of the diagonal occurs in the later phases of the development of projective concepts of space (Dolle, Bataillard & Guyon, 1973–74; Dolle, Bataillard, & Lacroix, 1974–75; Dolle, Vinter, & Germain, 1974–75; Olson, 1970). The representation of the diagonal involves the capacity to utilize deviations from the invariant dimensions of horizontal and vertical (Goldmeier, 1972). The diagonal or the oblique is a dynamic structure that creates a sense of tension in the representational field (Arnheim, 1954/1974) and enhances the representation of spatial recession into infinite space. The representation of the diagonal is a consolidation of perspective and an essential component of advanced concepts of projective space. Perspective within asymmetrical compositions utilizing the diagonal is another indication of the progress made in the modes of representation during the Baroque.

Because of the instability of the diagonal and the tendency for it to revert to the more stable invariant dimensions of horizontal and vertical, the representation of the diagonal requires the development of the sense of self as a unique and consistent reference point. As demonstrated by the psychological research on field independence (Witkin, 1965), the establishment of the self as a stable referent is a central factor in the ability to resist relying solely upon compelling perceptual cues immediately available in the environment. With the self as a stable and independent reference point, the individual is able to represent diagonal construction because he or she no longer needs to rely on the more compelling and stable perceptual dimensions of horizontal and vertical (Dolle, Bataillard, & Guyon, 1973–74; Dolle, Bataillard, & Lacroix, 1974–75; Dolle, Vinter, & Germain, 1974–75).

The sense of self as a stable reference point is not only a major factor in the representation of three-dimensional space, but is also central to the articulation of affects and emotional reactions. A "reflective self-awareness" is essential if affect is to become an important dimension of experience (Schafer, 1968). A sense of self is necessary for an appreciation of affective nuances and subtleties, particularly in an interpersonal matrix. Empathy and introspection (Kohut, 1959; Schafer, 1959) are essential components of the capacity to become aware of one's own feelings and to share in the feelings of others. Sensitivity to affective and interpersonal nuances, the capacity for empathy and assuming the role of others, is correlated with concrete operational thought and the ability to represent perspective (Feffer, 1959, 1967, 1970). It is consistent with developmental psychological theory that the use of concrete operational modes of representation and the consolidation of projective concepts of space (e.g., the use of the diagonal) in the Baroque should be accompanied by an increased interest in and a capacity for representing affects and emotions, particularly in interpersonal contexts. This increased emphasis on subjective experience in Baroque art is also consistent with greater emphasis in the society on individualism and the shift of responsibility for individual grace and salvation from the Church to personally within the individual.

In Baroque art, figures are no longer universal, external and ideal but are specific, personal, and unique, involved in particular everyday activities. A sense of time is introduced, either in the representation of a dramatic event or of a particular moment in a familiar sequence. The content of art is no longer distant, eternal, and universal but concerned with more subtle and personal experiences that an observer can come to know through empathy and introspection. The representation of emotion in Baroque art was initially bold and dramatic. Subsequently, subtle nuances of affects and feelings were represented through the sensitive modulation of chiaroscuro and color. Depiction of concrete manifest form and features was deeply enriched and extended by the representation of subtle affective tones. Artists sought to capture the inner psychological world of affects and emotions. Paintings were no longer an object to be perceived, but an experience to be shared. The artist, the depicted figure, and the observer, all became participants in a dynamic field.

The emphasis upon inner experiences, emotions, and affects indicates that the representation of concrete, manifest features and form are being extended to the representation of more abstract, internal dimensions and experience. In Piaget's developmental theory, this indicates that concrete operational modes of representation are being extended to formal operational modes that deal with abstract internal dimensions in addition to manifest form. This attention to inner form, structure, and meaning eventually led to Impressionism and its search for the internal constituent elements of light and color that comprise perceptual experiences. Impressionism sought to capture the inner form and structure of perceptual events. The search for the articulation and representation of inner form and structure, first in the Baroque and later in Impressionism, was the beginning of a shift to more formal operational, abstract modes of representation.

PARALLEL DEVELOPMENT IN RENAISSANCE AND BAROQUE ART AND SCIENCE

The struggles in art to discover the central vanishing point for the representation of recession in depth and for establishing integrated and coherent compositions coincided with controversies in natural philosophy about the earth as the center of the solar system and the possibility of the infinity of the universe. The development of linear perspective in art, like developments in Renaissance and Baroque science, was part of an evolving conception of space as homogeneous, isotropic, and infinite. A quantitative coordinate system provided the mathematical basis for the systematic integration of a multitude of objects within an embedding context of space in art and science.

These developments were part of a basic change in the conception of man's position in nature. The representation of depth and infinity in the picture plane involved a fundamental reconsideration of the individual's place in reality. The discovery of the central vanishing point within the picture plane occurred during the same time period that Nicholas Cardinal of Cusa and Giordano Bruno reconsidered the issues of infinity in natural philosophy, Copernicus developed a revolutionary reformulation of the organization of the planetary system, and Descartes developed a spatial coordinate system (Butterfield, 1957; Koyré, 1957; Panofsky, 1924/25, 1960). Alberti's development of the concepts of linear perspective and the Copernican reformulation of the organization of the solar system were expressions of an emerging quantification of space derived from modifications and revisions of a qualitative conception of space expressed, for example, in the formulations of Ptolemy. This new conception of space as homogeneous, isotropic, and infinite emerged in art in the late 15th and 16th centuries and in science throughout the 16th and 17th centuries. In developmental psychological terms, the development of linear perspective and the shift from a geocentric to a heliocentric conception of the universe involved a fundamental decentration from a basic egocentrism and a shift from a preoperational, intuitive mode of representation to a new, more advanced operational mode of representation involving a coordination of dimensions and the capacity for transformations with reversibility and conservation.

Riegl (1901) used the concepts of haptic (tactile) and optic (visual) modes of representation to describe developments within both Classic and Renaissance art and the long-term development from Ancient to Renaissance and Baroque art. Strikingly, the same categories have been applied by Van Hoorn to the contrast between Classical and Renaissance geometry. According to Van Hoorn (1972):

> Aristotle's description of space as the adjacent *boundary* of the containing body seems to allude to the definite two-dimensional character of space. Greek geometry, I would like to suggest, was perhaps so much confined to the plane because the Greeks possessed a *tactile-muscular intuition* of space. The visual intuition of space, so characteristic for the Renaissance, is essentially tridimensional. After all, even Euclid's *Elements* show that a science of solid geometry had hardly been developed in Greek Antiquity. (p. 99)

Van Hoorn qualifies his generalization about Aristotle by acknowledging that Aristotle considers both place and body as bounded by the three dimensions of length, breadth, and depth. But despite these considerations about concrete objects in the *Physics*, space, as discussed by Aristotle in *De Caelo* (On the Heavens), remains topological, spherical, and bounded.

New concepts of space evolved from a confluence of several different lines of development including a new instrument, the telescope; a mathematical rather than teleological concept of God; and a revival of Platonic philosophy in an eclectic theology that identified both God and space as infinitely extended (Koyré, 1957; Lovejoy, 1964).

During the Middle Ages and the early Renaissance, various aspects of Greek culture were rediscovered, not only in new—and occasionally contradictory—Aristotelian texts and their Islamic additions and amendments, but also in atomistic and Platonic philosophies over which Aristotelian thought had prevailed.[21] These philosophies placed a premium on mathematical (particularly geometrical) reasoning. The atomists had also held the belief that space was infinite, and the extent to which the atomists' philosophy influenced developments in the Renaissance is still a matter of historical debate.

Renaissance figures such as Nicholas of Cusa, Copernicus, Bruno, Kepler, and Galileo rejected successive elements of the Aristotelian system and substituted in their place a belief in an unbounded universe. Descartes and Newton finally conceived of the universe as explicitly infinite, insofar as they interpreted space mathematically. But earlier, Nicholas of Cusa, Copernicus, Bruno, and even Kepler used essentially Aristotelian methods of scholastic debate, along with a gradually increased emphasis on mathematical reasoning, to resolve traditional Medieval problems on the boundedness or the infinity of the universe, the relationship between the place of the universe and astronomical space, and the mathematical exactness of the geocentric scheme for the motion of heavenly bodies. Much of the debate turned, at the outset, on specifying the cosmological implications of God's perfection. Nicholas of Cusa (in *Learned Ignorance*, 1440), for example, argued that contrary to the closed world of Aristotle, the universe is boundless and that the earth moves (although he did not propose a heliocentric system). He based these ideas on the theological notions that God is everywhere and that the created world is inexact and imperfect. In the latter argument, Cusanus recalled Plato's view that reality is only an imperfect realization of the perfection of pure ideas. But his views had little immediate impact on or consequence for cosmology or astronomy (Koyré, 1957).

Renaissance philosophical thought concentrated on the dignity of man and the attempt to understand the whole of nature within a

---

[21] Koyré (1957, p. 5) observes that "the infinitist conceptions of the Greek atomists were rejected by the main trend, or trends, of Greek philosophical and scientific thought—the Epicurean tradition was not a scientific one—and that for this very reason, though never forgotten, they could not be accepted by the mediaevals." He adds, by way of amplification (p. 278, n7), that the scientific sterility of ancient atomism "lies, in my opinion, in the extreme sensualism of the Epicurean tradition; it is only when this sensualism was rejected by the founders of modern science and replaced by a mathematical approach to nature that atomism—in the works of Galileo, R. Boyle, Newton, etc.—became a scientifically valid conception."

unified explanatory system. Philosophers attempted to eliminate conceptions of nature based on transcendental influences such as the activities of spirits and demons or even the capricious intervention of God himself, and instead to seek the explanation of all natural phenomena within a system of nature that was self-sufficient and guided by basic principles and laws (Butterfield, 1957). Copernicus provided the initial structure for the eventual development of a comprehensive system of the universe that explained the movement of the earth and other planets. Copernicus in his great work, *de Revolutionibus Orbium* shifted the sun to the center of the universe and set the earth in motion among the other planets in order to solve a set of mathematical problems existing in the geocentric conception that Ptolemy had elaborated from the Aristotelian system. Copernicus was persuaded of the correctness of his heliocentric system partly on the basis of a mathematical aesthetic of simplicity; a heliocentric system allowed Copernicus to reduce the number of epicycles—ad hoc corrective suborbits that had been incorporated by Ptolemy to account for the irregular departure (and retrograde motion) of the planets from perfectly circular orbits.

The stability achieved in art in the development of linear perspective and in cosmology in Copernicus' reformulation of the structure of the universe was soon to be challenged. Concepts of linear perspective began to be questioned in art as Mannerist and Baroque artists attempted to find new ways to express volume and depth in deliberate experimentation with transformations of space. Linear perspective continued to be controversial; it was viewed as too technical and mechanical and concern was voiced about a loss of the individual emphasis of the artist because of dominant concerns for perspective space (Chastel, 1977). The same types of challenge of dogma were also reflected in science. Butterfield (1957, p. 108) discusses the revolutionary quality of the late 16th and early 17th century science as they recognized the need for a scientific revolution "not merely for an explanation of existing anomalies but for a new science and a new method." There were, for instance, continuing astronomical difficulties with Copernicus' conservative reformulation of the world system. Copernicus essentially had remained bound by many of the major philosophical and contextual assumptions of the Greeks and Medieval astronomy and cosmology such as the sphericity of the universe, the treatment of the world system planet by planet rather than as a unified and integrated system, and the continuing reliance on scholastic, as well as mathematical, arguments, all in relation to a teleological concept of God. Like Renaissance perspective, Copernican astronomy had the dual sense of recapitulation and rationalization of a traditional system, as well as of revolution. With the earth displaced from the center of the universe by the sun, it became possible to imagine other stars as the centers of other worlds in an infinite universe. Giordano Bruno, and then Galileo Galilei, were quick to seize on the implications of Copernicus' system that the stars must be extremely far away, that space is probably infinite in its extent and that there is no good reason to think of our own sun as the center of the only world in the universe. Bruno, toward the end of the 16th century, used the same intellectual strategy as Nicholas of Cusa—the scholastic method of considering the implications of God's perfection for cosmology and an increased emphasis on reason to correct the limitations of sensation. He argued that the universe is not simply boundless but is "of indefinite size and the worlds therein without number" (cited by Koyré, 1957, p. 49).

Kepler was forced by Tycho Brahe's systematic and detailed observations to abandon his planetary system of circular orbits of nested perfect geometric solids to formulate a planetary system based on elliptical orbits. Kepler's recomputations and formulations of elliptical orbits represented a search for a new foundation on which to construct a mathematical astronomy—based on a liberation not only from a bounded universe but a spherical one with circular orbits. For the first time in a millennium, there was an infusion of elements of Neo-Platonic and other philosophies rather than a further development along essentially Aristotelian lines. Kepler, in fact, stressed that the primary difference between his concepts of science and those of Aristotle was his emphasis on the importance of quantitative characteristics in understanding nature in contrast to Aristotle's use of qualitative distinctions (Burtt, 1931/1954). Rankings of intensity of qualities gave way to the accurate measurement of quantities and the development of the specification of exact functional relationships. Although Kepler made no reference to governing forces, he described precisely the motion of planets as a constant ellipse around the sun in which there was a direct proportion between the speed of the orbit around the sun and its average distance from the sun. In Kepler's formulations there was a shift from qualitative, ordinal differentiations to the quantitative measurement of an interval scale.

Although Kepler devised a more precise mathematical formulation for Copernicus' organization of the sun and the planets, Kepler considered infinity as an improper astronomical concept since it was not observable. Not even the unprecedented extensive use of mathematics and accurate astronomical observations of Tycho Brahe persuaded Kepler of the infinity of the universe. In addition, infinity implied a uniform distribution of stars, which did not seem to fit observations that the stars were quite far from the earth, yet clustered close to one another in the outermost reaches of the heavens. While it has been suggested that Galileo's telescopic observations in 1610 must have been decisive for the acceptance of the concept of an infinite universe because they showed a plethora of stars formerly unseen, these observations in fact only reassured Kepler of the lack of homogeneity in the distribution of stars in the universe. Moreover, the telescopic observations did not even move Galileo himself to a belief in the infinity of the universe. For the most part, he avoided the issue altogether, focusing instead on justifying the Copernican system and avoiding the heresy of Bruno's doctrine of a plurality of worlds in infinite space. While Galileo rejected a belief in a containing sphere or orb of fixed stars, he only went so far as to assert the indeterminacy rather than the infinity of the universe.

The acceptance of a concept of space as infinite and homogeneous required more than an awareness of internal contradictions in the Aristotelian system, problems in the details of Ptolemaic orbits, an infusion of Neo-Platonism, and novel telescopic observations. Descartes (1640) shifted the foundations of natural philosophy by negating the teleological arguments of scholastic philosophy, which rested on conflicting assumptions about the consequences of God's perfection. "Teleological conceptions and explanations have no place and no value in physical science, just as they have no place and no meaning in mathematics," Koyré has written describing Descartes' views. The world is, rather, "a strictly uniform mathematical world, a world of geometry made real . . ." (Koyré, 1957, p. 100–101). But Descartes did not view space as a void with bodies moving through it; instead space and matter are identical and extend indefinitely. Since "'place' and 'space' do not signify anything which differs *really* from the body that we say to be in some place" (Descartes quoted in Koyré, 1957, p. 103), Descartes thought that any location would have the attributes of length, breadth, and depth. These three dimensions could be used to treat space geometrically as one would a body. Space can be fully described by extension along three perpendicular axes, each indefinitely extended.

With the conceptualization of infinitely extensible Cartesian axes space became homogeneous, all points were unified within a single mathematical system based on interval scaling and measurement. Likewise in art, the picture plane became a single, unifying, coordinate system for representing the relative form, position, disposition, and motion of all objects in space. The coordinate system of linear perspective is a unified, quantified metric system that utilizes an interval scale in which the location and disposition of all objects can be defined within a consistent metric system emanating from a common, stable, and unifying reference point. The development of linear perspective in diagonal compositions and the relinquishing of a topological emphasis on boundaries and surfaces of objects indicated a consolidation of concepts of linear perspective in art, in which there was an even greater flexibility and power in the representation of infinite space. The unification in Cartesian coordinate geometry of algebraic symbols and geometric representation was also based on an interval scale and it gave a similar power and confidence to scientists in handling problems in astronomy and mechanics.

This shift in cognitive development from an intuitive preoperational to a concrete operational level involves a formalization and a quantification of previously intuitive qualitative constructs. The development of the ability to represent objects in perspective in art is analogous to the adoption of three-dimensional rectilinear space in physics. Both involve an operational level of representation with the capacity for transformation, reversibility, and object constancy. While Aristotle was interested in positions in space and thus with directions—up–down, left–right, before–behind—not only was his concept of space primarily concerned with the boundary of individual objects, but his directions were not reversible; up and down, for example, were considered as qualitatively different. Moreover, despite the awareness of left-right and before-behind, Aristotle's representation of position essentially had to do with the dimension of verticality. The development of directionality and reversibility in the three spatial axes was central in the development of linear perspective and was the culmination of the incorporation of Euclidean geometry and algebra into coordinate geometry in Cartesian and Newtonian physics. The development from an intuitive preoperational to a concrete operational level of representation describes the development from Galileo's qualitative view of infinite space and his use of geometrical analysis of motion, to Descartes' full-scale integration of these approaches through the mathematization of space as a single homogeneous entity of infinite dimension, capable of mapping all motions and positions in one integrated coordinate system. Descartes' synthesis provided a formal symbolic system not only for quantifying all positions and motions in space but also for manipulating those positions and motions in the abstract symbolic forms of algebra, rather than just the more literal metaphor of geometrical representations (Burtt, 1931/1954).

The conception of the universe as continuous and infinite, anticipated in the early 15th century by Nicholas of Cusa and eventually formalized in the 17th century by Descartes, involved a fundamental redefinition in natural science and philosophy of man's position in the universe. These changes in science and philosophy, as the development of linear perspective in art, were an essential expression of Renaissance humanism—the increasing recognition of the dignity of man and his role in establishing a systematic understanding of nature. In pre-Renaissance cosmology, the earth was in a diminished position in the structure of celestial concentric spheres. Aristotle's view of the cosmos, essentially restated by Ptolemy, Dante, and many others, was as a series of concentric spheres, one inside the other, with the earth as the motionless center far removed from God, but at the center of His attention. Nicholas of Cusa, in the 15th century, suggested that the earth was in motion and not at rest, but he did not develop the implication of these ideas. He also asserted that only God is infinite while the world is indefinite, but he opened the possibility for considering the infinity of the universe by explicitly denying that the world was finite and terminated by an outer shell. Nicholas of Cusa had a diverse and organized conception of the universe in which there is no hierarchical structure, but each component of the universe, by its own nature, contributed to the perfection of the whole (Koyré, 1957). Koyré (1957, p. 23) considers that "the spirit of the Renaissance breathes in the work of Cardinal Nicholas of Cusa." While some authors (e.g., Burtt, 1931/1954) stress the elevation of the importance and dignity of man in Medieval philosophy and others discuss the Copernican revolution as a blow to man's self-esteem in no longer being located at the center of the universe and God's attention, Lovejoy (1936/1964) offers an alternate interpretation:

It has often been said that the older picture of the world in space was peculiarly fitted to give man a high sense of his own importance and dignity. . . . Man occupied, we are told, this central place in the universe, and round the planet of his habitation all the vast, unpeopled spheres obsequiously revolved. But the actual tendency of the geocentric system was, for the medieval mind, precisely the opposite. For the centre of the world was not a position of honor; it was rather the place farthest removed from the Empyrean, the bottom of the creation, to which its dregs and baser elements sank. The actual centre, indeed, was Hell; in the spatial sense the medieval world was, literally diabolocentric. . . . The geocentric cosmography served rather for man's humiliation than for his exaltation, and . . . Copernicanism was opposed partly on the ground that it assigned too dignified and lofty a position to his dwelling-place. (pp. 101–102)

Copernicus created a transformation in mathematical astronomy, a new physics, a new conception of space and of man's relationship to God. Copernicus elevated the earth by placing it among, and equal to, the planets and thus undermined the Classical and Medieval hierarchical structure of the universe, in which the immutable celestial realm was contrasted with the terrestrial regions of change and decay. Copernicus' reformulation of the cosmos, begun as early as 1500 and eventually published in 1543, raised the earth from a lowly position to an integral part of the celestial system around the sun (Koyré, 1957), thereby he transformed man's conception of the universe and his relation to it (Lovejoy, 1936/1964). His formulations were in part an expression of the Renaissance's extensive philosophical reexamination of the dignity of man and the individual's role in a unified system of nature. His formulations were also part of the Renaissance attempt to replace dogmatic mystical and transcendental concepts with explanations of the general principles of nature in laws based on systematic observation. Copernicus highlighted the dignity of man by emphasizing the individual's capacity to understand the organization of nature.

In individual psychological development, the utilization of concrete operations that formalize intuitive cognitive constructs and modes is correlated with the differentiation of the individual's perspective from the perspective of others. The self becomes a stable and enduring reference point that is unique and differentiated from the perspective of others and eventually from the environment. It may be more than coincidence that Descartes, the inventor of coordinate geometry built around a single reference point, was also preoccupied metaphysically with exactly that issue: that the mind and soul are distinct and separate from all of material nature, although indeed, through its process of abstraction, the mind may develop a mathematics through which to describe patterns observed in nature. The correlation of the developing self-reflective awareness with the operational level of his geometric coordinate system is nicely expressed by Descartes' metaphysical pronouncement, "I think, therefore I am." Descartes, in *Meditations II*, discusses his search for a fixed, immovable "Archimedan point," his hope to "discover the one thing that is certain and indubitable." And Descartes goes on directly, of course, to establish his own existence as that certain and indubitable point.

Koyré (1957) discusses developments in science during this period as an expression of man's discovery of his consciousness and his essential subjectivity. Descartes' testimony to self-reflective awareness is not merely a slogan but a statement of his introspective method. Descartes even built such a self-awareness into the substance of his scientific theories about spatial perception. As Van Hoorn (1972) notes, Descartes considered that the dispositions of space are apprehended by reason, by an independent act of intellectual intention. It is striking that Descartes' coordinate geometry was a major synthesis in the development of a quantitative interval scaling of space and that Descartes was also a powerful spokesman for a meditative self-reflective method. Baroque painting, in the same era, likewise involved a full mastery of the coordinate system necessary for the representation of linear perspective and at the same time also reflected an interest in the representation of affects and feeling states (i.e., the subtleties of subjective experience and awareness.)

Descartes took the mathematization of space a step further than Copernicus and Kepler, who relied on mathematical simplicity only to formulate and justify the reversal of sun and earth in the world system and to chart planetary orbits more precisely. Descartes gave space a mathematical definition, and he demonstrated that all positions and motions in space could be treated by synthesizing algebraic and geometric methods with the assumption that space is describable by the metric of three perpendicular axes, where the coordinates of points, mapped on the axes around a central reference point, define all points in space. Newton adopted and developed Descartes' "mathematics" further by extending analytic geometry with the calculus—a mathematical method of analyzing instantaneous changes of location (i.e., speed) and instantaneous changes of speed (i.e., acceleration).

As space in Baroque art was unified and unlimited, so space was unified in Baroque science with an analytic geometry that mapped all positions and motions throughout infinite space. In addition, in Baroque art there was a change in the content of art from the universal and eternal forms of the Renaissance to the specifically temporal depiction of people and events at a particular moment. Likewise in science, early Renaissance geometrical models represented the static, unchanging qualities of the universe while, in contrast, Galileo developed the foundations of the dynamics of motion and Newton's (1687) magnificent *Mathematical Principles of Natural Philosophy* developed the calculus to treat instantaneous quantitative changes of position in the system of Cartesian coordinates as functions of instantaneous moments in time.

A conception of space as identical to matter and the laws of impact enabled Descartes to develop a unified mechanism for both planetary and terrestrial motion. Descartes explained planetary orbits as the result of the planets being swept along by a vortex of matter swirling around stars. While such a mechanism required the universe to be filled with matter, Newton denied that space and matter are co-extensive, although he continued to describe space by the infinitely extensible Cartesian axes. Newton believed in space as a void; and he demonstrated how the same force—gravity—accounts for falling bodies on the earth and keeps planets in their elliptical, Keplerian solar orbits and the moon revolving about the earth. While Newton assumed that space is infinite and is an indifferent or passive container of bodies, he did not assume its entire homogeneity because he believed there must be some center "at rest," (i.e., some absolute center, some basis for a fixed and immobile frame of reference). This view of space was compatible with his spiritual convictions, which, in accord with the Neo-Platonic philosophy and theology of his Cambridge milieu, distinguished matter and space and equated space with God's infinite spirit. But an absolute center of the universe was also established, Newton thought, by the fact that if space were homogeneous, it would be impossible to analyze circular motion that required a fixed center as a frame of reference. Newton's laws of motion are valid only in an inertial coordinate system that has its origin at the center of the solar system. In Koyré's words, a concept of absolute space, is indeed the necessary and inevitable consequence of the "bursting of the sphere," the "breaking of the circle," the geometrization of space, of the discovery or assertion of the law of inertia as the first and foremost law or axiom of motion. Indeed, if it is the inertial, that is, the rectilinear uniform motion that becomes—just like the rest—the "natural" *status* of a body, then the circular one, which at any point of its trajectory *changes* its direction through maintaining constant its angular velocity, appears, from the point of view of the law of inertia, not as a *uniform*, but as a *constantly accelerated* motion. But acceleration, in contradistinction to mere translation, has always been something absolute, and it remained so until 1915, when, for the first time in the history of physics, the general relativity theory of Einstein deprived it of its absoluteness. Yet as, in so doing, it reclosed the universe and denied the Euclidean structure of space, it has, by this very fact, confirmed the correctness of the Newtonian conception. (p. 169) (Italics, Koyré)

In other words, infinite Euclidean-Cartesian space was a transitional theory that could not sustain a concept of space as homogeneous and as infinite.

Newton made the metaphysical assumption that there must be some fixed or absolute pole around which all motions occur. But as Descartes had already realized, if rest and uniform motion are both natural states, there is no way to determine whether one's frame of reference is moving or at rest. Thus, as Newton's contemporary Leibniz pointed out, no experiment could be designed that could establish a fixed set of coordinates for "absolute space" because there was no way to differentiate between space as fixed or unmoving and space moving with constant linear motion (Jammer, 1954/1969). Nor was there any evidence of centrifugal forces (apart from those resulting from planetary motions around the sun) that alone could establish that the universe was in rotational motion around some fixed or absolute center. Nevertheless, the Newtonian view of absolute space remained an assumption in physics through the late 18th and early 19th centuries, although it had little impact on the study of physical phenomena until the late 19th century. Then, the notion of absolute space, describable by Euclidean geometry, began to be undermined by the combined impact of the development of non-Euclidean geometries; by studies of light and electromagnetic radiation that failed to demonstrate the immobile ether (a physical manifestation of absolute space) that had been the assumed vehicle for such wave phenomena; and by Einstein's reexamination of assumptions in physics regarding time, motion, mass, force, gravity, and the process of measurement. Theological conceptions had also become increasingly less concrete and more symbolic as the concept shifted from a God located in the heavens to God as all-pervasive. With God so removed from the heavens, it became far less crucial to consider whether the heavens had a perfectly spherical shape, or how, or if, they were bounded, or indeed to even have an absolute conception of space. It was now sufficient that God penetrated all of an infinite, all-containing, homogeneous space. It no longer seemed so important to have the earth at the center of God's attention and of the universe, or to posit God's location at an absolute center of the universe.

The Euclidean-Cartesian concept of space persisted as a transitional theory from the 17th through the 20th centuries and changed the conception of the shape of space from spherical to rectilinear. Spherical orbs and a spherical zone of fixed stars characterized cosmology not only through Copernicus but even through Galileo. Galileo ardently insisted on the boundlessness of the universe but yet believed that the fixed stars were located in

> a circle described about a determinate center and comprised within two spherical surfaces, to wit, one very high and concave, the other lower and convex betwixt which I would constitute the innumerable multitude of stars, but yet at diverse altitudes, and this might be called the sphere of the universe, containing within it the circles of the planets already by us described. (Quoted in Koyré, 1957, pp. 96–97)

A spherical universe corresponded with the emphasis on circular motion as the only sort of motion that is "natural" or occurs spontaneously in the heavens and maintains the planets in their non-deteriorating orbits. As Galilean boundless space was spherical in correspondence with the perfection of circular motion, Newtonian space was based on a rectilinear coordinate system in correspondence with the doctrine of linear inertia. Descartes and Newton believed that "natural" motion occurs in a straight line at a constant speed—bodies in motion tend to remain in motion at the same speed and in the same direction. In Newtonian space, bodies behave indifferently with respect to their location, as opposed to their action in Aristotelian space where earthy and watery substances strive toward the center, fiery and airy substances rise, and heavenly bodies, in virtue of their perfection, move in circular orbits. But in Cartesian and Newtonian space all bodies tend—no matter where they are—simply to stay put if at rest or to keep moving at the same speed along the same straight line. Newtonian space is therefore defined by infinitely extensible, perpendicular Cartesian axes that are the coordinates of natural motion, as the nested, bounded spherical orbs of the Aristotelian cosmos were the layers of a world in which circularity was perfectly natural.

The transition from the Aristotelian-Ptolemaic to the Copernican system was dependent upon valuing abstract mathematical arguments for the superiority of heliocentric orbits over the direct sensory experiences of an immobile earth. With the elaboration of the Copernican system by Kepler, Galileo, and Newton, cosmological concepts and systems were based less on immediate sensory experiences, common-sense phenomena, and ordinary appearances (Butterfield, 1957) and became instead more conceptual and symbolic. The same development occurred in art and science as sensorimotor-preoperational modes were replaced by preoperational, visual, intuitive modes, which gave way in turn to operational modes of representation that became increasingly more concerned with inner experience and form than with external, manifest concrete features. As Baroque art became interested in representing inner affective states and experiences, Baroque science became interested in powerful inner processes and structure, which determined outer form and action, such as magnetism, electricity, heat, optics, light, color, the combination and structure of matter, the dynamics of motion, and the elasticity of air in the interaction of temperature, pressure, and volume. These early attempts to understand inner processes and structures were the prologue for the later development of molecular theory (Hall, 1954/ 1966).

Thus, there were parallel changes in the modes of representation in art and science during the Renaissance and the Baroque. A fundamental change occurred in the structure of measurement and scaling from a qualitative, relative, comparative ordering or ranking to a quantitative interval scale in which there is an equivalence of measurement organized around a single unifying reference point. The representation of space was no longer based on a qualitative ordering of figures derived from visual experience, but now space was considered as homogeneous, infinite, and isotropic, with an equivalence of all points and directions in space. These developments and changes in the modes of representation in art and science involved the increased recognition of the importance of the role of the individual in understanding nature. This recognition of man's essential role as part of nature was expressed in the shift from a geocentric to a heliocentric conception of the universe in which man on earth was no longer in a lowly and debased position in the universe, but rather occupied a position equivalent to any other location in space. The individual was seen as having a unique position, which serves as a constant and stable reference point for organizing experiences and the understanding of nature. This unique reference point also includes the importance of utilizing personal experiences, such as meaning, emotions, and feelings, in understanding nature.

5
From Linear Perspective to Conceptual Art: Impressionism, Cubism, and Modern Art

IMPRESSIONISM AND POST-IMPRESSIONISM

The monumental discovery of linear perspective in the Renaissance continued to dominate art for almost 500 years. The discovery of perspective was based on an appreciation of the importance of defining a specified point of view and a central vanishing point. It introduced into art the importance of recognizing the role of the individual observer and subjective experience. Linear perspective was the mathematical codification of procedures for the representation, on a two-dimensional plane, of reality as it appeared to the viewer. Artists during Mannerism, and especially the Baroque period, consolidated the representation of depth and enriched the representation of subjective dimensions by discovering modes for effectively expressing action and emotion. In addition to depicting figures and scenes as they appeared to the viewer, paintings were now filled with tension and affect. Through the use of diagonal composition, chiaroscuro, and subtle variations in color, Baroque artists were able to represent inner psychological states and stimulate these experiences in the beholder.

Some art historians (e.g., Arnheim, 1954/1974; Gombrich, 1960) conceptualize the contributions of Mannerism, the Baroque, and Impressionism as revolutions against the precise canons and mathematical procedures developed during the Renaissance. Arnheim (1954/1974, pp. 134–135), for example, considers Impressionism a "radical countermovement," which sought to reject linear perspective and the representation of the idealized universal figure for a return to elementary shape and color after the "extreme exploitation of projective distortion." Others (e.g., Giedion, 1941/1967; Panofsky, 1924/25; Schapiro, 1932) prefer to conceptualize Impressionism as further progress in the representation of subjective dimensions that began in the Renaissance and was elaborated in Mannerism and the Baroque. Whether one considers the developments subsequent to the Renaissance to be revolution, evolution, or some combination of the two, Impressionism was a major revision in style that had continuity with developments that had taken place earlier in Mannerism and the Baroque. As with all major revisions, the discoveries of Impressionism not only maintained some continuity with prior developments, but also provided preparations for important modifications still to come. Whether viewed as a revolt against the cold, mechanical, mathematical canons of the Renaissance or as further development of the capacity to represent subjective experiences, Impressionism was a major shift in the mode of representation.

Impressionism emerged in the mid-19th century, typified by the works of Manet, Monet, Degas, Renoir, and culminated in the work of the Post-impressionists, such as Van Gogh, Seurat, and Cézanne. Rosenblum (1974, p. 189), in his analysis of the transformations in the late 18th century Neoclassic and Romantic art, demonstrates how the "destruction" of Renaissance and Baroque traditional perspective began around 1800, even before the work of Turner and Constable in 1820–1835 and Courbet and Manet in 1850–1860. Rosenblum discusses how Neoclassic Romantic works by David, Flaxman, Ingres, and Blake, with their pseudo-simplicity of pure line and perspective, actually contained radical deviations from the principles of perspective that created a personal spatial system within a pictorial flatness. But it was the paintings of Turner and Constable, in the first half of the 19th century, with their primary use of atmospheric factors, shading, and variations of color rather than form, that were major factors in the transition from the Baroque to Impressionism. Giedion (1941/ 1967, p. 69) compares Turner and Constable to Michelangelo: Michelangelo provided the bridge from Gothic spirituality to the "worldly universality of the Baroque," and Turner and Constable linked the late Baroque to the French Impressionists of the late 19th century. Turner and Constable extended the Baroque subtle variations of color, light, and atmosphere, with minimal articulation of form. Constable and Turner were major figures in the integration of atmospheric color and perspective—a vital part of the transition from the Renaissance to Impressionism (Fry, 1934). In Turner, color and light became the essence of the aesthetic experience; form was subordinate to the immediacy of the sensory experience of color and light. Constable, like Turner, also depicted perceptual impressions rather than scenes of nature. Constable took "real shape" for granted and modified it even at the risk of a loss of functional clarity in order to express momentary appearance (Gombrich, 1960). Turner carried this even further and dissolved the structure of objects in the momentary experiences of mist, light, and haze. Turner's use of color in his later work expresses an intense, subjective reaction to atmospheric conditions. For both Turner and Constable, the painting was no longer the depiction of a timeless scene but the representation of a momentary perceptual experience (see Figs. 71 and 72). The Impressionists carried this concept even further and attempted to represent objects and scenes purely on the basis of momentary sensory impressions of variations in light and color.

Instead of representing the external, manifest, physical features of the object, Impressionists sought to represent the basic, constituent elements of the object as expressed in the subtle details of the visual experiences it evoked. They attempted to go beyond the perception of the complete, composite, total figure they knew was there, and instead represented the elements and inner form that led to the immediate visual experience. Because of prior developments in the modes of representation that had taken place particularly in the late Baroque and in the works of Turner and Constable, the Impressionists were confident that they and the spectator could reconstruct an integrated totality from the representation of discrete visual elements. Impressionism, as a major revision in style, was possible only because a unified spatial system had already been achieved (Panofsky, 1924/25). The assurance offered by the integrated system for the representation of the constant and stable form of objects within unified three-dimensional space allowed the Impressionists to relinquish the representation of the manifest, external, physical form of the object and to experiment with the representation of minute, discrete, visual sensations of color and light. The emphasis on a subtle,

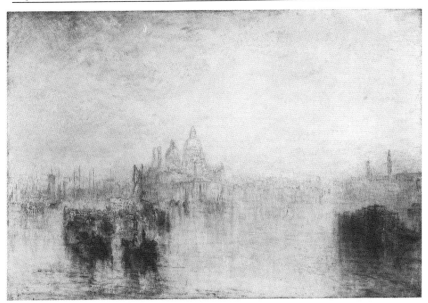

FIG. 71   Turner, *Venice, Santa Maria della Salute* (1844) (The Tate Gallery, London).

detailed analysis of the visual experiences of light and color enabled the Impressionists to capture aspects of the inner form and structure of nature.

Objects were decomposed into flecks of light and the individual minute particles that constitute the object in a particular atmospheric field. The object's form and its surrounding space were systematically ignored. Space was undifferentiated so both foreground and background were rendered in small, blurred flecks of light and color. Foreground and background became fused flat surfaces. In addition, objects were not represented with their own constant, intrinsic color, but color was contingent upon the light and atmosphere of a particular moment or circumstance. The Impressionists sought to represent the object in its most subjective form, in terms of its fundamental, sensory dimensions, uniquely experienced at a specific moment in a particular context. They struggled to capture aspects of their visual experience rather than the object they knew was there (Jaffe, 1969). The Impressionists were interested in understanding how isolated, fragmented visual experiences were organized to create images of substantial objects in three-dimensional space. When the beholder was close to the canvas, colors tended to blend and merge and objects lost their definition, but when the picture was viewed from a distance,

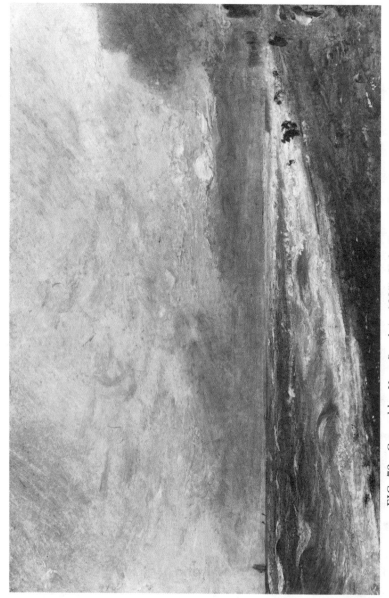

FIG. 72 Constable, *Hove Beach* (c. 1825) (Yale Center for British Art, Paul Mellon Collection).

the forms of the objects could be constructed. Objects in Impressionist paintings were primarily a series of minute, dissected, particles of visual sensory experiences and not clearly defined forms of concrete objects in three-dimensional space. Discrete independent patches of pure color were the major components of the picture rather than formal contours of the object with subtle gradations of color and light. The use of pure colors created a bold, sparkling effect in a picture plane that was intentionally reduced to a flat surface by the concentration on the sensory experiences of color and light.

The subject matter of Impressionist paintings was primarily scenes of nature. What matters most was not the figures and the meaning of scenes but a sensuous appreciation of the natural scene and its subtle perceptual variations. The Impressionists often painted water because its amorphous, unarticulated form is ideally suited for representing movement and the momentary, flickering reflections of light and color (see Fig. 73). Impressionist painters focused exclusively on making a coherent statement based on color and light, independent of meaning (Schapiro, 1932). They sought to capture the first impression without the interference of intellectual elements; it was an attempt to represent reality as it was experienced, not as it was known to be. Impressionists ignored the physical form of the object and tried to go beyond the external features to represent the constituent elements beneath the manifest form.

Some of the motivation for the Impressionist interest in representing the basic sensory qualities of nature was their contempt for the polite veneer of European society and the pomp and decadence of the French Academy. Artists such as Gauguin sought to disengage themselves from the pretense and pretext of a hypocritical society. The Impressionists reacted against the superficiality and hypocrisy of the Victorian era by portraying life in fundamental terms. Some art historians (e.g., Venturi, 1950, p. 218) describe this period from 1870–1900 as a "struggle for autonomy." This struggle was expressed in a number of ways. The Impressionists had agreed not to show their work at the official Salon of the French Academy. The group expressed a preference for "the irregular, the accidental, the spontaneous," instead of the "formal and hierarchical pageantry" of the Academy and the government (Baldwin, 1974, p. 6). They wanted to capture the moment, the flux, the instability, and the impermanence of the spontaneous event, which they considered the essence of life. Thus, a classic and highly conventional scene of a picnic was pre-

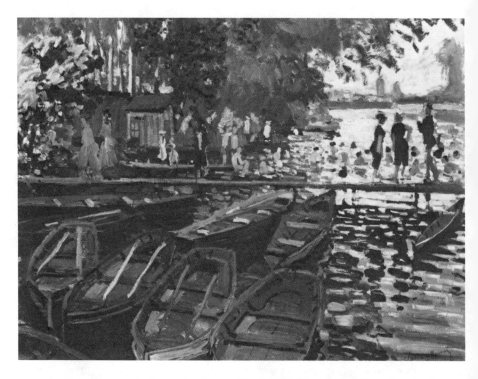

FIG. 73   Monet, *Bathers at La Grenouillère* (1869) (National Gallery, London).

sented in such a way as to violate contemporary sensibility by painting two women in the nude (Manet, *Luncheon on the Grass)* (Fig. 74). Toulouse–Lautrec portrayed the seamy side of Parisian life in his pictures of prostitutes and absinthe drinkers of Montmartre. In content and style, the Impressionists and Post-impressionists sought to present life as it was perceived and experienced, rather than as it was known and conceptualized.

The Impressionists were influenced by 18th-century Ukiyo-e Japanese prints that first came to France in about 1856 (Ives, 1974). Manet in particular was most impressed with the content and the structure of the Ukiyo-e sketches of Hokusai and other Japanese artists (Weisberg, Cate, Needham, Eidelberg, & Johnston, 1975). These Japanese print makers, like the Impressionists in their struggle with the French Academy, were rebelling against the court art and the art of the priesthood in Japan. Eighteenth-century Japan was a new era of stability and prosperity that fostered freedom of expression in an urban middle class. The Japanese prints reflected the life of the common

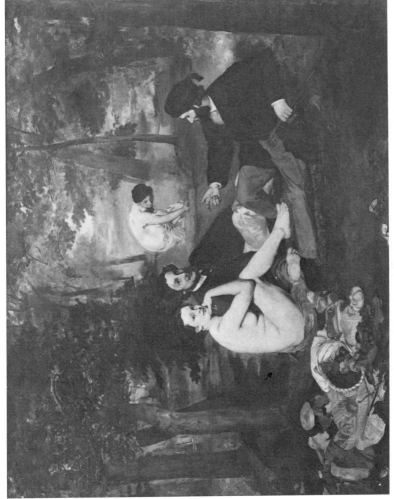

FIG. 74   Manet, *Luncheon on the Grass* (1863), Louvre, Paris (Giraudon).

man, his pleasures of the flesh and wanton women, and the excitement of the world of entertainment. The Impressionists were intrigued by both the subject matter and the flatness of these Japanese
prints (Hillier, 1954; Ives, 1974; Lane, 1962; Stern, 1969).

Impressionists were also influenced by the development of photography and the way a photograph seemed to excerpt a segment of an
ongoing flow of a natural event. They tried to capture this sense of a
momentary segment of nature in open compositions in which the
picture frame was only an arbitrary limit. Thus, Impressionist paintings, like the photograph and the 18th-century Japanese prints, had
arbitrary and indefinite edges.

While Manet never exhibited his work in the Impressionist exhibitions, he did participate in their discussions and was acknowledged as
the leader, at least in the early years of the group. Manet abandoned
the representation of perspective and of three-dimensional form
achieved through the modeling of light and shadow, for a subtle
harmony of colors in flat forms set in shallow backgrounds. He attempted to reduce the picture plane to a flat surface, and he used
limited and simplified backgrounds to highlight large, simple masses
and pure colors to represent the object. He sought to capture the
evanescent effects of reflections and flickering sunlight that created
the elusive, spontaneous experience of the moment (Hamilton, 1954).
In the mid-1860s, Monet, Renoir, and Degas followed Courbet's and
Manet's attempts to represent the immediate visual experience instead of the enduring, manifest, external form. They sought to represent the alterations of the natural color of objects that were created by
the momentary variations of color and light in atmospheric conditions. Monet, for example, painted endless series of the same subject
at different times of day and under different climatic conditions. He
painted 16 views of London Bridge and 26 views of Rouen Cathedral
(Fig. 75). Renoir and Degas also attempted to capture a moment in
time by representing a person at a special instant in a particular activity (see Fig. 76).

Beginning with Manet, the Impressionists struggled against age-old
conventions to create a new form of art. Colors were dealt with in a
delicate and sensitive fashion and the outline and the order of objects
remained relatively obscure behind the broad presentation of colors.
The Impressionists tried to remain detached from the manifest form
and definition of the object as a constant and consistent image. They
"concentrated their chief attention on lines, on forms, and on colours,

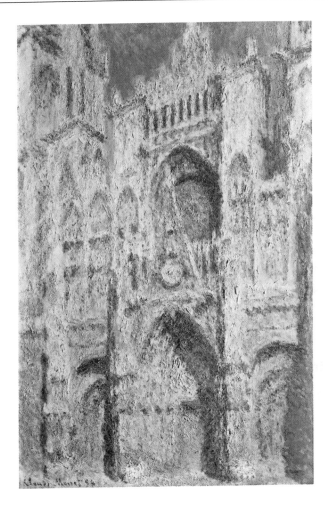

FIG. 75   Monet, *Rouen Cathedral* (1894) (The Metropolitan Museum of Art, The Theodore M. Davis Collection, Bequest of Theodore M. Davis).

rather than on the reality of the human beings and landscapes which their forms represented" (Venturi, 1950, p. 217). The Impressionists sought to construct a picture justified solely by its form and color "values rather than by its representational effectiveness." These new forces in art that "concentrated on the attainment of the autonomy of art . . . changed not only painting but also sculpture, architecture, music, literature, and even criticism" (Venturi, 1950, p. 218).

In developmental psychological terms, this struggle for autonomy was expressed in the Impressionists' attempt to free themselves from

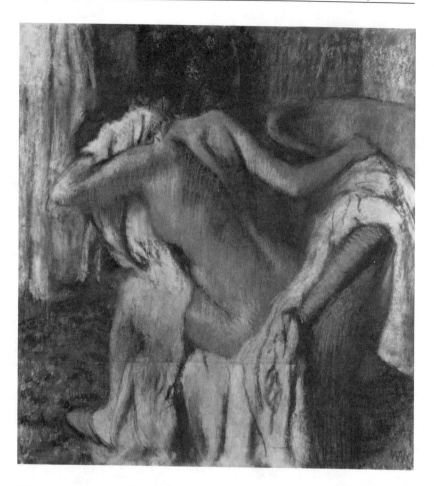

FIG. 76   Degas, *After the Bath* (1885) (National Gallery, London).

the constraints of the constant physical form of an object. They sought new modes for expressing the inner dimensions of objects that transcended external, manifest physical form and literal meaning. It was a struggle to go beyond conventional modes of experiencing and representing a generalized, perceptual totality, and to seek instead, within oneself, the inner form and nature of experience. In Piaget's terms, this was a continuation of the shift from a concrete operational to a formal (or abstract) operational level of representation that had started in Baroque art. Impressionism was a major step in the search for the representation of intrinsic, formal, abstract, symbolic form. To capture this inner form and structure, the Impressionists concentrated on the basic, discrete, sensory elements of which the object was composed. The canons of linear perspective and the manifest definition of the object were ignored and, instead, individual dabs of color captured isolated sensations of light and color. The subtle segments of isolated sensory events were an attempt to capture the inner form of the objects as well as the inner form of the artists' own experience. In order to relinquish representing the literal object, the Impressionists had to feel supremely confident that they and the beholder could reconstruct the appearance of the object from minute, sensory events. They were confident of their own and the spectator's capacity to construct an adequate image of an object from only partial information presented in the dissected sensory impressions. In developmental psychological terms, they were very much aware of the capacity for object constancy and conservation and thus did not feel compelled any longer to represent the well-defined, manifest form of a realistic object.

The dramatic change in the mode of representation developed by the Impressionists never endangered the stability of the spatial image and the solidity of objects because of the achievements of the Renaissance and the Baroque. Establishment of the operational modes of representation achieved in the Renaissance and the Baroque allowed for numerous transformations without threatening the basic definition of the object. The mathematical operations of linear perspective provided the basis for reversibility and conservation in the representation of objects and of space. Initially, these operations involved transformations of manifest, concrete dimensions and, therefore, the nature and degree of potential transformations were limited. With further development of the operational level of representation, progress was made toward transformations of more internal, abstract dimensions.

In many ways Impressionism was an extension of the subjectivism achieved in the Baroque. Baroque art was characterized by a relinquishing of the topological dimensions of boundaries and contours; figure and ground tended to merge as space became continuous and homogeneous. This conception of homogeneous space was extended in Impressionism by the search for the common properties and basic similarities of figure and ground. Impressionism found this basic structural similarity by treating all experience in terms of constituent, visual sensations. Space and object, figure and ground, were indistinguishable as they were decomposed and dissected into the basic structural units of discrete visual experiences. Objects and space were reduced to their fundamental sensory essence.

This interest in the basic constituents of the visual experience was similar to the scientific interests of the time—the measurement of sensory experiences and the investigation of the basic processes of vision and color perception (e.g., Fechner, Helmholtz). The dissection of visual experiences in art into basic components, this search for the inner form and structure of visual experiences, also occurred at the same time scientists were investigating and formulating the basic structural components of matter (e.g., Mendeleyev & Meyer, J. J. Thomson, Maxwell). Huyghe (1974) discusses Impressionism as part of the late 19th century reaction against the excessive materialism of Logical Positivism and its devotion to a concrete, literal conception of reality. Impressionism participated in the recognition that the form of nature is not concrete and inert but instead fluid and in constant flux. This new appreciation of the ephemeral qualities of the manifest form of nature not only occurred in art, but also in poetry (e.g., Verlaine), literature (e.g., Proust), and music (e.g., Debussy, Ravel). In art, firm lines were replaced by vague and fluid articulations, and in music Debussy and Ravel created a sense of shimmering iridescences and ripplings. Like the art of Baroque and Impressionism, Debussy, Ravel and others in music attempted to portray the experience of the moment. Composers rejected particular functions for given tones and, instead, began to consider harmonic aggregations and Schoenbergian perpetual variations that permitted "utilization of all chromatic possibilities and embraces in homogeneity all the constituent elements of musical discourse" (Brion-Guerry, 1977, p. 81).

In art and music, as in science during the late 19th century, there was also an increasing awareness of the importance of time as a vital dimension of experience and reality. Baroque art had already shifted from the timeless, eternal image, to capture a particular event. This was more fully extended as Impressionists sought to portray the very moment of an experience. As Monet was emphasizing the importance of time in his numerous paintings of Rouen Cathedral and London Bridge, Bergson in philosophy and Proust in literature were concerned with change over time—the fleeting, evanescent quality of nature and of life. Bergson was concerned with the "vital flow" and the "flux of the inner life" and Proust was preoccupied with man's confrontation with time (Huyghe, 1974, p. 22). In poetry, the line ceased to hold a precise meaning in any exact and restrictive way. As science finally relinquished concepts of absolute space and time, and as color and form became autonomous elements in paintings, the line in poetry evolved "toward autonomy, escaping the meaning that it holds; with Mallarmé and Valéry, it becomes reality in itself" (Brion-Guerry, 1977, p. 82). In art, literature, music, and science there was a search for something beyond the concrete, manifest form of nature— a search for the potentially infinite extension of the inner form and structure of nature.

Impressionism also attempted to bring the spectator more fully into the picture space. In the Renaissance, the composition was organized from a single, fixed point of view of a hypothetical spectator. Baroque art attempted to facilitate the spectator's identification with the mood and emotional tone of the figure in the painting and the artist's affective interpretation. Impressionism relied upon the spectator, instead of the artist, to integrate and organize the visual sensations. And there were also attempts to extend the picture space to include the space of the spectator. This had been done much earlier, for example, in Velasquez' *Maids of Honor* (see Fig. 65, p. 267), but not in Impressionism renewed attention was given to the spectator's role as an integral part of the picture field. Manet's *Bar at the Folies Bergère* (see Fig. 66, p. 268) and James Tissot's *The Milliner's Shop* (Fig. 77) exemplify attempts to draw the spectator into the picture. In Manet, the viewer becomes the patron at the bar and in Tissot one becomes the person for whom the shopkeeper is opening the door.

Impressionism was an integral part of the collective thought of its period; the modes of representation in art were an expression of the conceptual structure of its era. Impressionism not only expressed an interest in the discovery of the basic inner structure of reality underlying manifest form and function, but it also struggled to include a sense of time and the observer in the construction of reality. These were basic issues in Impressionism. They were extended in Post-impressionism and Cubism, and they culminated in the development of abstract art. Impressionism marked the beginning of the Modern era in art with its increasing attempt to define inner form and abstract structure, and to extend the representation of the three dimensions of space in a way that was consistent with emerging new conceptions of geometry and the fourfold spatiotemporal field that defines the observer as essential in any construction of reality.

The Post-impressionists continued the search for the representation of inner form and structure that had begun in Impressionism. Post-impressionists, such as Van Gogh, Seurat, Cézanne, Gauguin, and others, concentrated on the inner structure of

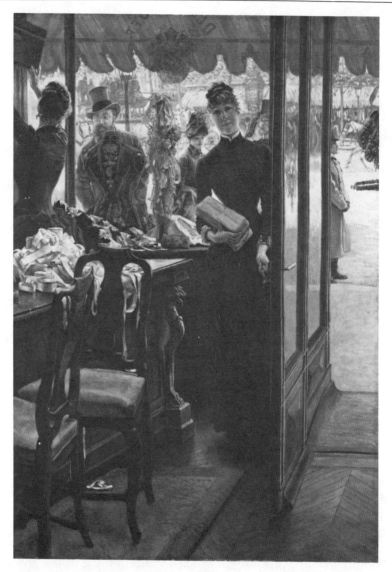

FIG. 77   Tissot, *The Milliner's Shop* (1883–85) (Art Gallery of Ontario).

geometric forms and patterns. They systematically reexamined the role of line, color, and geometric form in the representation of three-dimensional space. Arnheim (1954/1974, pp. 134–135) discusses Impressionism and Post-impressionism as "a return to elementary shapes and the elementary schemata of permanent structural norms . . . (so) conspicuous in the geometrical simplifications of

Seurat and Cézanne and the primitivism pervading much art of the early twentieth century." Actually, Van Gogh, Seurat, and Cézanne were not so much a part of a "primitivism" or "a return to elementary" form, but an integral part of the search for aspects of the internal structure of nature. They adopted the Impressionist interest in the inner structure of reality as expressed in the effervescent vitality of the visual sensations of light and color, but they also extended this interest in their fascination with intrinsic geometric form and structure.

Van Gogh was particularly interested in the expressive value of color and the tactile quality of thick brush strokes to express his emotional reactions to nature. But Van Gogh, like Cézanne, was also interested in the representation of space. Unlike Cézanne, however, Van Gogh was especially concerned about perspective and recession into space. He used exaggerated orthogonals and a steeply inclined foreground plane, for example, to transform an ordinary corridor (Fig. 78) into a recession into deep space (MOMA Catalogue, Cézanne, 1977).

Meyer Schapiro (1950), in contrasting Van Gogh with Cézanne, noted that Van Gogh

hastens the convergence, exaggerating the extremities in space, from the emphatic foreground to the immensely enlarged horizon with its infinitesimal detail. . . . Linear perspective was for him no impersonal set of rules, but something as real as the objects themselves, a quality of the landscape that he was sighting. This paradoxical device—both phenomenon and system—at the same time deformed things and made them look more real: it fastened the artist's eye more slavishly to appearances but also brought him more actively into play in the world. While in Renaissance pictures it was a means of constructing an objective space complete in itself and distinct from the beholder, even though organized with respect to his eye, like the space of a stage, in many of Van Gogh's first landscape drawings the world seems to emanate from his eye in a gigantic discharge with a continuous motion of rapidly converging lines." (pp. 29–30)

There has been recent controversy about Van Gogh's unique concepts of space. Heelan (1972), for example, has commented on paradoxes in Van Gogh's forms and his representation of space. Although the forms look intensely real, they are often distorted; there is a perspective system, yet it is most unusual. Space is organized with respect to the observer, but it is not constructed according to Euclidean rules, instead "foreground objects protrude but depth lines

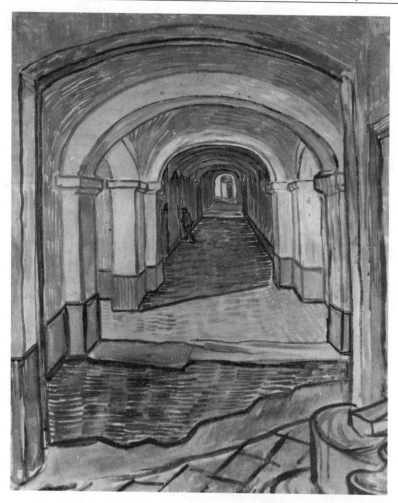

FIG. 78   Van Gogh, *Hospital Corridor at Saint Remy* (1889) (The Museum of Modern Art, New Abby Aldrich Rockefeller Bequest).

plunge to a finite horizon" (p. 478). Heelan concludes that Van Gogh represented spatial forms according to an unusual set of visual spatial rules—a mode of representation based on non-Euclidean geometry. Van Gogh experimented with a "strictly binocular visual comparison of depth and distance when all other clues to size, depth, and distance—such clues, for example, as those learned by moving around in the field of objects, by sighting, by touching them, by measuring them with rigid rulers—are inoperative" (Heelan, 1972, p. 482). Purely binocular vision results in a spatial experience that expresses a non-Euclidean hyperbolic geometry of a constant and systematic Gaussian curvature (Luneberg, 1947). In this hyperbolic space, near space protrudes in a convex bulge toward the observer and equally spaced frontal planar surfaces appear unequally spaced. In near space, frontal planar surfaces are more widely spaced (Pirenne, 1970); in distant space, planar surfaces appear concave and depth differentiation gradually disappears with distance. All objects at sufficient distance "from the observer will appear to be without depth on a sphere of infinite radius of which the observer is at the center" (Heelan, 1972, p. 483). Thus, depth lines plunge rapidly to a horizon at a finite distance from the observer while objects in near space appear to protrude convexly toward the observer. Heelan's analysis of a number of Van Gogh's paintings, particularly his *Bedroom at Arles* (1888) (Fig. 79), demonstrates both qualitatively and quantitatively that Van Gogh's representation of space involves "a systematic projection of hyperbolic space" (p. 483).The lack of a fixed viewpoint or eye level and the fact that "even single objects have multiple convergence points" indicate a deviation from classical perspective. But this apparently nonsystematic representation of perspective is actually "a unified representation of a homogeneous, though non-Euclidean, spatial structure," based on a hyperbolic geometry (Heelan, 1972, p. 484).

Heelan discusses Van Gogh's representation of space as based on "lived space" (e.g., Husserl, Merleau-Ponty, Sartre) which has a structure different from the homogeneity and isotropic equivalence of directions in Euclidean space. Lived space assimilates the metric structure of Euclidean space but also allows for qualitative differences; it maintains metric properties but allows for the possibility of privileged directions. The non-Euclidean geometry of lived space provides a new descriptive spatial language in which the fixed units of interval scaling of Euclidean space are replaced by ratio or proportional scaling. In Euclidean geometry, the three coordinates of space are defined in a scale of equal intervals from an arbitrary and fixed reference point. In lived space, the coordinates of space are defined in reference to the constant, but ever-changing, personally relevant reference point of the self as a unique point in space. Although one's position in space constantly varies, space is experienced and defined always in terms relative to this enduring and stable point. The ob-

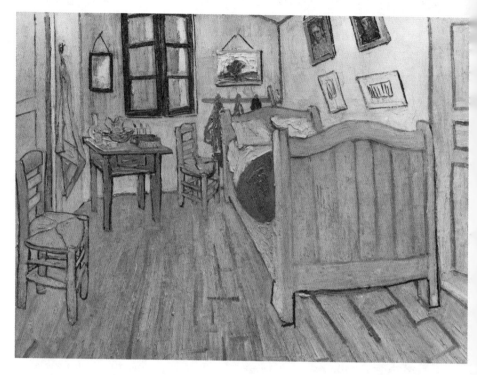

FIG. 79   Van Gogh, *Bedroom at Arles* (1888) (National Museum, Amsterdam).

server has become an integral part of the spatial field and thus there is
further emphasis upon the importance of relative, subjective experience in defining nature.

Ward (1976) takes exception to Heelan's interpretation and offers
the alternative explanation that Van Gogh's two-point perspective
constructions were a function of his artistic concerns and style, his
feelings about the subject matter, his difficulties seeing perspectively,
and the special problems inherent in the representation of space that
encompasses a wide visual angle. Ward (1976, p. 594) notes that Van
Gogh's "principal deviations from uniform perspective construction
. . . are a function of the shifting interaction with the room that is
inherent in the process of its depiction." Ward concludes that the
spatial distortions in a number of Van Gogh's paintings, particularly
those in the *Bedroom at Arles*, were created by Van Gogh's rotating the
plane of the drawing to different positions. Ward believes that it was
the series of realignments of the canvas within the room that complicated the spatial rendering of the scene. Hansen (1973, 1977,

p. 464), however, finds unconvincing Ward's alternative explanation that the deviations in Van Gogh's representations were based on his shifting of the canvas. Hansen points out how Van Gogh's fore-shortened shapes, "bounded by emphatically converging diagonals, as in a wide-angle view," are characteristic of a concern about the basic geometric structure of reality expressed by a number of Impressionist and Post-impressionist artists.

Seurat was also concerned about the basic geometric structure of nature and he sought to represent this in his meticulous construction of figures and scenes out of a multitude of tiny, isolated spots of color. Based on the contemporary interest in theories of optics and color vision, Seurat presented pure color in tiny dots that had an intensity and sparkle. Infinitely small spots of paint defined lines and forms; outlines and contours merged. In painting dots of pure color, Seurat demanded that the viewer, not the artist, blend the colors. He used opposition and contrast, rather than gradation, to achieve emotional climate and affective tone. Seurat, in 1866, at the last Impressionist exhibit, presented his *Grand Jatte* (Fig. 80) which, like Manet's *Luncheon* and many other Impressionist works, involved themes of nature and emphasized the visual sensations of color and light. But Seurat replaced the short, choppy brush-strokes of the Impressionists with a precise and organized placement of small dots that created a repetitive surface pattern as well as an illusion of three-dimensional space. In addition to an interest in the inner structure of light and color, Seurat was also concerned about the basic geometric form of objects and the basic geometric structure of space in the interaction of horizontals, verticals, and diagonals.

Seurat's compositions were tectonic and linear. His figures were flat, stilted silhouettes. While there is often a similarity in the compositional structure of Seurat and Cézanne (see *The Bathers* [Figs. 81 and 82], for example), Cézanne's figures had greater mass and volume, and space was more open. Cézanne's work was more painterly Wölfflin, 1915); he began to use diagonal structures and this painterly quality increased with time. Late in 1905, Cézanne wrote to Bernard of his concern about the black outline around figures and how he considered this a "fault which must be fought at all costs" because it did not exist in nature (Cézanne, 1976, p. 317). Cézanne opened the contours of objects and utilized the white space of the canvas as an integral part of the painting. This gave his work an even greater openness and vitality. Within the context of this painterly orientation,

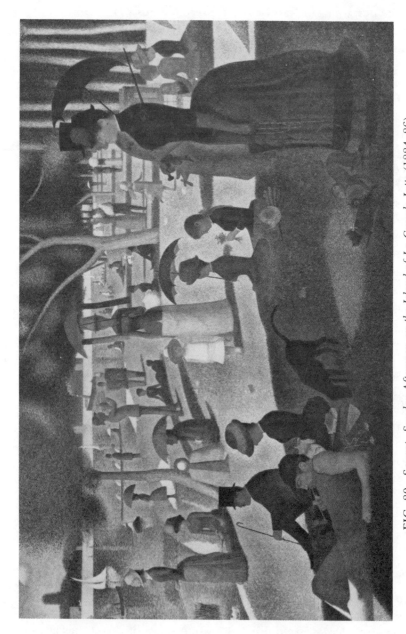

FIG. 80 Seurat, *Sunday Afternoon on the Island of La Grande Jatte* (1884–86) (The Art Institute of Chicago, Helen Birch Bartlett Memorial Collection).

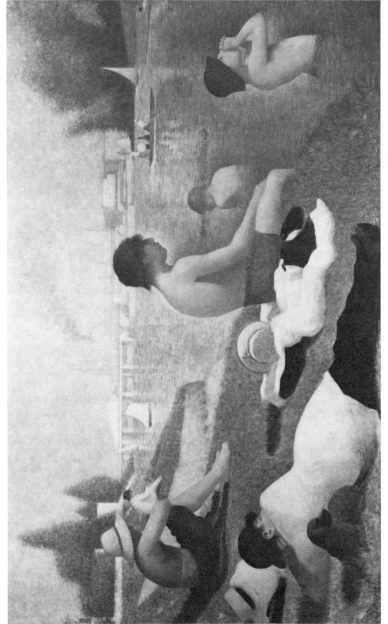

FIG. 81   Seurat, *Bathers* (1883–84) (National Gallery, London).

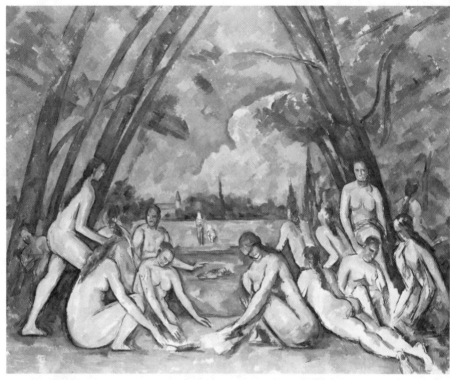

FIG. 82   Cézanne, *The Large Bathers*(1898–1905) (Philadelphia Museum of Art: W. P. Wilstach Collection).

Cézanne emphasized geometric structure and tectonics, supplemented by a "modulation" of color that enabled him to achieve volume and a substantiality of form. Cézanne's lines became more discontinuous, creating open edges and vague boundaries along which color planes were interconnected. This strong painterly orientation, combined with a continuous emphasis on fundamental geometric forms, provided the structure for Cézanne's increasingly abstract use of color.

Cézanne, early in his career, was influenced by the Impressionists' emphasis on the visual sensations of color and light. In fact, Cézanne presented three paintings at the first Impressionist exhibit in 1874. But, like Seurat, he became more and more interested in identifying and representing the basic geometric form and structure of reality. In the early 1880s, Cézanne became actively concerned with the geometric structure of space and tried to reduce forms to their basic geometric elements. He rotated objects toward the observer so that he could represent the basic form of each element. Recession into deep space was closed off to emphasize the fundamental geometric structure of a scene. Cézanne sought to represent the geometric structures of line and form that give nature an organization and coherence (Rubin, 1977). Gowing (1977, pp. 55–56) comments that Cézanne was the "turn from the logical mimetic theory of painting to another, one that is based on inherent meanings." Cézanne did not represent abstract geometric structures, but rather the natural geometric patterns of objects in their simplest, broadest, and most basic form. The most significant natural forms of cylinder, cone, and sphere were represented as simplified shapes without the limitation of a strict adherence to principles of linear perspective. Cézanne considered natural geometric patterns as the basic structure and the essence of objects (Kahnweiler, 1949)."Cézanne was trying, above all, to give an idea of the internal construction of the spaces before him" (Monnier, 1977, p. 113). Cézanne's early compositions were regulated by linear structure and a geometric plan; objects were situated in well-defined and clearly delineated space. But after 1895, the supportive framework of clearly defined space became less important and Cézanne stressed the natural geometric forms of objects. Also, space itself was represented in a succession of planes—another aspect of Cézanne's search for the basic geometric structure of reality (Monnier, 1977). Cézanne's representation of space and of basic, natural, geometric forms were among his most important contributions and provided the basis for Cubism and the subsequent interest of Modern art in the geometric and the abstract (Reff, 1977).

In order for Cézanne to capture the inherent geometric structure of nature, principles of perspective had to be violated to some degree. A table, for example, had to be partially rotated on its axis to emphasize its basic geometric form. In the process there was an inconsistency in the representation of perspective so that the table would slope toward the observer and objects would appear about to fall off the table and onto the floor. But perspective was altered only to the degree necessary to highlight sufficiently the basic form and structure of objects (see Figs. 83 and 84). Cézanne was also interested in preserving perspective as much as possible, for he wrote to Bernard (15 April, 1904) that "nature . . . is more in depth than surface" and "treat nature by means of the cylinder, the sphere, the cone, everything brought into proper perspective so that each side of an object or a plane is directed toward a central point" (Cézanne, 1976, p. 301). But

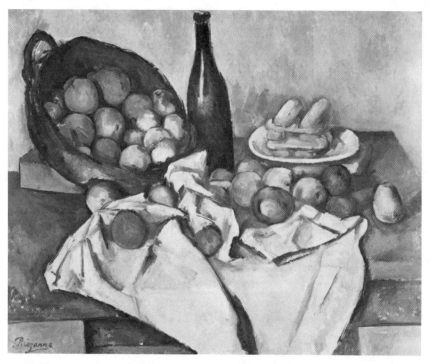

FIG. 83   Cézanne, *The Basket of Apples* (c.1895) (The Art Institute of Chicago, Helen Birch Bartlett Memorial Collection).

Cézanne "dismantled space" and overturned an order that had dominated Western painting for over 500 years. Space was "no longer a cube . . . inside which volumes are laid out in accordance with a pre-established arrangement." Unlike linear perspective, Cézanne's space was defined in terms of the natural geometric structure of objects and their extension into depth. The nature of basic geometric forms determined the conceptual structure of space (Brion-Guerry, 1977).

Cézanne's emphasis on representing basic geometric patterns began to create a system of constructions based on a combination of abstract forms. Objects were transformed into complex combinations of volumes; solids and voids were integrated into a unified structure (Brion-Guerry, 1977). Cézanne made extensive use of negative space—the bare portions of the canvas became as much a part of the picture as painted portions. Objects and space were transformed into complex combinations of volumes and basic geometric elements of the cylinder, the sphere, and the cone. Cézanne's exploration of basic geometric form and the integration of the void as an integral part of

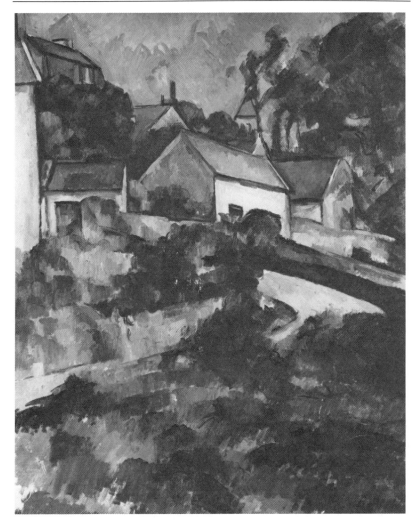

FIG. 84   Cézanne, *The Turning Road at Montgeroult* (1899) (Mrs. John Hay Whitney).

the painting were an essential step in the subsequent development of Cubism and abstract painting.

The integration of object and surrounding space was also facilitated by Cézanne's minimization of the outline contour of objects. Contours were no longer firm and continuous, and the forms of objects tended to merge with adjacent forms. The dissolution of contours allowed for a creation of "passages" between volumes and surrounding space. Objects could extend into the surrounding space while still maintaining their basic definition and integrity. As noted by Brion-Guerry (1977, p. 80) "the figures of the concrete world (persons, elements of landscape or still life) are no longer evoked in an imitation of form, which would only be a transcription of their volumetric materiality. Rather they are re-created beyond an external appearance, in the extensions of the latter, in its essentiality." The object is no longer a limited, immediately apparent value, but it transcends the visible natural world and becomes "a projection of the inner space of the one who re-creates it" (p. 81). Cézanne's search for a unified space enabled art to extend the representation of reality beyond its manifest, figurative appearance. "Space, which had been the place for the localization of the object, was to be entirely transformed with the abolition of that object, and this new space was to correspond to a new and autonomous pictorial reality" (Brion-Guerry, 1977, p. 82).

Cézanne's interest in basic, intrinsic, geometric form and his partial violation of the canons of linear perspective gave his figures a degree of flatness. He compensated for this flatness by using a "modulation" of color to achieve solidity, volume, and depth. Gowing (1977) discusses how Cézanne's use of color was an attempt to re-create the object that had been partially lost in the simplification of geometric form and the disintegration of contours. Cézanne also wrote to Bernard, "To read nature is to see it, as if through a veil, in terms of an interpretation in patches of color following one another according to a law of harmony. These major hues are thus analyzed through modulations. Painting is classifying one's sensations of color" (cited by Gowing, 1977, p. 57).

Color modulation involved the subtle gradations of hue around an object beginning with the highest saturation of color at the apex of the object and proceeding in small but discrete steps down the color spectrum as one moves away from the center of the object. Each new hue of color creates a new, subtle facet of the object that interlocks with other facets to create a sense of volume. Subtle gradations of hue around an object beginning at a climactic center, the point closest to the observer, create volume and a fullness of form. Cézanne (1976) wrote:

> in an orange, an apple, a ball, a head, there is a culminating point; and this point is always—in spite of the tremendous effect, light and shade and colour sensations—the closest to our eye; the edges of the objects flee towards a centre on our horizon (7/25/1904). (p. 306)

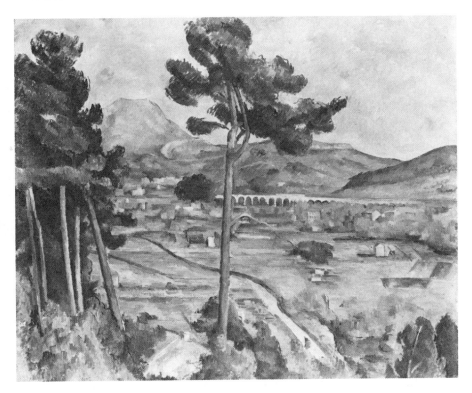

FIG. 85 Cézanne, *Mont Sainte-Victoire* (1885–1887) (The Metropolitan Museum of Art, Bequest of Mrs. H. O. Havemeyer, The H. O. Havemeyer Collection).

Color modulation allowed Cézanne to create volume and depth within the somewhat flattened intrinsic geometric form and structure. Depth was also achieved by utilizing the recession of cool colors and the advance of warm colors. Modulation of planes of color also expressed intervals of depth (see Fig. 85).

Color became an autonomous value in itself, independent of a reference to the object (Brion-Guerry, 1977). The use of color patches became increasingly abstract and "the objects and space that they represented were now translated into apparently immaterial relationships of color" (Gowing, 1977, p. 56). Color modulation created changes in the plane and the curvature of a surface. "Color contrasts become the internal life of art" (Gowing, 1977, p. 61). The structured sequences of color patches were a basic mode of representation for Cézanne in the last three or four years of his life. The sequential application of a spectrum of color in small graded patches, "according to a law of harmony," (Gowing, 1977, p. 63) was integrated with geometric forms and rectilinear structures. The modulation of hues of color created a volume of basic geometric forms. Cézanne, unlike the Impressionists, did not want to represent the fleeting moment, but rather the permanent dimensions of reality (Brion-Guerry, 1977) that exist beneath manifest appearance.

As discussed by Schapiro, the Impressionists and Post-impressionists including Cézanne and Matisse sought to dissect the scene "into surface patterns, the inconsistent, indefinite space, the deformed contours, the peculiarly fragmentary piecing of things at the edge of the picture, the diagonal viewpoint, the bright arbitrary color of objects, unlike their known local color" (Schapiro, 1932, p. 23). Both the Impressionist emphasis upon light and color and Cézanne's concentration on pattern and geometric form were attempts to reconquer the picture plane (Levy, 1943). Cézanne carried Impressionism further by capturing the inner dimensions of objects and scenes in terms of constituent geometric patterns and forms. The Post-impressionist schematized representation of geometric forms, like Impressionism's emphasis on the elements of visual sensation, was a progression toward a more abstract level of representation.

Cézanne was a central figure in the development of the new autonomy of art during the Impressionist and Post-impressionist period. No other individual artist had such an important role in this development (Novotny, 1937). Cézanne's discovery of a new mode for the representation of inner form and structure in geometrical patterns involved a shift from the concrete perceptual to the conceptual level of object representation. The Impressionists—and certainly Cézanne—were moving toward the use of more abstract, formal operations. Their paintings involved transformations of more internal, abstract dimensions rather than more external manifest ones. Cézanne sought to create "something solid and lasting," a new link in a chain of the modes of representing sensations (Cézanne, 1976; letter to Bernard, 1904). While Cézanne concentrated on geometric forms and patterns, he eventually sought to integrate this with light and color (Kahnweiler, 1949). As Cézanne stated:

> Drawing and colour are not at all distinct, everything in nature being coloured. One draws as one paints. Rightness of tone produces both light and the modelling of the object. The greater the colour harmony, the more precise the drawing. Contrasts and relationships of tone—that

is the whole secret of drawing and modelling. . . . A strong feeling for nature . . . is the necessary basis for every conception of art, the basis on which the grandeur and beauty of the art of the future must rest. And no less essential is the knowledge of the means of expressing our emotion. . . . See nature as cylinder, sphere and cone, the whole placed in perspective, so that each side of an object or plane is directed toward a central point. Lines parallel to the horizon give breadth—that is, a section of nature, or, if you prefer, of the spectacle which God the Father, omnipotent and eternal, unfolds before our eyes. Lines perpendicular to the horizon give depth. Now nature is for us more a matter of depth than of surface—whence the necessity of introducing into our vibrations of light, represented by reds and yellows, a sufficient number of bluish tones to give a feeling of air. (Cited by Venturi, 1950, pp. 127–128)

Cézanne presented the fundamental geometric forms that comprised the scene and demanded that the beholder integrate them into cohesive and coherent wholes. He sought to represent endless recessions of interwoven planes. Some art historians (e.g., Novotny, 1937) considered Cézanne's paintings "aloofness from mankind," "cold, rigid, almost repugnant," and difficult to comprehend. Novotny found Cézanne's human figures to have "an almost puppet-like rigidity" with expressions of "emptiness . . . bordering almost on the mask," and a complete lack of movement—a "rigidity which goes beyond their natural immobility" (p. 8). Novotny comments on Cézanne's peculiar representation of light as "neutral, somewhat timeless," indistinct, tending to fade away, failing to give "the impression of continuous lighting," and Cézanne's use of space as having transposed linear perspective in such a way as to reduce animation, attention, and feeling, and to give his objects "a kind of immateriality; despite the solidity of their corporeal and spatial structure" (p. 9). Novotny considers Cézanne's work lacking in the "form of expression of temperament . . . [as] the very antithesis of expressive art" (p. 10). However, it is these very characteristics, particularly Cézanne's rendering of space, "perspective . . . emptied of feeling, the peculiarities of . . . occasional changes of angle, [and] displacement of proportions," (p. 9) that Novotny considers a "turning point of the highest importance in the history of intellectual development" (p. 10). Novotny notes that in comparison with Impressionism, Cézanne's work emphasized a high degree of structural form. There is no earlier analogy to Cézanne's treatment of space. Cézanne reduced and attenuated perspective in favor of a new and unique relationship between pictorial planes and space. Cézanne's pictures were not flat and lacking in extension of depth, but it is difficult for the viewer to enter into the spatial constructions (Novotny, p. 11). Cézanne's pictorial structures were most unique; they emphasized the picture plane and the geometric forms of objects in the picture plane. The impressionist streaks and patches of color were used to elaborate and support the representation of the basic geometric "lapidary" forms that are the underlying structure of Cézanne's work. Cézanne's paintings were not based on the ordinary composition of objects and thus constituted, according to Novotny (p. 13), "the most revolutionary transformations in the history of the development of painting."

Meyer Schapiro (1962) considers Cézanne's art as lying between the veridical representation of objects and the harmony of color usually achieved in conventional paintings and the forms of abstract art. While Cézanne created realistic images of the visible world, his colors were not necessarily accurate for the particular object, but rather they were necessary for the harmony of the painting. In contrast to the Impressionist dissolution of objects in clusters of "twinkling" points of atmosphere and sunlight, Cézanne created a new sense of form and of space by placing successive segments of geometric patterns side by side. Objects on different planes and depths were juxtaposed, balanced, and unified into an organized pattern and composition. Cézanne sought a new sense of organization and structure that was not bound by the fixed canons of linear and atmospheric perspective. These canons had already been relinquished by the Impressionists in their search for representing inner form and structure based on the visual sensations of light and color. Cézanne also represented inner structure, but based on the geometric patterns that are the fundamental forms that constitute objects. It was through the specification of the geometric forms in the various planes that Cézanne was able to attain depth in the pictorial space in a unique and original fashion (Fry, 1932).

As early as 1913, Bell commented on a new movement founded on Cézanne's discovery of methods and forms that opened a horizon of unlimited possibilities for "thousands of artists yet unborn" (p. 207). Cézanne, like the Impressionists, was interested in nature, and he set out to create forms that would capture the structure of nature. For Cézanne, everything could be seen as pure form; form was the essence of an object. According to Bell (1913, p. 209), Cézanne's life was "a continuous effort to capture and express the significance of form" in order to represent the essence of an object. Cézanne sought to represent the object in its pure form, the thing in and of itself, devoid of context or association. Later, Bell (1922) described Cézanne as the bridge between Impressionism and Modern Art. Bell noted that "there is hardly one modern artist of importance to whom Cézanne is not father or grandfather, and that no other influence is comparable with his" (1922, p. 11). Much as Michelangelo bridged Gothic and Baroque, and Turner and Constable bridged Baroque and Impressionism, Cézanne linked Impressionism with Cubism, and in fact with all of Modern Art. Cézanne's contributions constituted a major shift in the mode of representation and, consequently, had profound impact on all Modern Art. Most immediately, Cézanne's style was evident in the development of Cubism, in the works of Braque, Picasso, and Gris. Picasso is known to have referred to Cézanne as "my one and only teacher," for Klee he was "the teacher par excellence," and Matisse is reported to have said that he was "the father of us all" (Reff, 1977, p. 13). Particularly important for the subsequent development of Modern Art were Cézanne's unique creation of form and space and the relation of line and color. Cézanne's emphasis on basic, intrinsic geometric forms, his development of color modulation to create form and volume, and his opening of the contours and creating passages between objects and planes so that they are interlocking provided the basis for much of the subsequent development in Modern Art beginning with Cubism.

CUBISM

Cézanne's articulation of fundamental geometric forms and patterns provided the theoretical basis for a paradigmatic change in the structure of pictorial representation—the simultaneous representation of multiple perspectives. In 1908, shortly after Cézanne's death, Picasso and Braque each independently introduced Cubism into painting. Both were greatly influenced by Cézanne's integration of the fundamental geometric forms of objects in a series of separate planes rather than the harmonious integration of figures around a central vanishing point (Cooper, 1972). Both Picasso and Braque found in Cézanne the basis for a new series of experimentations with the canons of linear perspective. Braque (1961; cited by Cooper, 1972) wrote:

> I said goodbye to the "vanishing point." And to avoid any projection toward infinity I interposed a series of planes, I set one on top of the

other, at a short distance from the spectator. It was to make him realize that objects did not retreat backwards into space but stood up close in front of one another. Cézanne has thought a lot about that. You have only to compare his landscapes with Corot's, for instance, to see that he had done away with distance and that after him infinity no longer exists. Instead of starting with the foreground I always began with the centre of the picture. Before long I even turned perspective inside out and turned the pyramid of forms upside down so that it came forward to meet the observer. (p. 4)

As early as 1894 *(The Kitchen Table)*, Cézanne had experimented with combining several different viewpoints to create a sense of rounded volume and substantiality in objects. He analyzed objects into basic geometric forms and simple planes and presented them from several viewpoints and an ambiguous perspective. Cézanne attempted to modify linear perspective without losing the basic coherence of the compositional structure. He sought "to give equal value to the mind and to the eye, to the permanent side of reality and to the transient effect, to volume and to flatness, to light effects and to the structure of space"—without linear perspective. He "built up forms and volumes and evoked space with color alone, avoiding linear definition. But in order to reconcile his awareness of depth and roundness with his desire to preserve the flatness of the picture-surface as a reality, Cézanne resorted to changes of perspective within the picture itself" (Cooper, 1971, pp. 19–20).

Cézanne was preoccupied with basic geometric structure and form (Kahnweiler, 1949), but objects in his paintings often appeared distorted because he shifted perspective within a single composition. He utilized modulations of color to achieve volume, and forms were organized into discrete areas. There was a contrast of forms in which objects were often realigned or reshaped. Picasso and Braque were fascinated by Cézanne's shifting perspective and his use of passages to maintain compositional integrity. Based on Cézanne's bold innovations, Picasso and Braque independently realized that they did not have to limit themselves to representations from a single, fixed vantage point, but could represent an object simultaneously from multiple perspectives—from several sides, above and below, and inside and outside. They no longer felt bound to the more or less veridical and realistic representation of an object's manifest features. Impressionism and Post-impressionism had already broken with the canons of linear perspective and the realistic representation of manifest form. Picasso and Braque each independently realized that by representing the primary characteristics of an object simultaneously from several different vantage points, various components and conceptions of the object, including its three-dimensional diversity, could be expressed and integrated within a single perceptual field. Braque is quoted (Cooper, 1972) as commenting to Vallier as follows:

> Traditional perspective gave me no satisfaction. It is scientifically ordered and never allows one to take full possession of things. It operates from a single vantage point, which is never abandoned. Now the viewpoint is a minor consideration. Imagine a man who spends his life drawing profiles, as though he would have one believe that man has only one eye. Once we reached this stage in our thinking—Picasso and I—everything changed. You have no idea of how much! I was above all attracted to making real the new sense of space that I felt—and this was a major force in Cubism. (p. 45)

Picasso and Braque completely abandoned the perceptual approach of linear perspective and the representation of reality from a single, fixed vantage point in favor of a more conceptual approach to representing various aspects and features of the object both in its immediately visible (and invisible) dimensions. These artists went beyond Cézanne's attempts to articulate basic geometric form and began to represent what they knew about the object as well as what was visible at a particular moment and from a particular view. Contours and boundaries were opened up, and separate volumes were integrated in interlocking planes. Through a series of variously oriented planes that interact and counteract with each other, various facets of objects were represented simultaneously, and elaborate arrangements of planes created volume and a new sense of space. For the first time since the Renaissance, art relinquished representation from a single, fixed vantage point for a systematic representation of multiple perspectives. An object was represented in numerous ways including what was seen of the object, what was known about the object, and what could be seen if the object were viewed from other vantage points. The Cubists not only broke away from the spatial illusion of perspective discovered in the Renaissance, but also from the emphasis on the classic, idealized, sterotyped form of objects, especially that of the human figure. While some critics discuss the influence of African art in Picasso's abandonment of normal anatomical features and proportions, the most significant aspect of Picasso's representation of the human body seems to have been a function of his change to a representation of objects from multiple perspectives (Cooper, 1971; Fry, 1966).

Picasso and Braque sought to create a new system for representing three-dimensional space independent of linear perspective. They wanted to penetrate closed forms (Kahnweiler, 1949) in order to achieve a fuller comprehension of the inner structure of objects. The background of the painting was limited so that the multiple facets of the object could be highlighted. Volume and mass were expressed through the analysis of forms and the integration of different aspects and facets. Volume within the object was represented as a series of interlocking cubes. Planes and forms opened up and interpenetrated each other so that the artist could discover inner structure (Cooper, 1971). The object was dissected in order to capture its inner composition.

In 1907, with his revolutionary painting *Les Demoiselles d'Avignon* (Fig. 86), Picasso integrated frontal, profile, and other views in a profound break with the Renaissance canons for realistic representation. While *Les Demoiselles* is not considered a fully Cubist painting, it marks a major turning point in the history of art leading into the "Cubist Epoch" (Cooper, 1971). In *Les Demoiselles,* Picasso flattened and simplified figures, gave them sharp contours, and compressed them into a very shallow pictorial space. He achieved an innovative form for representing space without the use of perspective, color, or light. The perceptual mode of representation of the Renaissance was abandoned and so also were the concrete manifest features of figures; instead, figures were given generalized, impersonal, mask-like geometric features. *Les Demoiselles* marked the birth of a new mode of representation to be developed more completely over the next seven years. Cubism is generally dated as beginning in 1907–1908 and continuing as an active style until 1925, though the major innovations were completed by 1914. Cubism, beginning with Picasso's *Les Demoiselles,* initiated "new approaches both to the treatment of space and to the expression of human emotions and states of mind" (Fry, 1966, p. 12). This painting marks Picasso's break with the two primary features that had characterized European art since the Renaissance: the spatial illusion of linear perspective and the representation of the classic human form.

In the early phases of Cubism, objects were dissected and surfaces became angular facets. The Cubists intially concentrated on achieving

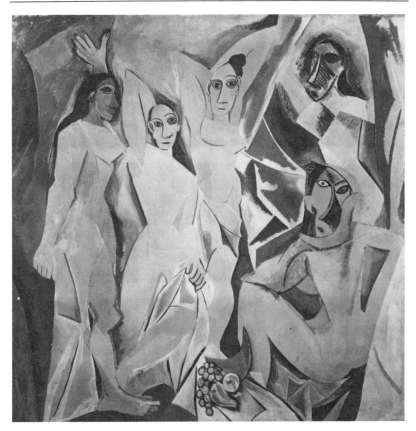

FIG. 86 Picasso, *Les Demoiselles d'Avignon* (1907) (The Museum of Modern Art, New York. Acquired through the Lillie P. Bliss Bequest).

a new representation of space in which form and volume were presented in a basic simplicity with little, if any, use of color. According to Giedion (1941/1967):

> Fragments of lines hover over the surface, often forming open angles which become the gathering places of darker tones. These angles and lines began to grow, to be extended, and suddenly out of them developed one of the constituent facts of space-time representation—the plane.
>
> The advancing and retreating planes of Cubism, interpenetrating, hovering, and often transparent without anything to fix them in realistic position, are in fundamental contrast to the lines of perspective which converge to a single focal point. (p. 437)

Cubism created a new kind of pictorial space based on the representation of basic geometric forms from multiple viewpoints and

markedly different angles. The simultaneous presentation of different viewpoints and discontinuous and interpenetrating planes replaced the representation of fixed appearance. The manifest external
form of objects was replaced by the representation of abstract inner
form. Objects, and their embedding space, could now be represented
by endless arrays of lines, planes, and color.

Cubism was a first major step in bringing into painting a self-
reflective awareness, a self-consciousness, about the act of painting.
Greco-Roman art had been based on a theory of vision, Renaissance
art had been founded on a theory of representation, and Cubism was
based on a theory of conception—on a self-reflective awareness of the
role of the individual (artist and observer) in the construction of nature. Cubism emphasized the arbitrary nature of one's perspective by
representing each of a number of perspectives by a different plane.
Cubism's multiple views of the same object was an attempt to represent the artistic process of looking at an object and studying its multiple aspects. Cubism evokes in the viewer a sense that no previous
painting has really represented "reality" because it was based on an
arbitrary choice of a unique but limited frame of reference or perspective. Cubism emphasized a self-reflective awareness of the subjective nature of the artistic process and the artist's role in choosing a
particular form of representation.

The development of Cubism is often discussed as a return to the
principles of an earlier mode of "conceptual" art that had occurred
during the Ancient period. Cooper (1971, p. 11) discussed Cubism as
"a return to the earlier conceptual principle, insofar as the artist assumed the right to fill gaps in our seeing, and to make pictures whose
reality would be independent of, but no less valid than, our visual
impressions of reality, and was thus stylistically the antithesis of Renaissance art." Ancient art was also described as "conceptual" by Bunim
(1940), who contrasted it with the "optical" mode of the Renaissance
in which objects were represented as they appeared to the spectator.
Ancient art, however, was not conceptual because it did not seek to
integrate the diversity of elements that were known or could be
known, about the object, but instead simply represented the object as
a concrete, literal entity as it existed in its manifest external form in
nature. Thus it seems more appropriate to think of Ancient art as
utilizing a concrete, rather than a conceptual mode of representation.
This early, literal, *concrete mode* in Ancient art should not only be
contrasted with the *optical mode* of the Renaissance but it should also

be differentiated from the *conceptual mode* begun in Cubism in which there was an attempt to represent the object in the multiple ways and forms it could potentially be known. The Cubists sought to portray a conception rather than a perception of reality, based on the awareness that we know and experience objects from many different perspectives (Fry, 1966).

Picasso (and Braque) used Cézanne's emphasis on geometric forms and shifting perspectives to represent "what he knew to be there and not what nature made him see at certain moments" (Cooper, 1971, p. 34). Picasso and Braque dissected material forms into their essential planes and volumes and challenged the Renaissance assumption that reality is perceived and conceptualized only as a continuous entity from a single, fixed perspective. Instead, Cubism stressed that reality must be defined from multiple segments taken from a variety of perspectives that must be integrated into a comprehensive conception. The Cubists sought to identify a basic underlying reality rather than manifest surface appearance (Gleizes & Metzinger, 1913) by representing forms in space from multiple perspectives in a series of discontinuous planes. Picasso and Braque, beginning in 1908, sought to explore further the form and structure of the representation of three-dimensional objects on a two-dimensional surface. Initially, they rejected light and color as means of creating form and sought to use geometric forms to understand the basic underlying three–dimensional structure of reality and to represent it on a two–dimensional surface (Kahnweiler, 1949) (see Figs. 87 and 88).

In the earlier phase of Cubism (Analytic Cubism), planes were used in a variety of ways to represent fragments of objects, the exterior and interior of objects, and manifest and imagined or fantasied aspects of objects. Objects were made tangible by the interaction and juxtaposition of facets in the picture plane and the composition of the painting was given coherence by the structure of vertical, horizontal, and diagonal lines. In Analytic Cubism, commonplace objects were simplified into basic geometric shapes that were constructed into intersecting and interpenetrating planes. The manifold aspects of an object were dissected and reintegrated in a representation of multiple features from many different angles. Color was neglected in favor of a preoccupation with the beauty of pure geometric form. In an elaborate arrangement of facets and planes, the boundary and contour of forms were opened up so the inner form and structure of objects could be penetrated (Cooper, 1971). Artists attempted to present the

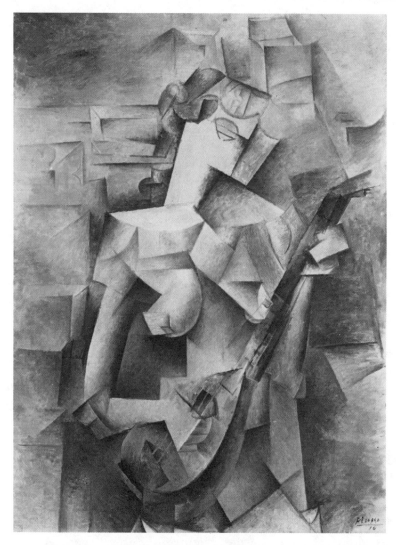

FIG. 87   Picasso, *Girl with Mandolin* (Fannie Teller) (early 1910) (Museum of Modern Art, New York, Nelson A. Rockefeller Bequest).

essential information about figures and objects and to create a visual reality in a non-mimetic mode of representation. Color was cautiously introduced into Cubism by Picasso in 1910. Cubism quickly moved toward greater abstraction, and objective content was only faintly apparent in the structure of lines, facets, and planes. Cubism struggled to maintain a balance between the representation of a tangible reality and the purely spatial structure (Cooper, 1971).

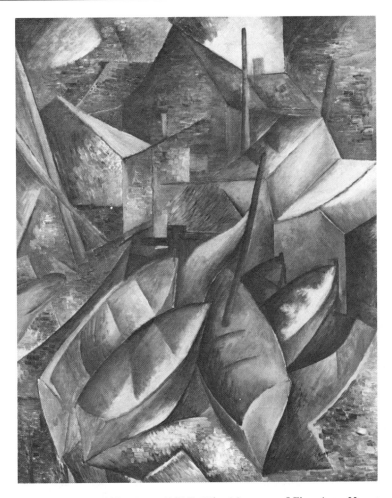

FIG. 88 Braque, *Fishing Boats* (1909) (The Museum of Fine Arts, Houston, John A. and Audrey Jones Beck Collection).

In the later phase of Synthetic Cubism, beginning around 1911, the emphasis on planes was augmented by the collage, in which a variety of materials added a tactile dimension. The overlapping and inter-locking pieces of material also heightened the flat, spatial ambiguity. Subsequently, color was added to the collage, first tentatively, spar-ingly, as an integral part of the object, but eventually color became diverse, intense, and independent of the natural color of objects. Color and light came to have existence in their own right, indepen-dent of form. The break with realistic (local) color was yet another step in demonstrating the arbitrary nature of painting. It was another assertion of artists' potential freedom from veridical naturalistic representation. The representation of the diversity of objects by lines, angles, facets, and interacting planes was enriched by independent dimensions of light, color, and textural variations. Curvilinear forms were also introduced, and there was a move toward breaking completely with literal representation, dealing instead with abstract forms that referred to external and internal features of objects in nature.

Cubism replaced the system of linear perspective that had dominated European art since the Renaissance. Cubism defined a new method of pictorial representation that enabled artists to integrate what they knew about an object as well as what they saw. Color, light, form, and volume became separate, independent, pictorial elements that allowed for multiple ways of representing the complexity and diversity of reality. Painting found a new freedom—it was no longer bound to a realistic representation from a single, fixed perspective. Objects were no longer defined by the surface and boundaries of closed forms, but instead a variety of colored planes were utilized to represent a synthesis of various dimensions and conceptions of objects (Fry, 1966). Cubism initiated a major revolution in the history of Western art.

Arnheim (1954/1974) disagrees with the interpretation that Cubism was, at least partially, an attempt to present a fuller conception of an object by combining various aspects and perspectives. He comments:

> The beholder is presumably to fly on the wings of his mind from one perspective view to the other, or to find himself at different locations simultaneously. By such mental acrobatics the viewer himself would perform the dynamics actually inherent in the work. In fact, of course, he is looking not at the three-dimensional object but at a flat picture of it, in which the aspects clash in deliberate contradiction. (p. 132)

Arnheim (1954/1974, p. 302) considers Cubism an attempt "to portray the modern world as a precarious interplay of independent" coherent units by intentionally setting up "visual clashes, contradictions and mutual interferences." He views Cubism as seeking to express a fundamental disorder that exists in the incompatibility inherent in space when self-contained, separate units are not part of a continuous whole but rather interact blindly and irrationally. Arnheim stresses that only the delicate balancing of innumerable forces and angles can provide a semblance of unity, not unlike the delicate balance needed to cope with ambiguity and contradiction in contemporary thought and social relations.

Gombrich (1960) in a similar vein, considers Cubism "the last desperate revolt against illusion" (p. 281). Cubism, to Gombrich, was an attempt to destroy the coherent image of reality achieved in the integration and coordination of clues according to perspective. By presenting contradictory clues of perspective, shading, and texture, Cubism attempted to counter and destroy the "transforming effects of an illusionist reading" (p. 282) of linear perspective. Gombrich views Cubism as a constant tease and temptation to destroy the single, best possible presentation in linear perspective by introducing contradictory clues that "resist all attempts to apply the test of consistency" (p. 282). Through frequent shifts in figure and ground and numerous other devices, the Cubists sought to "baffle our perception" (p. 284). In Cubism, each hypothesis about the nature of a three-dimensional object is rejected because of contradictory clues in the picture so that "our interpretation can never come to rest" (p. 283). Divergence between outline and silhouette, and transparent forms piled one upon the other, create ambiguity about the sequences of objects and the definition of coherent forms. According to Gombrich, the function of representational clues in Cubism is not to inform us about the nature of objects, but to "narrow down the range of possible interpretations till we are forced to accept the flat pattern with all its tensions" (p. 286).

Both Arnheim and Gombrich consider Cubism a desperate revolt against linear perspective because they consider it as presenting conflicting clues that do not add to the viewer's knowledge about the nature of objects and of space, but only create a flat pattern with tension and contradiction. This view of Cubism is consistent with the theoretical orientation that Arnheim and Gombrich use to approach the history of art, an orientation based on perceptual theory and research. Arnheim, using Gestalt theories of perception, and Gombrich, integrating the experimental perceptual research of Gibson (1950), Held (1965), Hochberg (1972), and others, analyze the perceptual dimensions of modes of representation in art. Their analysis of the history of art based on perceptual theory and research has provided considerable understanding of the development of modes of representation, particularly an appreciation of the monumental discovery of linear perspective in the Renaissance that enabled artists to create a complex, highly realistic, three-dimensional visual experience on a two-dimensional surface. Perceptual theory has been valuable for understanding the development of modes of representation of the manifest features and appearance of objects in a cohesive and integrated conception of space. But perceptual theory is limited for understanding the more conceptual modes of representation begun in Post-impressionism and Cubism. In terms of perceptual theory, Cubism has to appear as a desperate revolt against the coherent image achieved in one-point perspective. From a theoretical model based on perceptual processes, Cubism must be considered inconsistent and contradictory, destructive to the illusion of perspective, baffling to our perceptions, and demanding the viewer to engage in mental acrobatics and flights of fancy. A theoretical model based on perceptual theory is insufficient for an analysis of the modes of representation in Cubism and much of modern art that followed. A theory of perception is insufficient for articulating the continuity between the modes of representation in Cubism with earlier modes of representation. The more conceptual mode of representation in Cubism, as well as the earlier modes of representation in the history of art, however, can be viewed as integral aspects of a complex developmental process if one considers them from a cognitive theoretical model based on the development of modes of representation. Piaget stresses that perception and representation are interrelated processes, but he insists on the distinction between the passive, automatic, perceptual reading of a situation and the active, constructive, cognitive processes of representation. Representations are clearly based upon perceptual input, but the cognitive processes of representation go beyond innate perceptual processes. Because perception and representation are interrelated, analysis of the development of style in the history of art from a theory of representation is consistent with the insights gained from an analysis based on perceptual theory, but representational theory provides a broader, more extended and encompassing theoretical model. An analysis of the history of art based on representational theory provides a basis for understanding the concrete, optical, and conceptual modes of representation as well as the interrelationships among these modes. Representational theory provides the theoretical basis for the establishment of a continuity between the concrete representations of Ancient Art, the realistic representation of manifest and concrete objects in Renaissance Art, and the more abstract and symbolic modes of representation of Modern Art. Representational theory provides a comprehensive model for understanding the shifts from concrete to optical to conceptual modes in the history of art as shifts from preoperational to concrete to formal (or abstract) cognitive operational schema.

From the vantage point of a theory of representation, the conceptual modes of representation of Cubism must be considered a logical extension and enrichment of the level of representation achieved in the Renaissance. These developments in the history of art reflect a shift in modes of representation based on concrete operations to those based on formal operations. These developments involve a change in emphasis from manifest, concrete, external form to more abstract internal dimensions of an object, as well as a change from the representation of reality from the unique, fixed, single vantage point to an appreciation of multiple perspectives. According to Piaget (1970a), developmentally more advanced modes of representation require the resolution of a second level of egocentricity and the eventual realization that reality is not experienced in a single, generalized, universal form, but from many different and possibly equally valid perspectives. The multiple perspectives of Cubism are a search for the abstract form and intrinsic structure of objects, based on the recognition that experiences of reality are relative, multifaceted, and fundamentally indeterminate and ambiguous. While an object can certainly be recognized and represented from a particular perspective, Cubism attempted to acknowledge that concrete events and facts are constantly open to multiple interpretations. A full understanding and representation of reality must include the recognition of concrete objects or events, but also the recognition that different individuals, or one individual over time, can experience the same objects or events differently. An essential dimension in the development of modes of representation is the extension of the representation of the manifest form of objects from a particular vantage point to the appreciation that the object can also be experienced from multiple perspectives. It is important to stress that the representation of multiple perspectives in Cubism could not have taken place without the prior attainment of representations of the manifest form of objects from a single vantage point. Linear perspective was an essential step in the eventual development of the representation of multiple perspectives. But the multiple perspectives of Cubism must be considered a major extension in the development of modes of representation because it indicates progress, in Piaget's terms, from the egocentricity of a unitary, fixed, subjective vantage point, to an appreciation of multiple subjectivity. Cubism was not a struggle to break away from the illusion of linear perspective, but a natural extension of the representation of an object beyond the confines of a fixed, unitary conception of reality.

Some authors (e.g., Hamilton, 1956; Laporte, 1949, 1966; Levy, 1943) concluded that the simultaneous representation of multiple perspectives in Cubism, shortly after the Einstein-Minkowski conceptualization of the space-time continuum, introduced the element of time into art. Cooper (1971), however, disagreed because neither Picasso nor Braque imagined himself as a spectator walking among or around the objects being represented. Instead, Cooper concludes, the Cubists were trying to express the inner dimensions and structure of objects, both what was seen and visible as well as what was unseen but known to be there. Cooper is correct, for what is unique about the nature of representation in Cubism is not the introduction of time, but rather a shift from concepts of space based on Euclidean rectilinear geometry to concepts of space based on the integration of a number of different geometries, only one of which is the three-dimensional linear coordinate system of Euclidean geometry. El Lissitzky (1925) is noted to have commented (Descargues, 1976, p. 9) that "perspective bounded and enclosed space, but science has since brought about a fundamental revision. The rigidity of Euclidean space has been annihilated by Lobachevski, Gauss and Riemann." The Cubists were informed about the concepts of non-Euclidean geometries and used them as a rationale for representing deformed objects (Gleizes & Metzinger, 1913). Euclidean geometry had dominated both art and science since the late Renaissance, but in the mid-19th century, mathematicians (Lobachevski, Bolyai, Gauss, and Riemann) developed non-Euclidean geometries and concepts of n-dimensional space (Reichenbach, 1928/1957). And with the development of Cubism, art for the first time since the Renaissance reflected a new conception of space in which linear perspective was only a limited case within the infinite potentialities of non-Euclidean geometries (Chipp, 1968). This fascination with non-Euclidean, n-dimensional geometries was a dominant aspect of mathematical and scientific thought throughout the late 19th and early 20th centuries. The implications of these new geometries had an essential role in the development of Cubism in France (e.g., Apollinaire, 1949; Gleizes & Metzinger, 1913) and Futurist and Suprematist Art (e.g., Malevich) in Russia during the early 20th century (Henderson, 1975).

Linear perspective had provided a method for representing a predefined point of view that was specific, fixed, and unambiguous. Cubism abandoned linear perspective and sought to represent objects from multiple points of view simultaneously, from all sides of the object, above and below, inside and out. The Cubists in art, as the geometricians in mathematics, examined the fundamental assumptions and methods of representing space. The simultaneous representation of multiple perspectives in art was consistent with the contemporary recognition that reality could be experienced from a complex, infinite, and equally valid series of perspectives. According to Giedion (1941/1967, p. 437), "this new representation of space was accomplished step by step, much as laboratory research gradually arrives at its conclusions through long experimentation; and yet, as always with real art and great science, the results came up out of the subconscious suddenly." As we will discuss in more detail at the close of this chapter, it is impressive that Cubism occurred in the same period as Einstein's revolutionary formulations of the special and general theory of relativity in 1905 and 1915 that destroyed the concepts of absolute space and time and the concept of a privileged frame of reference for viewing the universe. It is equally impressive that as early as 1909–10, Arnold Bennett experimented with a new approach to the novel in his trilogy, *The Clayhanger Family,* in which he presented the same series of events as experienced from three different perspectives, and that during the later stages of Cubism, from 1914–1924, an emphasis on ambiguity and multiple or shaded meanings developed in literature in the work of T. S. Eliot, Ogden and Richards, Empson, and others.

Cubism provided the final break with the Renaissance tradition that had prevailed for 500 years; it replaced illusionism with a new interpretation of reality (Fry, 1966). Many of the contributions in art, literature, philosophy, and science at the beginning of the 20th century are characterized by an abandonment of fixed and absolute concepts of space and time and a fixed and pre-defined position for viewing nature. Instead, there was increasing awareness of equivalence of multiple perspective and the multidimensional, multifaceted, essentially ambiguous and ultimately indeterminate quality of our understanding of nature. Cubism continued to diminish the distinction between the viewer as subject and the painting as object, and to bring them into a unified field. Cubism achieved a fuller integration of the spectator and the painting by demanding that the viewer share in the dynamics inherent in the multiple perspectives and that the viewer construct, from the multiple planes, a unified conception of the object (Arnheim, 1954/1974). Artists became increasingly aware of their role in the construction of reality.

MODERN ART

There is general agreement that Cubism was the key to the development of modern art (Arnason, 1968; Rosenberg, 1975). Cubism moved beyond the representation of external manifest features of an object from a fixed point in space and at a particular moment in time. Cubism was the transition from an art of perception and mimesis to an art of conception and abstraction (Cooper, 1971; Fry, 1966; Gablik, 1976; Rosenberg, 1975). Paintings were no longer just to be looked at, but now they had to be understood (Cooper, 1971). The representation of external manifest form was replaced by the simultaneous representation of multiple viewpoints. There was also a dissociation of the pictorial elements of line, plane, shape, and color that permitted each of these dimensions to contribute to a representation of nature based on new principles. Reality was no longer defined as unitary and fixed but rather as complex and multifaceted, with everchanging meaning. Because art was no longer restricted to surface appearance and manifest form, a whole new universe of lines, planes, colors, and endless patterns could be explored. Cubism in art, like Einstein's theory of relativity in science, challenged the existing concepts of a fixed and predetermined frame of reference and of absolute space and absolute time. It became increasingly clear that the fundamental dimensions of nature had to be viewed from many, equally valid, vantage points.

These discoveries led, in part, to the realization that the experience and conception of reality is influenced by the relative position of the observer. Nature was no longer simply to be observed, but was a construction based on a particular vantage point. It was no longer possible to simply accept the surface appearance of phenomena as completely valid since there could be multiple ways of describing manifest characteristics. In order to understand phenomena, one had to identify the intrinsic structure and the organizational principles that underlie manifest appearance. It was a natural and logical extension of the general comparability of multiple perspectives to search for the fundamental, internal, abstract dimensions that underlie and are the basis of multiple viewpoints. This emphasis on internal structure became, to use Foucault's (1970) term, a major "cultural episteme" of our time. Structuralism became a central focus in multiple fields of endeavor. Structuralism involves the identification of the inherent principles of organization that define the relationships among elements and their potential transformations in hierarchically organized systems. This interest in underlying structural principles of organization has had a major impact in the physical, social, and biological sciences, and in art, literature, linguistics, anthropology, psychology, and the history of art. In all these disciplines increasing emphasis has been placed on the need to identify and understand the principles of structural organization that define the interrelationships and potential transformations of elements that determine variations of surface phenomena.

Cubism sought to identify and represent underlying structure and inner form. While Cubism maintained ties with the stable, constant, concrete manifest form of the object, it represented the object as a multifaceted experience in an essentially indefinite context. Cubism maintained a balance between manifest features and a degree of abstraction and transformation, but it also opened the way for the representation of more abstract and formal dimensions. The representation of multifaceted manifest form as well as aspects of internal form and underlying structure provided the basis for the development of abstract, nonrepresentational art that attempts to specify the basic internal structures and principles that unify and integrate multiple, manifest features.

As discussed by Walter Benjamin (1977), it is difficult, if not impossible, to appreciate historical trends within contemporary culture because one needs the distance of time to understand which trends will eventually become the major contributions of any historical epoch. Thus, any formulation and analysis of trends in contemporary art must, to some degree, be myopic and distorted by the *Weltanschauung* and individual values and priorities. In contrast, a historical analysis over time has the benefits of the leveling and sharpening of major and minor trends that become apparent only within the ruins of history (Benjamin, 1977). Based on developmental psychological theory, however, one major direction in Modern Art has been the further development of the representation of inner structure and organization—the abstract and symbolic dimensions that lie beneath the manifest, concrete features of a specific object. While Cubism began to represent the inner form and structure of specific objects, Modern Art has tried to capture the basic abstract dimensions inherent in all objects and in the process of painting itself. Art has grown increasingly autonomous of specific objects in nature, searching instead for basic, universal, inner forms and underlying structural principles. In developmental psychological terms, there has been a major shift from modes of representation based on concrete operations and manifest features to modes of representation based on formal operations that deal with abstract relations and internal structures. In Modern Art, artists seek to represent pure form and balance, independent of content and context. Nonobjective art utilizes formal, logical, geometric forms to represent underlying structural principles such as harmony, balance, order, sequence, progression, regularity and randomness. The use of "pure form aims more directly at the hidden clockwork of nature" (Arnheim, 1954/1974, p. 147). Gablik (1976), based on developmental psychological concepts, provides an excellent analysis of the search in Modern Art for the representation of inner form and structure. Painting is no longer founded on a theory of vision as in the Archaic and Greco-Roman period, or on a theory of representation as in the Renaissance and the Baroque, but now on a theory of conception and symbol formation.

Kandinsky and Mondrian, two primary figures in the transition from Cubism to Modern Art, provided the final break with mimetic art and the representation of a concrete manifest object (Apollinaire, 1949). Kandinsky had been most impressed with Monet's *Haystack* that he saw in Moscow in 1895 and he is reported to have "wondered if it would not be possible to go further in this direction" (cited by Stratton, 1977, p. v).

Kandinsky (1913) wrote:

That it was a haystack the catalogue informed me. I could not recognize it. This nonrecognition was painful to me. I considered that the painter had no right to paint indistinctly. I dully felt that the object of the picture was missing. And I noticed with astonishment and confusion that the picture not only draws you but impresses itself indelibly on your memory and, completely unexpectedly, floats before your eyes even to the last detail. All this was unclear to me, and I could not draw the simplest conclusions of this experience. But what was entirely clear to me—was the unsuspected power of the palette, which had up to now been hidden from me, and which surpassed all my dreams. Painting acquired a fairy–power and splendor. And unconsciously the object was discredited as an indispensable element of a painting (cited by Herbert, 1964; p. 26).

Kandinsky was part of the Munich Secession of the late 1890s in which younger artists sought to break away from "academy–dominated organizations and exhibitions" and find "standards of simplified abstraction and beauty . . . (free) from the mechanized, industrial world" (Stratton, 1977, p. vi). Kandinsky was also very influenced by the Fauvist liberation of color and eventually by abstraction which permitted him to express his spirituality and "inner self." Kandinsky wrote (cited by Stratton, 1977, p. vii) "I value only those artists . . . who consciously or unconsciously . . . embody the expression of their inner life." Kandinsky sought to leave the art of the objective world to discover a new method and a new subject matter based only on the artist's "inner need" and subjectivity. His quest to dematerialize the object and to relinquish the last vestiges of natural representation was central to the major artistic revolution toward a theory of non-objective art (Stratton, 1977). Kandinsky eventually developed a geometric style in which the forms of the triangle, circle, and pyramid were predominant in a search for a "reasoned and conscious . . . constructive" (Kandinsky, 1911/1977, p. 57) method in which form is adapted "to its inner meaning" as it "springs from the soul" of the artist (p. 55–56).

Kandinsky emphasized the properties of color, line, and shape, while ignoring subject matter and surface appearance. He emerged from the German Expressionist movement of the later 19th and early 20th centuries which, like French Impressionism, was interested in emotions and experiences rather than the fixed manifest forms of nature. German Expressionism and French Impressionism were both reactions against the idealized and romantic interpretations of nature and the classical themes that dominated art in the 19th century. German Expressionism, like French Impressionism, was a reaction against the stifling artistic climate of the established academies. They both sought to identify the underlying structure of objects. But instead of attempting to identify intrinsic structures in the experiences of light and color, Expressionists sought this structure in geometric forms and basic composition. Influenced by Impressionism, Post-impressionism, and Cubism, they attempted to depict the underlying spirit and structure of nature and man in generalized forms. By 1914, Kandinsky was arranging geometric shapes in carefully planned and logically ordered sequences. He was also utilizing colors to express feelings with little preconception or intention. He sought to express emotional experience and the deep personal sense of reality within ourselves, rather than the rational naturalistic world (see Fig. 89).

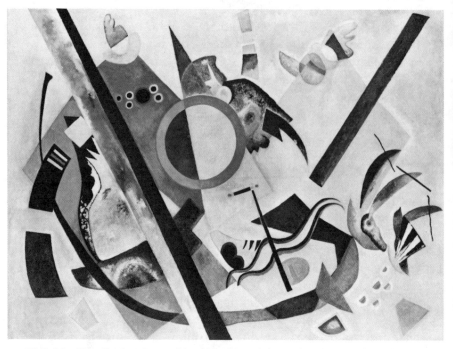

FIG. 89   Kandinsky, *Composition No. 238: Bright Circle* (1921) (Yale University Art Gallery, Gift of Collection Société Anonyme).

Mondrian also renounced all manifest representational elements and instead used only basic geometric forms such as horizontal and vertical straight lines, right angles, squares and rectangles, and primary colors (red, yellow, and blue) and non-colors (black, white, and grey). He constructed two-dimensional designs of balance and order in an asymmetrical organization of line, color, shape, and area (see Fig. 90). Mondrian (1951, p. 15) noted that "true reality is attained through dynamic movement in equilibrium . . . that equilibrium can only be established through the balance of unequal but equivalent oppositions." Rosenberg (1975, p. 42) discusses how Mondrian's abstractions "carried Cubism to the logical conclusion of absolutely flat and non-representative compositions" that provided the basis for Abstract Art. Landscapes were translated into horizontals and verticals, objects were compressed into straight lines, and nuances of nature were replaced by quantitative harmonies. Mondrian sought to use art to define the essential dimensions of nature, and he was very much aware that his work was only the beginning of abstraction in art.

Arnheim (1954/1974) agrees with the emphasis in Modern Art on

FIG. 90   Mondrian, *Fox Trot B* (1929) (Yale University Art Gallery, Gift of Collection Société Anonyme).

the appreciation and study of the interplay between shape, color, shading, and content. But he is concerned that the subject matter not be dismissed as unimportant because content is correlated with abstract and formal patterns and can provide a concrete embodiment of an abstract theme. Arnheim notes that there has always been abstraction in representational art. Even in representational mimetic art, the simplest line is symbolic and expresses meaning. As Panofsky (1924/ 25) insisted, the process of depicting a three-dimensional object on a two-dimensional surface is essentially an abstract, symbolic process. But abstract, non-mimetic art focuses exclusively on the underlying abstraction that has always been present but essentially ignored in representational art. Abstract art emphasizes the inner abstract, symbolic dimensions that transcend any particular object and yet establishes that basic common structures that are inherent in, and serve to unite, all objects. As Mondrian stated in 1937, "we are now at the turning point of this culture; the culture of particular form is approaching its end. The culture of determined relations has begun . . . nonfigurative art demands an attempt of . . . the destruction of particular form and the construction of a rhythm of mutual relations, of mutual forms or free lines" (cited by Herbert, 1964, p. 121–122). Abstract art is no longer tied to a concrete, literal reality, but is now dealing with hypothetical constructs. Art has moved "beyond objects to a series of possibilities, alternatives or speculative hypotheses" (Gablik, 1976, p. 86). There has been a shift from an art of perception to an art of conception (Cooper, 1971); from an art of actuality to an art of potentiality.

Kasmir Malevich sought to represent the "supremacy of pure feeling or perception" independent of the context of natural forms. Malevich (1927), like Kandinsky and Mondrian, considered "The visual phenomena of the objective world . . . meaningless; the significant thing is feeling, as such, quite apart from the environment in which it is called forth. . . . The appropriate means of representation is always the one which gives fullest possible expression to feeling as such and which ignores the familiar appearance of objects. . . . Feeling is the determining factor. . . . The one and only source of every creation" (cited by Herbert, 1964, pp. 93–95). Malevich entirely eliminated content and context, and worked exclusively with pure form, space, line, color, and design. Malevich began to distort the invariant organization of geometric form with subtle variations of corner angles to produce warped rectangles and squares. He sought to express the most subtle variations of color, shape, and line through differentiations of size, shape, angle of inclination, and minor modulations of texture and tone (see Fig. 91). The subtle variations of abstract forms and dimensions created a sense of tension and potential, what Malevich called an "exhilaration of distortion" (cited by Gablik, 1976, p. 86).

Artists (e.g., Kelly, Serra, Mangold) attemped to alter and distort the basic Gestalt tendency to complete invariant geometric forms (Pragnanz) of incomplete circles and squares, while others (e.g., Bochner, Hinman, Rockburne, LeVa, and LeWitt) sought unique modes of composition in the structural principles of centrality and symmetry. In highly systematic and logical ways, they altered the basic shape and structure of fundamental geometric forms through complex combinations. Gablik (1976) discusses Bochner's precise placement of edges

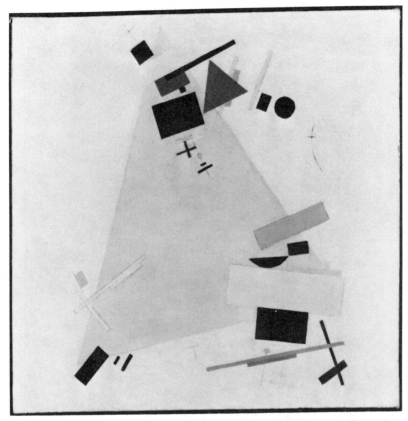

FIG. 91   Malevich, *Dynamic Suprematism* (1915–1918) (Tate Gallery, London).

and lines as an attempt to find patterns that alter the fixed, invariant structure of horizontal and vertical. Invariant geometric structures such as horizontal and vertical, parallel, circular forms and right angles give a sense of regularity, strength, stability, and even rigidity. Alterations of these invariant structures give the composition a dynamic tension and a sense of action and vitality. Other artists worked with other abstract concepts such as gravitational force, chance, randomness, and impermanence.

Barnett Newman argued for the need of painting "to replace scenes, images, symbols with abstract figures that had the materiality of things and events. The essential was the idea/object, and, to attain that, any suggestion of appearance and even abstractions derived from nature . . . had to be resolutely purged" (cited by Rosenberg, 1975, p. 52). Newman emphasized the physical dimensions of paint-

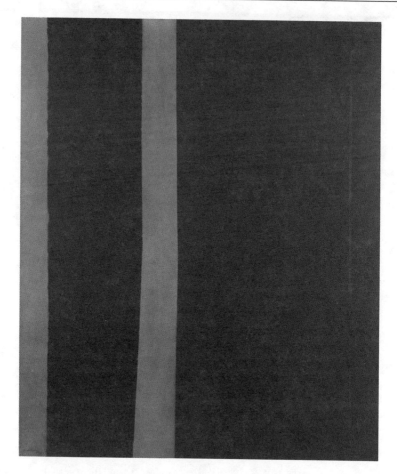

FIG. 92   Newman, *Adam* (1951–1952) (The Tate Gallery, London).

ing and he removed all content and permitted the spectator to view
his painting as simply an organization of colored planes and lines, as a
reality defined only by the title given to the work (see Fig. 92). Rosenberg discusses Newman's art as a search for underlying, symbolic,
abstract structures, for the inner form and dimensions of reality,
based on Jewish mysticism and primitive and Greek mythology.

Paul Klee provided an excellent summary of the purpose and goals
of Abstract Art. He wrote:

> We used to represent things visible on earth. . . . Now we reveal the
> reality of visible things, and thereby express the belief that visible reality
> is merely an isolated phenomenon latently outnumbered by other

realities. Things take on a broader and more varied meaning, often in seeming contradiction to the rational experience of yesterday. . . . In the end a formal cosmos will be created out of purely abstract elements of form quite independent of their configurations as objects, beings, or abstract things like letters or numbers. . . . An apple tree in bloom, its roots, the rising sap, its trunk, the cross-section with the annual rings, the blossom, its structure, its sexual functions, the fruit, the core with its seeds. A complex of stages of growth. In the highest sense, an ultimate mystery lies behind the ambiguity which the light of the intellect fails miserably to penetrate (cited by Miller, 1946, pp. 12–13).

Abstract Art is yet another phase in the search for the inner form and the principles of structural organization that began earlier in Impressionism, Post-impressionism, and Cubism, in their interest in fundamental sensory experiences and geometric forms. Abstract Art completely broke the tie with external manifest features in its search for underlying form and structural principles. It sought to define basic structural principles of order, sequence, and regularity and to maintain these structures despite major alterations and transformations of invariant geometric forms and patterns. In developmental psychological terms, Abstract Art involves a full relinquishing of concrete operations and manifest forms; art is now based primarily on formal operations, abstract principles, and symbolic forms. The search in Abstract Art for the principles of underlying structural organization inherent in all objects is only one of the most recent developments in a lengthy and complex developmental sequence that has progressed from the interest in Archaic art to capture the actual object, to the Renaissance search for the modes to realistically represent the outer, manifest appearance of objects, to Impressionism's search for the underlying sensory factors that determine the surface appearance of objects, to the Cubists' investigation of the inner structural form and composition of specific objects. When the line became independent of the contour of objects and art became free of mimesis and of having to represent a concrete, literal reality, manifest form and concrete operations gave way to underlying structure and formal operations. This provided art with a new-found autonomy and freedom. A shift occurred from the perceptual to the conceptual, from outer to inner form, from surface to underlying structure, and from concrete detail to abstract form.

The search for inner structure and form in art is consistent with the contemporary "cultural episteme" expressed in multiple fields of inquiry in the physical, biological and human sciences, including psychoanalysis. In fact, it is not the Surrealists' use of symbols, supposedly from the world of dreams, that is the congruence between modern art and psychoanalysis, but it is the search in art for inner form and structure beneath the manifest surface that is similar to Freud's fundamental discovery, at the beginning of the 20th century, of the unconscious, and his later structural theory of id, ego, and superego.

The emphasis in Abstract Art on basic geometric form and structural principles, however, resulted in a "dehumanization" in art (Ortega y Gasset, 1925/1972). Excessive abstraction and the lack of human form and content in Abstract Art expresses the impersonal, alienated anomie of our technological society. Subsequent developments in art may require an integration of abstract forms and manifest features, in which each aspect has full expression in its own right and contributes to a greater synthesis. Later levels of representation do not simply replace earlier levels of representation, but they are extensions and integrations of earlier levels. Later levels of representation are more conceptual and abstract while earlier levels are more concrete, immediate, and direct. Thus aspects of earlier modes of representation can serve to enrich and vivify later levels by adding affective dimensions and personal meanings (Blatt, 1974). Subsequent to the articulation of the basic principles of Cubism, Picasso integrated the representation of multiple perspectives with the representation of the manifest features of the human form, thereby achieving a synthesis of several different levels of representation (see Fig. 93). Likewise, Welliver's use of color, according to the principles of color relativism of Josef Albers, establishes vivid naturalistic representations based on a synthesis of abstract principles with manifest form. Welliver's use of color is relatively independent of the characteristic of the object and its local color, and is determined primarily by the principles of color relativism and the relationship of color to the representation of volume and depth. The value of color tones and their juxtaposition and integration into a unified composition are the primary factors creating spatial depth and volume. The integration of the principles of color relativism with aspects of manifest form and general principles of perspective gives Welliver's work a rich vitality and meaning. His work is based upon a synthesis of a diversity of representational modes, including abstract principles of color and concrete and manifest form (Welliver, 1978; personal communication) (See Fig. 94). It is the integration and synthesis of the

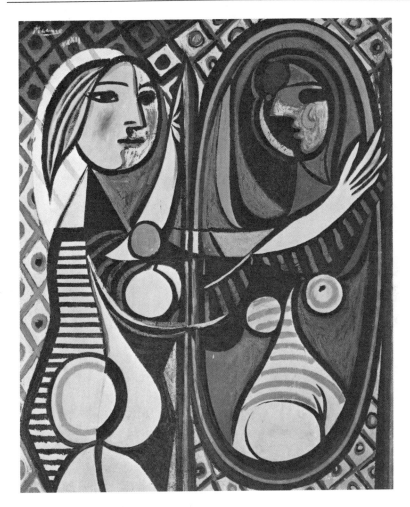

FIG. 93   Picasso, *Girl Before a Mirror* (1932) (The Museum of Modern Art, New York. Gift of Mrs. Simon Guggenheim).

multiple levels of representation that may serve to reduce the "dehumanization" of Abstract Art (Ortega y Gasset, 1925/1972).

A second major direction expressed in Modern Art has been the search for ways of representing reality as stable and predictable, and yet, at the same time, as relative, indeterminate, variable, and ever-changing. Newtonian absolutism expressed in a unitary conception of space with a fixed center was revised in physics by Einsteinian concepts of relativity and indeterminacy within a spatiotemporal field. At the same time, in the first quarter of the 20th century, art began to

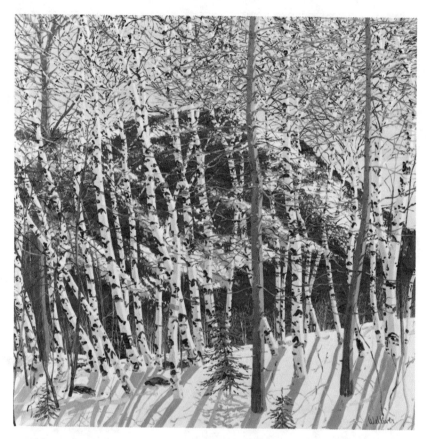

FIG. 94   Welliver, *The Birches* (1979) (Permission of Neil Welliver and The Metropolitan Museum of Art, Gift of Dr. and Mrs. Robert Carroll).

relinquish the representation of reality from a single, fixed perspective. As discussed earlier, Cubists represented objects as a multifaceted, complex series of interpenetrating planes and perspectives. Some critics and art historians (e.g., Apollinaire, 1949; Gardner, 1975; Laporte, 1949, 1966; Levy, 1943) consider Cubism as suggesting the addition of time to spatial representation, since objects appear to be represented not as seen at any one moment, but in a temporal sequence. They argue that the representation of multiple views of the object requires movement by the viewer through some temporally sequential positions. As discussed by Henderson (1975), in an extensive analysis of the impact of the development of non-Euclidean geometries and concepts of relativity on art, it is clear that Cubism did not introduce concepts of time and relativity into art. Henderson bases this conclusion in part on the fact that the Cubists were uninformed about Einstein's theoretical contributions of 1905 and the concepts of his General Theory of Relativity. Henderson, in an otherwise excellent presentation of these issues, makes the basic assumption that art is influenced by the concepts of science rather than viewing both art and science as only different expressions of the same fundamental "cultural episteme." Art and science are both expressions of a general cognitive mode that pervades the culture and is expressed in all its intellectual endeavors. Nevertheless, while the Cubists did not introduce the concept of time into art (Cooper, 1971; Henderson, 1975), their representation of multiple perspectives provided the basis for the subsequent extension of the concepts of space in art to include a temporal dimension in a fourfold spatiotemporal field.

One of the early attempts to include the dimension of time in art was the work of the Futurists. Based on the techniques developed in Cubism, the Futurists tried to represent movement by depicting the various positions of a figure moving through space. The Futurists used the Cubist multifaceted, interpenetrating planes to represent the frantic activity and excitement of modern industrial society. As illustrated by Balla's *Swift Paths of Movement and Dynamic Sequences* (1913) (Fig. 95), the Futurists were inspired by movement, speed, crowds, work, factories, airplanes, automobiles, and locomotives. Artists such as Balla, Boccioni, Carra, and Russolo sought to represent speed, science, mechanization, and dynamism. Cooper (1971, p. 165) comments that Futurism showed "a surprising awareness of modern scientific ideas in its references to the deformation and multiplication of images of moving things on the retina and to the vital principle of opposition between static and dynamic elements." Traditional modes of pictorial representation were considered invalid because they failed to capture the flux and dynamic properties of reality. The Futurists were influenced by Cubism's representation of mass and volume, but they felt Cubism failed to capture the dynamic movement and activity that was an inherent aspect of reality (Cooper, 1971). In 1910, Boccioni wrote of Futurism:

> Everything moves, everything runs, everything turns swiftly. The figure in front of us is never still, but ceaselessly appears and disappears. Owing to the persistence of images on the retina, objects in motion are multi-

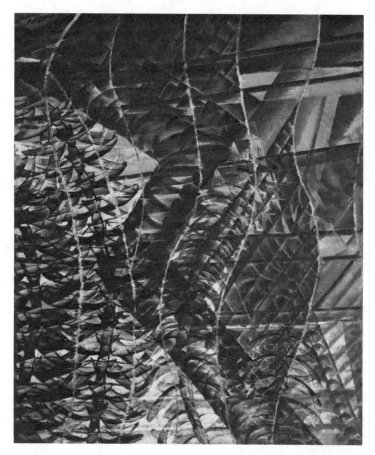

FIG. 95   Balla, *Swift Paths of Movement and Dynamic Sequences* (1913) (Museum of Modern Art, New York).

plied and distorted, following one another like waves through space. Thus a galloping horse has not four legs: it has twenty, and their movements are triangular. (cited in Goldwater & Treves, 1945, p. 435)

Duchamp's series of paintings entitled *Nude Descending a Staircase,* begun as early as 1911, is an excellent example of the attempt to represent movement (Fig. 96). Duchamp utilized the multiple facets of Cubism to try to capture movement in the sequential stages of an action as the figure progresses through a succession of evolving movements. Duchamp, through a coordinated series of transformations of an object in motion, sought to introduce time and motion into painting. Duchamp was probably greatly influenced by the well-known

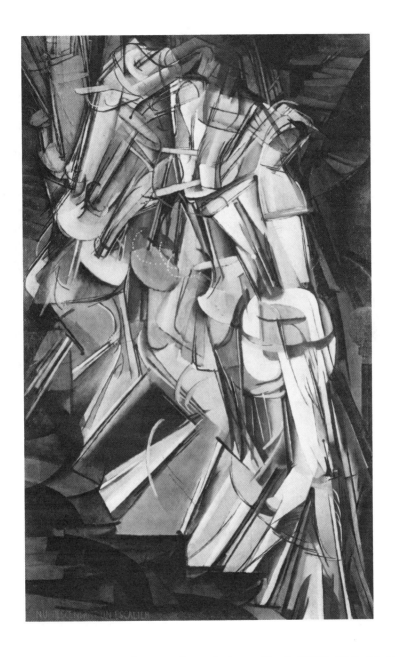

FIG. 96   Duchamp, *Nude Descending a Staircase, No. 2* (1912) (Philadelphia Museum of Art: The Louise and Walter Arensberg Collection).

experiments of Eadweard Muybridge on movement in 1887 in which he took a series of photographs of animals and people in various stages of an action in order to illustrate and study the different phases of a regular sequence of action over brief, uniform intervals of time.

Jackson Pollock's action paintings (Fig. 97) can be understood as another attempt to introduce motion and time into painting by inviting the spectator to identify with the movement in the painting (Rosenberg, 1964) and the artist's activity in the creation of the work (Gombrich, 1960). Although Pollock's paintings depict activity and the various stages of movement, they remain static and fail to integrate movement and time into painting. In order to create movement in painting, at least two visual images must exist at succeeding points in time. Kahnweiler (1949) notes that though the representation of movement and time would tremendously enrich art, it may be impossible to represent movement in the plastic arts. He cites Picasso as commenting that movement could be included in art only by the introduction of a clock mechanism or by the presentation of a rapid succession of images such as in a motion picture.

According to developmental psychological concepts, the representation of time must be based on the coordination of the movement of independent objects, or of an object and the self, moving at different velocities. Movement, according to Piaget (1927/1969a), is different from simple displacement or change in position. Displacements can occur spatially, which can create a beginning sense of time. But this sense of temporal sequence or duration can easily be confused with spatial order or the spatial path traversed. A full sense of time can be constructed within the representational field only by the coordination of two or more objects moving at different velocities (Piaget, 1927/1969).

Agam, in his optic and kinetic art, has created a technique that introduces temporal elements of sequence, progression, and continuity into painting, by demanding that the observer view the painting through a series of positions. The painting is experienced sequentially from an infinite array of equally valid perspectives. By a complex coordination of abstract geometric forms with color, Agam created a spatiotemporal field whereby the painting is experienced in an endless series of different ways, explicitly contingent on the position and movement of the observer. With this technique, Agam has created a painting in which the viewer is an integral part of a spatiotemporal field; the painting can only be defined in relation to

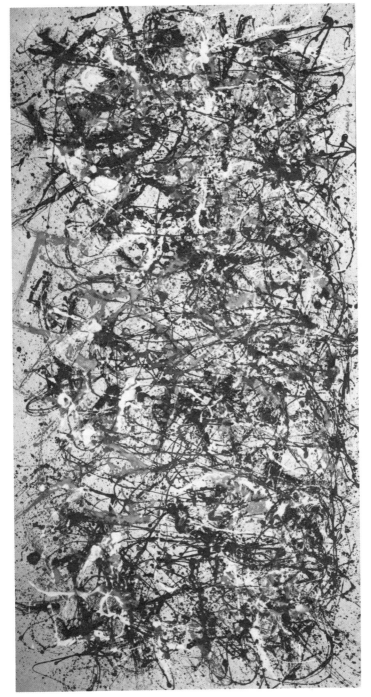

FIG. 97 Pollock, *Autumn Rhythm* (1950) (The Metropolitan Museum of Art, George A. Hearn Fund).

the observer. By forcing the observer to move through an endless series of positions while viewing the work, Agam introduced temporal concepts into painting—concepts of duration, sequence, and continuity. Not only are there an infinite number of equally valid perspectives, but each viewer, depending on the sequence and speed of his or her motion around the painting, has a uniquely different experience. The activity of the spectator in interaction with a basically fixed object creates the sense of time and an unending series of actual and potential transformations. The picture space is fully integrated with the viewer's space, thereby creating a relativistic, indeterminate, infinite spatiotemporal field.

In Agam's work, there has clearly been a shift from the static representation of the manifest features of an object from a fixed point of view to the representation of an object that participates in an interactive process with the relative position and motion of the observer. There is constant interaction between the abstract forms and colors in the painting and the movement of the observer. In developmental psychological terms, topological concepts of space, with an emphasis on the boundary and contour of manifest forms, and projective-Euclidean concepts of space, with a fixed coordinate reference system, have been integrated within a Riemannian-Einsteinian spatiotemporal field. The observer and nature exist in dynamic flux in a spatiotemporal field based on the relativity of positions and movement. Andre Malraux (1966) contrasts the simple impact of a static picture with the dynamic quality of Agam's work. Agam achieves both simultaneous and consecutive contrast in endless variations by forcing the viewer to move around the work, to become part of the picture space, in order to discover the infinite possibilities contained in the painting. The viewer becomes a fundamental element in the aesthetic experience. There is an endless sequential function and interaction of forms, which, like life itself, does not isolate one movement from the other but, rather, creates experiences of succession, progression, and continuity. Malraux (1966) notes that for Agam

> the work is not complete when the artist finishes it, but rather continues its dynamic life after the confrontation with the beholder's eye; it forces the beholder into activity in order to let him get to know its potentialities and qualities. The picture obliges the spectator to move around and to discover its qualities . . . while walking from one end of the picture to another, discovering a new composition from each point of view, parallel to the preceding one, and intercepting the following one (p. 5).

Agam comments that it is the "all-inclusive (that) is . . . the essence of form's sense and completion. . . . Form is composed of an unending totality of forms" (cited by Malraux, 1966, p. 4).

Agam has created a spatiotemporal field in which the spectator dynamically participates in the work (see Fig. 98). Agam (1962), in extensive commentary on his work, discusses his search for an inner truth that is infinite, and autonomous of concrete, physical reality. He is disinterested in a concrete object within a static structure in which the viewer passively observes the work from a single position. In reaction against the static nature of painting, Agam has created a type of painting that exists in both space and time as an infinite number of situations, and that results in an unending series of discoveries. Agam encourages the spectator to participate in and discover the essence and the organic unity of the work. Agam seeks to create a painting that has an organic reality—an enduring identity, but one altered to some degree by multiple and multifaceted contacts with the observer. The artistic work has a life of its own, an organic unity with continuity despite the endless changes the individual experiences in interaction with it. There is harmony in the picture in which autonomous forms are linked to one another in a variety of clearly determined fundamental relationships. But the nature and forms of these relationships will vary and change depending on the position and movement of the observer. The movement of the observer creates a sense of continuity and evolution in which various experiences flow one into the other, creating an organic unity. The painting, rather than being a single structure or a combination of structures in a static relationship of forms and colors, now has sequence and continuity, like music, literature, and even life itself. Forms are not placed in a single position within a composition, but in several positions within the structure of the painting, so that each form has multiple aspects. The viewer discovers the work progressively, but is always left with the feeling that things still remain hidden and yet accessible in the complexity of the various permutations and combinations within the work. Agam's paintings can be transformed infinitely and the various themes or elements are juxtaposed one against the other or within one another as thesis, antithesis, and synthesis. The direction and speed of the spectator's movements transform the composition. Forms and themes appear, disappear, reappear and blend, modify, and interact successively, while still retaining their original identity. Agam (1962) summarizes his artistic goals as follows:

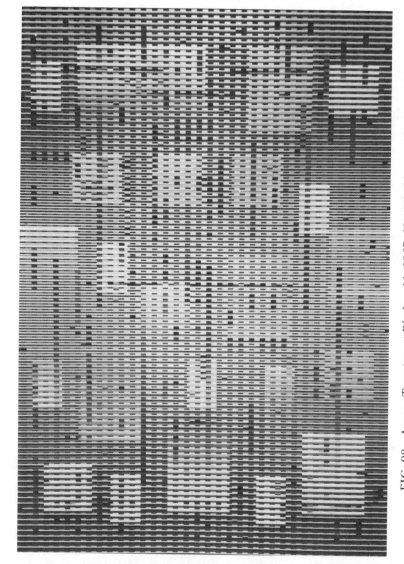

FIG. 98   Agam, *Transparent Rhythms 11* (1967–68) (Hirshhorn Museum and Sculpture Garden, Smithsonian Institution, Washington, D.C.).

The organic law that governs the combination of forms in the pictorial space of transformable painting is based on a quite different principle from the one which is at the basis of painting as it has existed until now. Whereas in the latter expressiveness is determined by relations between the elements, which relations are first of all fixed (including the space between the forms, which has an expressive value of equal importance) the relations between forms in transformable painting are significant, expressive and valid, *whatever* their situation in the pictorial space and their position relative to one another. In my transformable works, I have verified and proved by endless experiments the validity of the multiple reciprocal plastic relations, both in regard to their position and in regard to their relative reciprocity (for example, a certain form will appear as large next to a smaller one and as small next to a larger one). . . . In transformable painting, chance and the unforeseen are an integral part of the work, which becomes metamorphosed as it evolves; as in life, we are in situations whose mutual relations are unforeseen. Thus the transformable painting integrates a "slice of life" in which chance becomes incorporated. (pp. 104, 107)

The task in art, for Agam, is to be able to express contradictory inclinations in a simultaneous and coherent way, to give the work the potential to express multiple ideas simultaneously. The essence is to allow things to coexist, to be experienced as totality, and to vary over time and still have duration and continuity—to have continuity as well as change. Agam's transformable art is based on a conception of a spatiotemporal universe in which aspects of reality are both stable and enduring, as well as relative, indeterminate, and infinite. Concrete operational thought has been enriched by modes of representation based on formal operations and abstract, propositional thought. Projective-Euclidean concepts of space have been integrated within a Riemannian-Einsteinian relative, spatiotemporal field. It is fascinating to note that contemporary modes of representation in art, such as the transformable paintings of Agam, are based on the same assumptions and concepts that are predominant in our current cultural context and are expressed in other cognitive endeavors, including science, literature, and philosophy.

PARALLEL DEVELOPMENT IN
POST–RENAISSANCE ART AND SCIENCE

Linear perspective survived, as did Cartesian analytic geometry and Newtonian mechanics, well into the 19th century. In the mid- to late-19th century, the Impressionists in art began to look beneath the external and manifest form of objects to concentrate on the basic, discrete sensory elements of which objects were composed. The canons of linear perspective and the manifest definition and form of the object were ignored and, instead, in individual dabs of color the Impressionists sought to capture isolated visual sensations of light and color. This attempt in art to analyze visual experience into its constituent sensory elements had its parallel in the sciences, especially in theories of matter. Just as art turned from manifest features to internal structure, so beginning in the Baroque, scientists concentrated less on macroscopic mechanics and focused instead on micromechanical models. Impressionism was a further development of the subjectivity of the Baroque, and matter theory was a further development of the implications of Newtonian mechanics. Objects were successively deprived, on a microscopic scale, of their sensory, manifest, macroscopic properties. For instance, the combustibility of a substance no longer depended on its containing a material of combustion endowed with specific qualities of color and texture, but instead combustibility was the result of the more abstract characteristics of its quantitative combining potential. The heat of a substance was seen as corresponding to the kinetic energy in the motion of the individual molecules that constituted the substance. By the end of the 19th century, manifest features of systems, such as pressure, volume, and temperature that had been articulated in 17th century science, began to be defined as functions of internal, invisible constructs such as particle number and speed. Likewise, the periodic table displayed chemical and physical properties as a function of a quantitative measure, atomic weight (Gillispie, 1960). Thus both in science and art there were attempts to define the structure underlying manifest form and to become free of the fixed, rigid, and concrete image of reality that had been established in art in the development of linear perspective and in science in the concepts of Newtonian mechanics.

The mid- to late-19th century Impressionists began to question and break away from centuries-old traditions of "realistic" representation and the techniques of linear perspective at about the same time as geometricians such as Lobachevski and Riemann began to reexamine fundamental assumptions of Euclidean geometry—assumptions on which the physical treatment of terrestrial and celestial mechanics had been equally long established and confidently based. The Impressionists tried to ignore the traditional modes of spatial representation and to turn instead to an analysis of the experience of light and color, or, as in the case of Van Gogh, to represent objects as seen in space solely through binocular vision, which led to a pictorial space assimilated to a hyperbolic geometry. This development in art, analogous to developments in science, is perhaps most clearly apparent in the work of Cézanne—the primary transitional figure between Impressionism and the entirety of Modern Art. Instead of simply ignoring linear perspective for a concern with light and color, Cézanne explicitly sought a new spatial analysis through an attempt to depict objects and space in terms of their underlying geometric structures. While the Impressionists and Post-impressionists sought to abandon the techniques of linear perspective that were based on Euclidean concepts of space for new ways of representing experience, geometricians were considering alternatives to Euclid's fundamental assumption, his fifth postulate, which essentially stated that infinitely extended parallel lines do not converge. This assumption was a major support of the rectilinear, infinite conception of space, and geometricians found that other equally valid assumptions led to developments such as spherical and hyperbolic geometries (Cassirer, 1950).

Mathematicians such as Gauss, Riemann, Lobachevski, and Bolyai, in the second half of the 19th century, relinquished Euclidean geometry as the sole system for treating mathematical problems. They concluded that a logically consistent geometry does not require Euclid's fifth postulate, the assumption that infinitely extended parallel lines never converge—perhaps they even might meet if space were curved. Having concluded that logically consistent geometries could be developed by postulating nonrectilinear coordinate systems, Lobachevski and Riemann, among others, began to explore non-Euclidean geometries, without, however, making any assumptions about their relevance to the solution of actual physical problems. This mathematical development was completed by the time scientists, beginning with Michelson and Morley, failed in various experimental attempts to establish the presence of a stationary ether. They had sought evidence of such an ether—the physical manifestation of absolute space—that served as the vehicle for electromagnetic radiation (e.g., light). At the same time, for philosophical and experimental reasons, Einstein began to develop the implications of his intuition that a relativistic view of space was valid (Eddington, 1966).

Einstein not only argued that a relativistic view of both space and time must be assumed, but further pointed out that space and time are indissociable, that they together constitute a space-time field that cannot be described readily by the perpendicular axes of Euclidean geometry. He began with the principle of relativity because he thought no experiment could establish whether an observer moves uniformly or remains at rest. He reasoned that studies of motion simply assumed an observer at rest in space for the sake of mathematical convenience. Just as space is not absolute, so time has no absolute measure. Statements about time depend on the frame of reference to which they refer. Einstein pointed out in 1905, in the special theory of relativity, that an absolute frame of reference at rest and an absolute time reference cannot be determined, and he also realized in the general theory of relativity of 1915 that one cannot distinguish whether an experience of acceleration is due to one's frame of reference undergoing accelerated motion or to the proximity of a large gravitating mass because they would have indistinguishable effects. Because mass deflects light rays and electromagnetic radiations, and because light rays and electromagnetic radiations are the means by which the geometry of space is established, the shape of space must be nonrectilinear insofar as masses distributed through it deflect such radiations from linear paths. Moreover, if the distribution of mass is changing in time, then the geometry of space changes in time. Thus, the Einsteinian concept of a space-time field defines the shape of space as nonrectilinear and as changing in time. But even the Newtonian differentiation of space and mass (or body)—the former being simply the container of the latter—becomes untenable when one further element is introduced: The law that energy and matter are interconvertible ($E = mc^2$). This law implies that mass and energy are two manifestations of the same thing. Mass represents a vast concentration of energy while, on the other hand, energy—such as the gravitational field—represents a distribution of matter.

In the late 19th and early 20th century, Ernst Mach and others launched a reexamination and critique of Newton's concepts of absolute space, and later Einstein's theoretical speculations in 1905 led to the disavowal of an absolute frame of reference for the relativistic assumption of equally valid, multiple frames of reference. Space and time, indissociably united, constitute a spatiotemporal field that cannot be described adequately by the perpendicular axes of Cartesian geometry. Space and time are now more integrated than the static, separate Newtonian concepts of absolute space and absolute time. Descartes to some degree recognized the importance of time in any conception of space, yet Newton's absolutes of space and time prevailed until the latter part of the 19th century. In the Einsteinian spatiotemporal field, the individual's perspective is no longer a unique and singular point of reference, but now there is the possibility of multiple perspectives—a relativity of perspective. One realizes the relativity of one's viewpoint to one's own time period, and becomes aware of the arbitrariness of perspectives held in particular historical epochs and cultural matrices. Cubism, beginning in 1908, shortly after Einstein's initial contributions in physics in 1905 and Minkowski's discussion of the space-time continuum in 1908, opened the modern epoch in art by relinquishing unitary, linear perspective and seeking instead to represent objects and space in terms of multiple perspectives. While Cubism did not introduce the concept of time into art, it did assume multiple perspectives are available simultaneously, with respect to any object. The Cubists' attempt to represent multiple perspectives was basically similar to the attempts in physics to define equally valid frames of reference.

Modern Art extended the developments of Impressionism, Post-impressionism, and Cubism in at least three aspects. As in science, a distinctive concern with space and its "realistic" representation was replaced by other issues. First, there were attempts to extend the fixed representation of simultaneous multiple perspectives by incorporating concepts of time. Artists struggled to introduce into the representational process concepts of the space-time field and the quantum principle of indeterminism or uncertainty by creating the conditions in which observations of works of art are a function of the action and position of the observer. Second, Modern Art also moved toward an increasing level of abstraction in which the painting itself is the object to be perceived and comprehended, rather than being an attempt to represent something else. In a similar way, non-Euclidean concepts of space are less perceptually based and more abstract and conceptual. Space has become entirely a scientific concept with no claim to illuminate everyday perception or commonsense understanding, just as the painting has become an object in its own right, not a window for, or mirror of, a readily comprehensible segment of nature. Non-Euclidean concepts of space are not based on immediately perceived objects or motions but on the abstract structuring of geometric systems and the use of abstract mathematics descriptive of physical phenomena in order to determine the appropriate geometric system. Finally, Modern Art has emphasized the development of a sense of a subjective self-consciousness in the viewer. Artists have forced viewers to become increasingly aware of their roles in constructing an experience of nature. Paintings are no longer simply viewed, they must now be understood. Similarly, concepts of relativity and the principle of uncertainty are based on a fundamental self-consciousness about the process of scientific observation and the recognition that the questions being asked depend on the historical context, the underlying assumption, and the conditions of observation. The scientist *selects* a geometrical representation of space; the selection of a system that corresponds with equations for the physical phenomena being studied is made on the basis of relevance for the particular context (Reichenbach, 1928/1957; Watson, 1938).

The various changes in art begun in the Modern period and the changes in science from Newtonian to Einsteinian concepts are illustrations of a basic transition in cultural episteme from concrete operational modes of representation to formal operational levels. This transition not only involves greater levels of abstraction but also a shift from an interest in systems of relationships to a consideration of the relations among systems of relationships. It involves a transition from a system of measurement based on an arbitrary unit of measurement and an arbitrary reference point (an interval scale) to systems of measurement and scaling based on quantitative metrics established with an experientially and numerically relevant zero or reference point which creates an equality of ratios in addition to an equality of intervals (a ratio scale). It is precisely such considerations that have occurred in the analysis and questioning of basic assumptions apparent in the development of non-Euclidean geometries and Einsteinian relativity theory and in modern concepts of art.

No development in art can ever be regarded as final; art is an "open, unfinished, ever-alterable process of development" (Hauser, 1953/1959, p. 248). Progress in the revisions of the modes of representation in art is likely to continue to be correlated with the revisions of the cognitive structures with which we understand and conceptualize our universe. The development of modes of representation within the history of art in Western Civilization has followed a natural order of development from relatively undifferentiated, unarticulated, and unintegrated forms to more complex levels of organization that are increasingly differentiated, articulated, and integrated. This process is a particular characteristic of cognitive development both in individual and cultural development. The sequences in the development of modes of representation in the history of painting, progressing from Paleolithic to contemporary time, are expressions of the concepts and cognitive structures predominant within each cultural epoch. Art, literature, philosophy, and science are parallel and interrelated expressions of the predominant cognitive structure of each cultural period. And these cognitive structures have developed over the cultural epochs in a natural developmental sequence.

We, like our predecessors in all epochs in the history of civilization, however, cannot be certain how our concepts of the universe—of space, time, and causality—will develop and evolve. We can only understand our universe through the cognitive structures that are a part of our cultural heritage and are available to us within our current cultural context. We, as participants and observers throughout the history of civilization always have been, are restricted within our cultural epoch by the conceptual tools available to us (Kleinbauer, 1971). As Hauser (1953/1959, p. 236) has noted, the art historian is constrained by the "limits set by the artistic aims of his time; his concepts of form and categories of value are bound up with the modes of seeing and the criteria of taste of a certain age." We are unable to reflect on subsequent levels of development that may exist beyond our current levels of representation until new constructs and cognitive structures are expressed in the artistic, philosophic, and scientific endeavors of our culture. While we cannot know how our subsequent conceptions will evolve, we can be certain that our concepts of the universe, including our conceptualizations of ourselves and our modes of representation, will become increasingly differentiated, articulated, and integrated. With new knowledge and changed social conditions, new constructs and modes of representation will evolve in our culture, and they will be expressed simultaneously in multiple cognitive endeavors including art, science, and literature. We will then become aware of the potential within each of us to understand and comprehend our reality, our universe, and ourselves in an even more differentiated, articulated, integrated, and comprehensive way.

References

Abel, T. A comparison of two-dimensional and tri-dimensional designs of high school Pueblo American Indians in New Mexico. *Transactional Mental Health Research Newsletter*, 1981, *22*, 9–15.

Ackerman, J. S. Art history and the problems of criticism. *Daedalus*, 1960, *89*, 253–263.

Ackerman, J. S. A theory of style. In M. C. Beardsley & H. M. Schueller (Eds.), *Aesthetic inquiry: Essays on art criticism and the philosophy of art*. Belmont, Mass.: Dickenson, 1967 (1962).

Agam, Y. Yaacov Agam: *Texts by the Artist* (Agam par lui-meme). Neuchâtel, Switzerland: Editions du Griffon, 1962.

Ainsworth, M. D. *Infancy in Uganda; infant care and the growth of love*. Baltimore, Md.: Johns Hopkins University Press, 1967.

Alberti, L. B. Della pittura. In J. R. Spencer (Trans.), *On Painting*. New Haven, Ct.: Yale University Press, 1956 (1435).

Aldred, C. *Akhenaten, Pharoh of Egypt: A new study*. London: Thames & Hudson, 1968.

Antal, F. Remarks on the method of art history: I. *Burlington Magazine*, 1949, *91*, 49–52.(a)

Antal, F. Remarks on the method of art history: II. *Burlington Magazine*, 1949, *91*, 73–75.(b)

Antal, F. Reflections on classicism and romanticism. *Burlington Magazine*, 1953, *96*, 159.

Apollinaire, G. *The cubist painters; aesthetic meditations, 1913*. New York: Wittenborn, Schultz, 1949.

Arnason, H. H. *History of modern art: painting, sculpture, architecture*. New York: Abrams, 1968.

Arnheim, R. Comments and discussion. In D. R. Olson & S. Pagliuso (Eds.), From perceiving to performing: An aspect of cognitive growth. Special issue: *Ontario Journal of Educational Research*, 1968, *10*, 203–207.

Arnheim, R. *Art and visual perception: A psychology of the creative eye*. Berkeley: University of California Press, 1974 (1954).

Artz, F. B. *The mind of the Middle Ages, A.D. 200–1500; An historical survey*. (3rd ed.). New York: Knopf, 1959.

Artz, F. B. *Renaissance humanism, 1300–1550*. Kent, Ohio: Kent State University Press, 1966.

Auerbach, E. *Mimesis; the representation of reality in western literature* (W. R. Trask, Trans.). Princeton, N.J.: Princeton University Press, 1953 (1946).

Baldwin, C. Impressionism. In *The Impressionist Epoch.* New York: Metropolitan Museum of Art, 1974.

Baltrušaitis, J. *Anamorphic art* (W. J. Strachan, Trans.). New York: Abrams, 1977.

Barnhart, E. N. Developmental stages in compositional construction in children's drawings. *Journal of Experimental Education,* 1942, *11,* 156–184.

Bartlett, F. C. *Thinking; an experimental and social study.* New York: Basic Books, 1958.

Bell, C. *Art.* New York: A. Stokes Co., 1913.

Bell, C. *Since Cézanne.* London: Chatto & Windus, 1922.

Bell, S. M. The development of the concept of the object as related to infant-mother attachment. *Child Development,* 1970, *41,* 292–311.

Benjamin, W. *The origin of German tragic drama* (J. Osborne, Trans.). London: New Left Books, 1977.

Bennett, A. *The Clayhanger family: I. Clayhanger, II. Hilda Lessways, III. These Twain.* London: Methuen, 1925 (c. 1910).

Berenson, B. *The Italian painters of the Renaissance.* London: Phaidon; distributed by Garden City Books, New York, 1956.

Berger, P. L., & Luckmann, T. *The social construction of reality.* New York: Doubleday, 1966.

Bergson, H. *Time and free will.* (F. L. Pogson, Trans.) New York: Macmillan, 1959 (1912).

Berlyne, D. E. The influence of the albedo and complexity of stimuli on visual fixation in the human infant. *British Journal of Psychology,* 1958, *49,* 315–318.

Bernheimer, R. (H. W. Janson, Ed.) *The nature of representation: A phenomenological inquiry.* New York: New York Univ. Press. 1961.

Bettelheim, B. *The empty fortress.* New York: Free Press, 1967.

Beyen, H. G. *Pompejanische Wanddekoration* (2 vols.). The Hague, 1938.

Blatt, S. J. Levels of object representation in anaclitic and introjective depression. *Psychoanalytic Study of the Child,* 1974, *29,* 107–157.

Blatt, S. J. Narcissism and egocentrism as concepts in individual and cultural development. *Psychoanalysis and Contemporary Thought,* 1983, *6,* 291–303.

Blatt, S. J., & Feirstein, A. Cardiac response and personality organization. *Journal of Consulting and Clinical Psychology,* 1977, *45,* 115–123.

Blatt, S. J., Quinlan, D. M., & D'Afflitti, J. Magnification and diminishing of image size and their effects on psychological states. *Journal of Abnormal Psychology,* 1972, *80,* 168–175.

Blatt, S. J., & Ritzler, B. A. Thought disorder and boundary disturbances in psychosis. *Journal of Consulting and Clinical Psychology,* 1974, *42,* 370–381.

Blatt, S. J., & Wild, C. M. *Schizophrenia: A developmental analysis.* New York: Academic Press, 1976.

Brachert, T. A musical canon of proportion in Leonardo da Vinci's *Last Supper* (C. P. Casparis, Trans.). *Art Bulletin,* 1971, *53*(4), 461–466.

Breuil, H. *Four hundred years of cave art.* (M. E. Boyle, Trans.). Paris: Montignac, 1952.

Brion-Guerry, L. The elusive goal. In W. Rubin (Ed.), *Cézanne: The late work.* New York: Museum of Modern Art, 1977.

Britsch, G. *Theorie der bildenden Kunst* (E. Kornmann, Ed.). Munich: Bruckmann, 1926.

Brunner-Traut, E. Aspective. Epilogue to H. Schafer, *Principles of Egyptian art* (J. Baines, Ed. and Trans.). Oxford: Clarendon Press, 1974.

Brunswik, E. Ontogenetic and other developmental parallels to the history of science. In H. M. Evans (Ed.), *Men and moments in the history of science.* Seattle: University of Washington Press, 1959.

Bunim, M. *Space in medieval painting and forerunners of perspective.* New York: Columbia University Press, 1940.

Burckhardt, J. C. *The civilization of the Renaissance in Italy.* (S. G. C. Middlemore, trans.) (3rd ed., rev.). London: Phaidon Press, 1950 (1860).

Burnham, J. W. *The structure of art* (Assisted by C. Harper & J. Benjamin Burnham.) New York: Braziller, 1971.

Burtt, E. A. *The metaphysical foundation of modern science.* New York: Doubleday, 1954 (1931).

Butterfield, H. *The origins of modern science: 1300–1800.* New York: Free Press, 1957.

Carpenter, G. C., Tecce, J. J., Stechler, G., & Friedman, S. Differential visual behavior to human and humanoid faces in early infancy. *Merrill-Palmer Quarterly,* 1970, *16,* 91–108.

Carter, B. A. R. Perspective. In H. Osborne (Ed.), *The Oxford companion to art.* Oxford: Clarendon Press, 1970.

Cassirer, E. *Substance and function, and Einstein's theory of relativity.* (W. C. Swabey & M. C. Swabey, Trans.). Chicago: The Open Court Publishing Company, 1923 (1910).

Cassirer, E. *Language and myth* (S. K. Langer, Trans.). New York: Dover Publications, Inc., 1946.

Cassirer, E. *The problem of knowledge.* New Haven: Yale University Press, 1950.

Cassirer, E. *The philosophy of symbolic forms* (Vol. 1) (R. Manheim, Trans.). New Haven, Ct.: Yale University Press, 1955.

Cassirer, E. *The individual and the cosmos in Renaissance philosophy.* (M. Domandi, Trans.). Oxford: Blackwell, 1963 (1927).

Cassirer, E., Kristeller, P. O., & Randall, J. H. (Eds.). *The Renaissance philosophy of man.* Chicago: University of Chicago Press, 1948.

Cézanne, P. *Letters* (4th ed., rev. & enl.) (J. Rewald, Ed., M. Kay, trans.). New York: Hacker Art Books, 1976.

Chastel, A. Lecture at World Congress, 1977 (cited by Kleinbauer).

Chipp, H. B. *Theories of modern art.* Berkeley: University of California Press, 1968.

Chomsky, N. *Language and mind* (Enl. ed.). New York: Harcourt Brace Jovanovich, 1972 (1968).

Clark, K. *Civilization: a personal view.* New York: Harper & Row, 1969.

Clarke-Stewart, K. A. Interactions between mothers and their young children: Characteristics and consequences. *Society of Research in Child Development Monograph,* 1973, *38.*

Cocking, R. A., & Segal, I. *The concept of decalage and representational thinking.* Paper delivered at Wheelock Conference, Boston, Mass., 1975.

Cooper, D. *The cubist epoch.* New York: Phaidon, 1971.

Cooper, D. *Braque: The great years.* Chicago: The Art Institute of Chicago, 1972.

Croce, B. *Aesthetic as science of expression and general linguistic.* (D. Ainslie, Trans.). New York: Noonday Press, 1953.

Davis, M. D. *Piero della Francesca's mathematical treatises.* Ravenna: Longo, 1977.

Décarie, T. G. *Intelligence and affectivity in early childhood.* New York: International Universities Press, 1965.

Descargues, P. *Perspective* (I. M. Paris, Trans.). New York: Abrams, 1976.

Descartes, R. *Discourse on Method and the Mediations.* (F. E. Sutcliffe, Trans.). New York: Penguin, 1968.

Dilthey, W. *Philosophy of existence: Introduction to Weltanschauugslehre.* (W. Kluback & M. Weinbaum, Trans.). New York: Bookman Assoc., 1957 (1927).

Doesschate, G. ten. *Perspective; fundamentals, controversials, history.* Nieuwkoop: B. de Graaf, 1964.

Dolle, J. M., Bataillard, C., & Guyon, J. *La construction représentative de l'espace volumétrique chez l'enfant. Bulletin de Psychologie,* 1973–1974, *27,* 578–589.

Dolle, J. M., Bataillard, A., & Lacroix, F. Apprentissage opératoire de la représentation graphique d'une figure volumétrique. *Bulletin de Psychologie,* 1974–1975, *28,* 956–964.

Dolle, J. M., Vinter, S., & Germain, Y. Schemes de préhension-exploration et construction représentative de formes spatiales chez l'enfant entendant et malentendant d'age scolaire. *Bulletin de Psychologie,* 1974–1975, *28,* 836–843.

Dörig, J. Sculpture, painting and other arts. In *Greek art and architecture.* New York: Abrams, 1976.

Durkheim, E. *The elementary forms of religious life: A study in religious sociology* (1912). London: Allen & Unwin, 1976.

Dvořák, M. *Idealism and naturalism in Gothic art* (R. J. Klawiter, Trans.) South Bend, Ind.: University of Notre Dame Press, 1967 (1918).

Eddington, A. *The theory of relativity and its influence on scientific thought.* New York: Oxford University Press, 1922.

Eddington, A. *Space, time and gravitation; an outline of the general relativity theory.* Cambridge, England: The University Press, 1966.

Edgerton, S. Y. Jr. *The Renaissance rediscovery of linear perspective.* New York: Basic Books, 1975.

Eliade, M. *The myth of the eternal return* (W. R. Trask, Trans.). Princeton: Princeton University Press, 1971 (1954).

Elkind, D. *Children and adolescents: Interpretive essays on Jean Piaget.* (2nd ed.). New York: Oxford University Press, 1974 (1970).

Escalona, S. Emotional development in the first year of life. In M. J. E. Senn (Ed.), *Transactions of the Sixth Conference on problems of infancy and childhood.* New York: Josiah Macy, Jr. Foundation, 1953, 11–92.

Falmagne, R. J. *Reasoning: Representation and process.* Hillsdale, N.J.: Lawrence Erlbaum Associates, 1975.

Fantz, R. L. Pattern vision in newborn infants. *Science,* 1963, *140,* 296–297.

Fantz, R. L., & Nevis, S. Pattern preferences and perceptual-cognitive development in early infancy. *Merrill-Palmer Quarterly,* 1967, *13,* 77–108.

Federn, P. *Ego psychology and the psychoses.* New York: Basic Books, 1952.

Feffer, M. The cognitive implications of role-taking behavior. *Journal of Personality,* 1959, *27,* 152–168.

Feffer, M. Symptom expression as a form of primitive decentering. *Psychological Review,* 1967, *74,* 16–28.

Feffer, M. Developmental analysis of interpersonal behavior. *Psychological Review,* 1970, *77,* 197–214.

Feffer, M., & Gourevitch, V. Cognitive aspects of role-taking in children. *Journal of Personality,* 1960, *28,* 383–396.

Feffer, M., & Suchotliff, L. Decentering implications of social interactions. *Journal of Personality and Social Psychology,* 1966, *4,* 415–422.

Ficino, M. *Five questions concerning the mind* (1476). (J. L. Burroughs, Trans.). In E. Cassirer et al. (Eds.), *The Renaissance philosophy of man.* Chicago: University of Chicago Press, 1948.

Focillon, H. *The life of forms in art.* (2nd English ed., enl.) (C. B. Hogan & G. Kubler, Trans.). New York: Wittenborn, Schultz, 1948 (1934).

Foss, M. *The idea of perfection in the western world.* Princeton, N.J.: Princeton University Press, 1946.

Foucault, M. *The order of things: An archaeology of the human sciences.* London: Tavistock Publications, 1970.

Fraiberg, S. Libidinal object constancy and mental representation. *Psychoanalytic Study of the Child,* 1969, *24,* 9–47.

Franciscis, A. de. *La Villa Romana di Uplontis.* Recklinghausen: Verlag Aurel Bongers, 1975.

Frankfort, H., Frankfort, H. A., Wilson, J. A., & Jacobsen, T. *Before philosophy, the intellectual adventure of ancient man; an essay on speculative thought in the ancient Near East.* Baltimore, Md.: Penguin Books, 1949.

Frankfort H. A. (Groenewegen). *Arrest and movement; An essay on space and time in the representational art of the ancient Near East.* Chicago: University of Chicago Press, 1951.

Frankfort, H. A. (Groenewegen), & Ashmole, B. *Art of the ancient world: Painting, pottery, sculpture, architecture from Egypt, Mesopotamia, Crete, Greece, and Rome.* New York: Abrams, 1971.

Frankl, P. *The Gothic; literary sources and interpretations through eight centuries.* Princeton, N.J.: Princeton University Press, 1960.

Freud, A. *Normality and pathology in childhood: Assessments of development; The writings of Anna Freud, vol. 6.* New York: International Universities Press, 1965.

Freud, S. Inhibitions, symptoms and anxiety. In *The standard edition of the complete psychological works of Sigmund Freud* (Vol. 20). London: Hogarth Press, 1959 (1926).

Friedlaender, W. F. *Caravaggio studies.* Princeton, N.J.: Princeton University Press, 1955.

Friedlaender, W. F. *Mannerism and anti-mannerism in Italian painting*. New York: Columbia University Press, 1958.

Fry, E. F. *Cubism*. New York: McGraw-Hill, 1966.

Fry, R. E. *Cézanne*. London: Hogarth Press, 1927.

Fry, R. E. *Vision and Design*. London: Chatto & Windus, 1928.

Fry, R. E. *Cézanne, a study of his development* (2nd ed.). London: L. & V. Woolf, 1932.

Fry, R. E. *Reflections on British painting*. New York: Macmillan, 1934.

Fuchs, W. Hellenistic art. In *Greek art and architecture*. New York: Abrams, 1976.

Gablik, S. *Progress in art*.London: Thames & Hudson, 1976.

Gabo, N. The constructive idea in art. In *Circle* (N. Gabo, J. L. Martin, & B. Nicholson, Eds.). London: Farber & Farber, 1937.

Gadol, J. *Leon Battista Alberti: universal man of the early Renaissance*. Chicago: University of Chicago Press, 1969.

Galassi, P. *Before photography*. New York: Museum of Modern Art, 1981.

Garcia, R., & Piaget, J. Physico-geometric explanations and analysis. In Piaget, J. with the collaboration of Garcia, R. *Understanding Causality* (D. & M. Miles, Trans.). New York: Norton, 1974.

Gardiner, A. *Egypt of the Pharaohs*. Oxford: Clarendon Press, 1961.

Gardner, H. *The quest for mind: Piaget, Levi-Strauss and the structuralist movement*. New York: Vintage, 1972.

Gardner, H. *Gardner's art through the ages* (6th ed., revised by H. de la Croix & R. G. Tansey). New York: Harcourt Brace Jovanovich, 1975 (1926).

Garner, W. R. *Uncertainty and structure as psychological concepts*. New York: Wiley, 1962.

Gay, P. *Style in history*. New York: Basic Books, 1974.

Gibson, J. J. *The perception of the visual world*. Boston: Houghton Mifflin, 1950.

Gibson, J. J. Pictures, perspective and perception. *Daedalus*, 1960, *89*, 216–227.

Gibson, J. J. *The senses considered as perceptual systems*. Boston: Houghton Mifflin, 1966.

Giedion, S. *The eternal present: The beginnings of art*. New York: Pantheon Books, 1962.

Giedion, S. *Space, time, and architecture: The growth of a new tradition*. Cambridge, Mass.: Harvard University Press, 1967 (1941).

Gillispie, C. *The edge of objectivity*. Princeton, NJ: Princeton University Press, 1960.

Gioseffi, D. Optical concepts. In *Encyclopedia of world art* (Vol. 10). New York: McGraw-Hill, 1965.

Gioseffi, D. Perspective. *In Encyclopedia of world art* (Vol. 11). New York: McGraw-Hill, 1966.

Gleizes, A., & Metzinger, J. *Cubism*. London: T. F. Unwin, 1913.

Godol, L. On intuitional arithmetic and number theory (1933). In M. Davis (Ed. and trans.), *The undecidable: Basic papers on undecidable propositions, unsolvable problems and computable functions*. Hewlett, N.Y.: Raven Press, 1965.

Goldmeier, E. Similarity in visually perceived forms. *Psychological Issues,* 1972, *8,* (1) (1936).

Goldwater, R. J., & Treves, M. (Eds). *Artists on art, from the XIV to XX century* (2nd ed., rev.). New York: Pantheon Books, 1945.

Gombrich, E. H. *The story of art.* New York: Phaidon Publishers, Oxford University Press, 1950.

Gombrich, E. H. *Art and illusion; a study in the psychology of pictorial representation.* New York: Pantheon Books, 1960.

Gombrich, E. H. Psycho-analysis and the history of art. *International Journal of Psychoanalysis,* 1954, *25,* 401–411. Also in *Meditations on a hobby horse, and other essays on the theory of art.* London: Phaidon Press, 1963.

Gombrich, E. H. *Norm and form; studies in the art of the Renaissance.* London: Phaidon Press, 1966.

Gombrich, E. H. Style. *International Encyclopedia of the Social Sciences,* 1968, *15,* 352–362.

Gombrich, E. H. The evidence of images: I. The variability of vision. In C. S. Singleton (Ed.), *Interpretation: Theory and practice.* Baltimore: Johns Hopkins Press, 1969, 35–68.(a)

Gombrich, E. H. *In search of cultural history.* London: Oxford University Press, 1969.(b)

Gombrich, E. H. Norm and form: The stylistic categories of art history and their origin in Renaissance ideals. In *Norm and form: Studies in the art of the Renaissance.* London: Phaidon Press, 1971, pp. 81–98.

Gombrich, E. H. The "what" and the "how": Perspective representation and the phenomenal world. In R. Rudner & I. Scheffler (Eds.), *Logic and art; essays in honor of Nelson Goodman.* Indianapolis: Bobbs Merrill, 1972.

Gombrich, E. H. Mirror and map: Theories of pictorial representation. *Philosophical Transactions of the Royal Society of London,* 1975, *270,* 119–149.

Gombrich, E. H. Lecture, University College, University of London, 1977.

Goodman, N. *Languages of art: An approach to a theory of symbols* Indianapolis: Bobbs-Merrill, 1968.

Gould, S. J. *Ontogeny and phylogeny.* Cambridge, Mass.: Harvard University Press, 1977.

Gowing, L. The logic of organized sensations. In W. Rubin (Ed.), *Cézanne: The late work.* New York: Museum of Modern Art, 1977, 55–73.

Grant, E. Cosmology. In D. C. Lindberg (Ed.), *Science in the Middle Ages.* Chicago: University of Chicago Press, 1978.

Graziosi, P. *Paleolithic art.* New York: McGraw-Hill, 1960.

Gregory, R. L. *Eye and brain; the psychology of seeing.* New York: McGraw-Hill, 1966.

Grünbaum, A. *Philosophical problems of space and time.* New York: Knopf, 1963.

Guttman, S. A. Psychoanalysis and science: The concept of structure. *Annual of Psychoanalysis,* 1973, *1,* 73–81.

Hagan, M. A. A new theory of the psychology of representational art. In C. F. Nodine & D. F. Fisher (Eds.), *Perception and pictorial representation.* New York: Praeger, 1979.

Haith, M. M. Response of the human newborn to visual movement. *Journal of Experimental Child Psychology*, 1966, *3*, 235–243.

Hall, A. R. *Scientific revolution: 1500–1800*. New York: Becon, 1966 (1954).

Hamilton, G. H. *Manet and his critics*. New Haven, Ct.: Yale University Press, 1954.

Hamilton, G. H. Cézanne, Bergson and the image of time. *College Art Journal*, 1956, *19*, 2–12.

Hansen, R. This curving world: Hyperbolic linear perspective. *Journal of Aesthetics and Art Criticism*, 1973, *32*, 147–161.

Hansen, R. A rejoinder to John Ward. *The Art Bulletin*, 1977, *59*, 464–465.

Hartmann, H., Kris, E., & Loewenstein, R. Comments on the formation of psychic structure. *Psychoanalytic Study of the Child*, 1946, *2*, 11–38.

Hartt, F. Art and freedom in the Quattrocentro Florence. In L. F. Sandler (Ed.), *Essays in memory of Karl Lehman*. New York: New York Univ. Press, 1964.

Hartt, F. *History of Italian Renaissance art: Painting, sculpture, architecture*. New York: Abrams, 1969.

Haskins, C. H. *The Renaissance of the twelfth century*. Cambridge, Mass.: Harvard University Press, 1927.

Hauser, A. *The philosophy of art history*. New York: Knopf, 1959 (1953).

Hauser, A. *The social history of art* (S. Godman & A. Hauser, Trans.) (4 vols.). New York: Vintage Books, 1960 (1951).

Hauser, A. *Mannerism; the crisis of the Renaissance and the origin of modern art* (2 vols). London: Routledge & Kegan Paul, 1965.

Havelock, E. A. *Preface to Plato*. Cambridge, Mass.: Belknap Press of Harvard University Press, 1963.

Haynes, D. *Greek art and the idea of freedom*. London: Thames and Hudson, 1981.

Head, H. *Studies in neurology* (2 vols.). London: Frowde, Hodder & Stoughton, Ltd., 1920.

Hebb, D. O. *The organization of behavior; a neuropsychological theory*. New York: Wiley, 1949.

Heelan, P. A. Toward a new analysis of the pictorial space of Vincent Van Gogh. *The Art Bulletin*, 1972, *54*, 478–492.

Held, J. S., & Posner, D. *Seventeenth and eighteenth century art: Baroque painting, sculpture, architecture*. New York: Abrams, 1971.

Held, R. Object and effigy. In G. Kepes (Ed.), *Structure in art and in science*. New York: Braziller, 1965.

Henderson, L. D. *The artist, "The fourth dimension," and non-Euclidean geometry. 1900–1930: A romance of many dimensions*. Unpublished doctoral dissertation, Yale University, 1975.

Herbert, R. L. *Modern artists on art:* Ten unabridged essays. Englewood Cliffs, New Jersey: Prentice-Hall, 1964.

Hertz, R. Cited in R. Needham, *Right and left: Essays on dual symbolic classification*. Chicago: University of Chicago Press, 1973 (1909).

Hildebrand, A. von. *The problem of form in painting and sculpture* (M. Meyer & R. M. Ogden, Trans. and rev.). New York: G. E. Stechert & Co., 1907 (1893).

Hillier, J. R. *Japanese masters of the colour print; a great heritage of oriental art.* London: Phaidon, 1954.

Hochberg, J. E. Effects of the Gestalt revolution: The Cornell symposium on perception. In D. C. Beardslee & M. Wertheimer (Eds.), *Readings in perception.* Princeton, N.J.: Van Nostrand, 1965 (1958).

Hochberg, J. E. The representation of things and people. In E. H. Gombrich, J. Hochberg, & M. Black, *Art, perception and reality.* Baltimore: Johns Hopkins University Press, 1972.

Holländer, H. *Early medieval* art (C. Hiller, Trans.). New York: Universe Books, 1924.

Home, H. J. The concept of mind. *International Journal of Psycho-analysis,* 1966, *47*, 42–49.

Hoorn, W. Van. *As images unwind.* Amsterdam: University Press, 1972.

Hubel, D. H., & Wiesel, T. N. Receptive fields of single neurones in the cat's striate cortex. *Journal of Physiology,* 1959, *148*, 574–591.

Huyghe, R. Shifts in thought during the Impressionist Era: Painting, science, literature, history and philosophy. In *Impressionism: A centenary exhibition.* Paris: Imprimerie moderne du Lion, 1974, 14–33.

Inhelder, B., & Piaget, J. *The growth of logical thinking from childhood to adolescence; an essay on the construction of formal operational structures.* (A. Parsons & S. Milgram, trans.). New York: Basic Books, 1958 (1955).

Inhelder, B. & Piaget, J. *The early growth of logic in the child: Classification and seriation.* New York: Harper & Row, 1964 (1959).

Inhelder, B., Sinclair, H., & Bovet, M. *Learning and the development of cognition.* Cambridge, Mass.: Harvard University Press, 1974.

Ittelson, W. H. *Visual space perception.* New York: Springer, 1960.

Ives, C. F. *The great wave: The influence of Japanese woodcuts on French prints.* New York: Metropolitan Museum of Art, 1974.

Ivins, W. M. *On the rationalization of sight.* New York: DaCapo, 1973 (1938).

Ivins, W. M. *Art and geometry; a study in space intuitions.* Cambridge, Mass.: Harvard University Press, 1946.

Jacobson, E. *The self and the object world.* New York: International Universities Press, 1964.

Jaeger, W. W. *Paideia: The ideals of Greek culture* (Vol. 1) (G. Highet, Trans.). New York: Oxford University Press, 1937.

Jaffé, H. L. C. *The world of the impressionists.* Maplewood, N.J.: Hammond, Inc., 1969.

Jakobson, R. Linguistics and poetics. In T. A. Sebeok (Ed.), *Style in language.* Cambridge, Mass.: MIT Press, 1960.

Jammer, M. *Concepts of space: The history of theories of space in physics.* Cambridge, Mass.: Harvard University Press, 1969 (1954).

Janson, H. W. Introduction to R. Bernheimer, *The nature of representation: A phenomenological inquiry.* New York: New York Univ. Press, 1961.

Janson, H. W. *The History of Art* (Revised Ed.) New York: Abrams, 1969.

Kagan, J. *Change and continuity in infancy.* New York: Wiley, 1971.

Kahnweiler, D. H. *The rise of cubism* (H. Aronson, Trans.). New York: Wittenborn, Schultz, 1949.

Kandinsky, W. *Concerning the spirituality in art* (1911). New York: Dover, 1977.

Kant, I. *Critique of pure reason* (Transl. N. K. Smith). London (1871). Macmillan & Co., 1929.

Kaplan, B. The study of language in psychiatry. In S. Arieti (Ed.), *American Handbook of Psychiatry* (1st ed., Vol. *3*). New York: Basic Books, 1966.

Karmel, B. Z. Complexity, amounts of contour, and visually dependent behavior in hooded rats, domestic chicks, and human infants. *Journal of Comparative and Physiological Psychology*, 1969, *69*, 649–657.

Karmel, B. Z., Hoffman, R. F., & Fegy, M. J. Processing contour information by human infants evidenced by pattern-dependent evoked potentials. *Child Development*, 1974, *45*, 39–48.

Kennedy, J. M. *A psychology of picture perception*. San Francisco: Jossey-Bass, 1974.

Kitto, H. D. F. *The Greeks*. Baltimore: Penguin Books, Inc., 1951.

Klein, W. *Vom Antiken Rokoko*. Vienna: Holzel, 1921.

Kleinbauer, W. E. *Modern perspective in western art history; an anthology of 20th-century writings on the visual arts*. New York: Holt, Rinehart, & Winston, 1971.

Koffka, K. *Principles of Gestalt Psychology*. New York: Harcourt Brace Jovanovich, 1935.

Köhler, W. *Gestalt Psychology*. New York: Liveright, 1947.

Kohut, H. Introspection, empathy, and psychoanalysis. *Journal of the American Psychoanalytic Association*, 1959, *7*, 459–483.

Koyré, A. *From the closed world to the infinite universe*. Baltimore: Johns Hopkins University Press, 1957.

Krautheimer, R., & Krautheimer-Hess, T. *Lorenzo Ghiberti*. Princeton, N.J.: Princeton University Press, 1970.

Kris, E. *Psychoanalytic explorations in art*. New York: International Universities Press, 1952.

Kris, E., & Kurz, O. *Legend, myth & magic in the image of the artist: an historical experiment*. New Haven, Ct.: Yale University Press, 1979 (1934).

Kristeller, P. O., & Randall, J. H. General introduction. In E. Cassirer, P. O. Kristeller, & J. H. Randall (Eds.), *The Renaissance philosophy of man*. Chicago: University of Chicago Press, 1948.

Kubler, G. *The shape of time; remarks on the history of things*. New Haven, Ct.: Yale University Press, 1962.

Kuffler, S. W. Neurons in the retina: Organization, inhibition, and excitation problems. *Cold Spring Harbor Symposium in Quantitative Biology*, 1952, *17*, 281–292.

Kuhn, T. *The Copernican revolution: Planetary astronomy in the development of Western thought*. New York: Vintage, 1962 (1957).

Kuhn, T. *The structure of scientific revolutions*. (2nd ed., enl.). Chicago: The University of Chicago Press, 1970 (1962).

Lacan, J. *The language of the self; the function of language in psychoanalysis* (A. Wilden, Trans.). Baltimore: Johns Hopkins Press, 1968.

Lacan, J. *Ecrits: A selection* (A. Sheridan, Trans.). New York: Norton, 1977.

Lane, M. *Introduction to structuralism* (M. Lane, Ed.). New York: Basic Books, 1970.

Lane, R. D. *Masters of the Japanese print, their world and their work.* Garden City, N.Y.: Doubleday, 1962.

Laporte, P. M. Cubism and science. *Journal of Aesthetics and Art Criticism,* 1949, *7,* 243–256.

Laporte, P. M. Cubism and relativity. *The Art Journal,* 1966, *25,* 246–248.

Laurendeau, M., & Pinard, A. *Causal thinking in the child; a genetic and experimental approach.* New York: International Universities Press, 1962.

Laurendeau, M., & Pinard, A. *The development of the concept of space in the child.* New York: International Universities Press, 1970.

Leroi-Gourhan, A. *Treasures of prehistoric art* (N. Guterman, Trans.). New York: Abrams, 1967.

Levi-Strauss, C. *Structural anthropology* (C. Jacobson & B. G. Schoepf, Trans.). New York: Basic Books, 1963.

Levy, G. R. The Greek discovery of perspective: Its influence on Renaissance and modern art. *Journal of the Royal Institute of British Architects,* 1943, 51–57.

Levy, G. R. *The gate of horn: The study of the religious conceptions of the stone age and their influence upon European thought.* London: Faber & Faber, 1948.

Levy, G. R. *Religious conceptions of the stone age and their influence upon European thought.* New York: Harper & Row, 1963.

Lindberg, D. C. The science of optics. In D. C. Lindberg (Ed.), *Science in the middle ages.* Chicago: University of Chicago Press, 1978.

Lissitzky-Küppers, S. *El Lissitzky: Life, letters, texts* (1925) (Transl., H. Aldwinckle and M. Whittall) Greenwich, Conn.: New York Graphic Society, 1968.

Loewald, H. W. Perspectives on memory in psychology versus metapsychology: Psychoanalytic essays in memory of George Klein. *Psychological Issues,* 1976, *9*(4), 298–325.

Loewy, E. *The rendering of nature in early Greek art* (J. Fothergill, trans.). London: Duckworth & Co., 1907 (1900).

Lohman, A. *Some relationships of self-object differentiation to empathic responsiveness and self esteem.* Unpublished doctoral dissertation, University of Michigan, 1969.

Lovejoy, A. O. *The great chain of being.* Cambridge, Mass.: Harvard University Press, 1964 (1936).

Luneberg, R. K. *Mathematical analysis of binocular vision.* Hanover, N.H.: The Dartmouth Eye Institute, 1947.

Luneberg, R. K. Metric studies in binocular visual space. *Journal of the Optical Society of America,* 1950, *11,* 627.

Mach, E. *Erkenntnis und Irrtum. Skizzen zur Psychogie der Forschung.* Leipzig: Barth, 1905.

Mahler, M. S. *On human symbiosis and the vicissitudes of individuation.* New York: International Universities Press, 1968.

Mahler, M. S., Pine, F., & Bergman, A. *The psychological birth of the human infant: Symbiosis and individuation.* New York: Basic Books, 1975.

Malevich, K. *The non–objective world.* (H. Dearstyne, Trans.). Chicago:

P. Theobald, 1959 (1927).

Malraux, A. *The voices of silence* (S. Gilbert, Trans.). Garden City, N.Y.: Doubleday, 1954.

Malraux, A. *Notes to an exhibition of the works of Yaacov Agam.* New York: Marlborough-Gerson Gallery, May, 1966.

Manetti, G. The dignity and excellence of man. (1452) In E. Cassirer et al. (Eds.), *Renaissance philosophy of man.* Chicago: University of Chicago Press, 1948.

Mauss, M. *The gift, forms and functions of exchange in archaic societies* (I. Cunnison, trans.). Glencoe, Ill.: Free Press, 1954 (1950).

Meiss, M. *Painting in Florence and Siena after the Black Death.* Princeton, N.J.: Princeton University Press, 1951.

Miljkovitch, M. Development of the representation of space in normal children: The drawing of a village. Paper presented at a meeting of Society for Personality Assessment, Phoenix, Arizona, March 1979.

Miller, G. A., Galanter, E., & Pribram, K. H. *Plans and the structure of behavior.* New York: Holt, Rinehart, & Winston, 1960.

Miller, M. (Ed.) *Paul Klee.* New York: Museum of Modern Art, 1946.

Minkowski, H. Space and time (1908) In the *Principle of relativity* (A. Sommerfeld, Ed). (Transl. W. Perrett & G. B. Jeffery) New York: Dodd, Mead & Co., 1923.

Modell, A. *Object love and reality: An introduction to a psychoanalytic theory of object relations.* New York: International Universities Press, Inc., 1968.

Mondrian, P. *Plastic art and pure plastic art (1937), and other essays, 1941–1943.* New York: Wittenborn, Schultz, 1951.

Monnier, G. The late watercolors. In W. Rubin (Ed.), *Cézanne: The late work.* New York: Museum of Modern Art, 1977.

Moore, W. E. *Social change* (2nd ed.). Englewood Cliffs, N.J.: Prentice-Hall, 1974 (1963).

Museum of Modern Art. *Notes to Exhibit: Cézanne: The late work.* New York: Museum of Modern Art, 1977.

Muybridge, E. *Complete human and animal locomotion* (1887). New York: Dover, 1979.

Needham, R. (Ed.). *Right and left; essays on dual symbolic classification.* Chicago: University of Chicago Press, 1973.

Newell, A., & Simon, H. A. *Human problem solving.* Englewood Cliffs, N.J.: Prentice-Hall, 1972.

Newton, I. *Mathematical principles of natural philosophy.* Berkeley, Calif.: Univ. of California Press, 1966 (1687).

Noble, J. V. *The techniques of painted attic pottery.* New York: Watson-Guptill, 1965.

Novotny, F. *Cézanne.* Vienna: Phaidon Press, 1937.

Olson, D. *Cognitive development; the child's acquisition of diagonality.* New York: Academic Press, 1970.

Olson, D. On the relations between spatial and linguistic processes. In J. Eliot & N. J. Salkind (Eds.), *Children's spatial development.* Springfield, Ill.: Thomas, 1975.

Ortega y Gasset, J. The dehumanization of art. In A. Brown (trans.), *Velaz-*

quez, Goya, and the dehumanization of art. New York: Norton, 1972 (1925).

Osgood, C. *Method and theory in experimental psychology.* New York: Oxford University Press, 1953.

Overton, W. General systems, structure and development. In K. F. Riegel & G. C. Rosenwald (Eds.), *Structure and transformation.* New York: Wiley, 1975.

Panofsky, E. Die perspektive als "symbolische form." *Vorträge der Bibliothek Warburg,* 1924/25, 258–330. Leipzig and Berlin, 1927.

Panofsky, E. *Albrecht Durer.* Princeton, N.J.: Princeton University Press, 1943.

Panofsky, E. *Early Netherlandish painting.* Cambridge, Mass.: Harvard Univ. Press, 1953.

Panofsky, E. The history of the theory of human proportions as a reflection of the history of styles. In *Meaning in the visual arts; papers in and on art history.* New York: Doubleday, 1955a.

Panofsky, E. Art as a humanistic discipline. In *Meaning in the visual arts; papers in and on art history.* New York: Doubleday, 1955b.

Panofsky, E. *The Codex Huygens and Leonardo da Vinci's art theory.* Westport, Ct.: Greenwood Press, 1971 (1940).

Panofsky, E. *Renaissance and renascences in western art.* New York: Harper & Row, 1972 (1960).

Parsons, T. & Bales, R. F. *Family; socialization and interaction process.* Glencoe, Ill.: Free Press, 1955.

Paul, I. H. Studies in remembering the reproduction of connected and extended verbal material. *Psychological Issues,* 1959, *1*(2).

Peckham, M. *Man's rage for chaos.* Philadelphia: Chilton Books, 1965.

Pepper, S. C. *World hypotheses; a study in evidence* Berkeley: University of California Press, 1961 (1942).

Perry, W. G. Forms of intellectual and ethical development in the college years: A scheme. New York: Holt, Rinehart, & Winston, 1970 (1968).

Pevsner, N. The architecture of mannerism. In H. Spencer (Ed.), *Readings in art history,* 1969, 119–148.

Piaget, J. *The child's conception of physical reality.* (M. Gabain, Trans.). New York: Harcourt Brace, 1930 (1927).

Piaget, J. *The psychology of intelligence* (M. Piercy & D. E. Berlyne, Trans.). London: Routledge & Kegan Paul, 1950.

Piaget, J. *The construction of reality in the child.* (M. Cook, Trans.). New York: Basic Books, Inc., 1954 (1937).

Piaget, J. *The origins of intelligence in children.* New York: International Universities Press, 1956.

Piaget, J. *Judgement and reasoning in the child.* (M. Warden, Trans.). London: Routledge & Kegan Paul, 1962(a) (1928).

Piaget, J. *Play, dreams and imitation in childhood.* (C. Gattegno & F. M. Hodgson, Trans.). New York: Norton, 1962(b) (1945).

Piaget, J. *The language and thought of the child.* (M. Warden, Trans.). New York: Harcourt Brace, 1963 (1926).

Piaget, J. *The child's conception of the world.* (J. & A. Tomlinson, Trans.). London: Routledge & Kegan Paul, 1965 (1929).

Piaget, J. *Six psychological studies* (D. Elkind, Ed., A. Tenzer, Trans.). New York: Vintage Books, 1968.

Piaget, J. *The child's conception of time.* (A. J. Pomerans, Trans.). New York: Basic Books, 1969(a) (1927).

Piaget, J. *The mechanisms of perception.* (G. N. Seagrim, Trans.). New York: Basic Books, 1969(b) (1961).

Piaget, J. Introduction. In M. Laurendeau and A. Pinard (Eds.), *The development of the concept of space in the child.* New York: International Universities Press, 1970a.

Piaget, J. *Structuralism* (C. Maschler, Ed. and Trans.). New York: Basic Books, 1970b.

Piaget, J. *Genetic epistemology* (E. Duckworth, Trans.). New York: Norton, 1971.

Piaget, J. *Understanding causality* (with the collaboration of R. Garcia) (D. & M. Miles, Trans.). New York: Norton, 1974.

Piaget, J. *The development of thought: Equilibration of cognitive structures* (A. Rosin, Trans.). New York: Viking Press, 1977.

Piaget, J., & Inhelder, B. *The child's conception of space.* (F. J. Langdon & J. L. Lunzer, Trans.). New York: Norton, 1967 (1948).

Piaget, J., & Inhelder, B. *The psychology of the child* (H. Weaver. Trans.). New York: Basic Books, 1969.

Piaget, J., & Inhelder, B. *Mental imagery in the child; a study of the development of imaginal representation.* (P. A. Chilton, Trans.). New York: Basic Books, 1971 (1966).

Piaget, J., Inhelder, B., & Szeminska, A. *The child's conception of geometry.* London: Routledge & Kegan Paul, 1960.

Pico della Mirandola, G. Oration on the dignity of man. (1486) (E. L. Forbes, Trans.). In E. Cassirer et al. (Eds.), *Renaissance philosophy of man.* Chicago: University of Chicago Press, 1948.

Pirenne, M. H. The scientific basis of Leonardo da Vinci's theory of perspective. *British Journal for the Philosophy of Science,* 1952–1953, *3*, 169–185.

Pirenne, M. H. Review of "Perspectiva Artificialis; per la storia della prospettiva; spigolature e appunti" by D. Gioseffi. *The Art Bulletin,* 1959, *41*, 213–217.

Pirenne, M. H. *Optics, painting and photography.* Cambridge: Cambridge University Press, 1970.

Pliny, The Elder. *Natural history* (H. Rachman, Trans.). 1938.

Pollitt, J. J. *The art of Greece, 1400–31 B.C.: Sources and documents.* Englewood Cliffs, N.J.: Prentice-Hall, 1965.

Pollitt, J. J. *Art and experience in classical Greece.* Cambridge: Cambridge University Press, 1972.

Pollitt, J. J. *The ancient view of Greek art: Criticism, history and terminology.* New Haven: Yale University Press, 1974.

Popper, K. *The poverty of historicism.* Boston: Beacon Press, 1957.

Popper, K. *The logic of scientific discovery.* New York: Basic Books, 1959.

Praz, M. *Mnemosyne: The parallel between literature and the visual arts.* Princeton, N.J.: Princeton University Press, 1970.

Quinones, R. *The Renaissance discovery of time.* Cambridge, Mass.: Harvard University Press, 1972.

Rapaport, D. On the psychoanalytic theory of thinking. In R. P. Knight & C. R. Friedman (Eds.), *Psychoanalytic psychiatry and psychology.* New York: International Univ. Press, 1950.

Rapaport, D., & Gill, M. The points of view and assumptions of metapsychology. *International Journal of Psychoanalysis,* 1959, *40,* 153–162.

Read, H. E. *The philosophy of modern art.* London: Faber & Faber, 1952.

Reff, T. Painting and theory in the final decade. In *Cézanne: The late work.* New York: Museum of Modern Art, 1977.

Reichenbach, H. *Philosophy of space and time.* New York: Dover, 1957 (1928).

Richter, G. M. Perspective, Ancient, Mediaeval and Renaissance. In *Scritti in Onore di Bartolomea Nogara raccolti in occasione del suo LXX anno.* Rome: Città del Vaticano, 1937.

Richter, G. M. *Perspective in Greek and Roman Art.* New York and London: Phaidon, 1970.

Richter, J. P. (Ed.). *The literary works of Leonardo da Vinci.* Oxford: Oxford University Press, 1939.

Riegl, A. *Spätrömische Kunstindustrie.* Wien: Osterreichischte Staatsdruckerei, 1927 (1901).

Riemann, B. Über die hypothesen welche du geometrie zu grunde liegen (H. Weyl, Ed.). Berlin: 1923. In A. Grünbaum, *Philosophical problems of space and time.* New York: Knopf, 1963.

Rochlin, G. *Griefs and discontents; the forces of change.* Boston: Little, Brown, 1965.

Rosenberg, H. *The anxious object; art today and its audience.* New York: Horizon Press, 1964.

Rosenberg, H. *Art on the edge: Creators and situations.* New York: Macmillan, 1975.

Rosenberg, J., Slive, S., & Kuile, E. H. ter. *Dutch art and architecture: 1600–1800.* England: Penguin Books, 1972 (1966).

Rosenblum, R. *Transformations in late eighteenth century art.* Princeton, N.J.: Princeton University Press, 1974.

Rosenwald, G. C. Epilogue: Reflections on the universalism of structure. In K. F. Riegel & G. C. Rosenwald (Eds.), *Structure and transformation.* New York: Wiley, 1975.

Roth, D., & Blatt, S. J. Spatial representations and psychopathology. *Journal of the American Psychoanalytic Association,* 1974, *22,* 854–872.

Rubin, W. *Cézanne: The late work.* New York: Museum of Modern Art, 1977.

Ruskin, J. *Modern painters, by a graduate of Oxford* (New ed., 5 vols.). New York: Lovell, 1873.

Salapatek, P., & Kessen, W. Visual scanning of triangles by the human newborn. *Journal of Experimental Child Psychology,* 1966, *3,* 155–167.

Saussure, F. de. *Course in general linguistics* (C. Bally & A. Sechehaye, Eds.; W. Baskin, Trans.). New York: Philosophical Library, 1959.

Schaefer-Simmern, H. *The unfolding of artistic activity, its basis, processes, and implications.* Berkeley: University of California Press, 1948.

Schäfer, H. *Principles of Egyptian art.* (J. Baines, Ed. and trans.). Oxford: Clarendon Press, 1974 (1919).

Schafer, R. Generative empathy in the treatment situation. *Psychoanalytic Quarterly,* 1959, *28,* 347–373.

Schafer, R. *Aspects of internalization.* New York: International Universities Press, 1968.

Schapiro, M. Matisse and impressionism. *Androcles,* 1932, *1,* 21–36.

Schapiro, M. Nature of abstract art. *Marxist Quarterly,* 1937, *1,* 77–98.

Schapiro, M. *Vincent Van Gogh.* New York: Abrams, 1950.

Schapiro, M. Style. In A. L. Kroeber (Ed.), *Anthropology today.* Chicago: University of Chicago Press, 1953; and reprinted in M. Philipson (Ed.), *Aesthetics today.* Cleveland: World Pub. Co., 1961.

Schapiro, M. *Cézanne.* New York: Abrams, 1962.

Scribner, S. Developmental aspects of categorical recall in a West Africa society. *Cognitive Psychology,* 1974, *6,* 475–494.

Segull, R. A., Campbell, D. T., & Herskovitz, M. J. Cultural differences in the perception of geometric illusions. *Science,* 1963, *139,* 769–771.

Seltman, C. Art and society, *The Studio,* 1953, 98–114.

Shearman, J. K. *Mannerism.* Harmondworth, Eng.: Penguin, 1967.

Sieveking, A. *The cave artists.* London: Thames & Hudson, 1979.

Simson, O. G. von *Sacred fortress: Byzantine art and statecraft in Ravenna.* Chicago: University of Chicago Press, 1948.

Smyth, C. H. *Mannerism and maniera.* Locust Valley, N.Y.: J. J. Augustin, 1962.

Sontag, S. *Against interpretation.* New York: Farrar, Straux & Giroux, 1961.

Stern, H. P. *Master prints of Japan: Ukiyo-e Hanga.* New York: Abrams, 1969.

Stevens, S. S. Mathematics, measurement, and psychophysics. In S. Stevens (Ed.), *Handbook of experimental psychology.* New York: Wiley, 1951.

Stratton, R. Preface to Kandinsky, W., *Concerning the spirituality in art.* New York: Dover (1911), 1977.

Sypher, F. W. *Four stages of Renaissance art: Transformations in art and literature, 1400–1700.* Garden City, N.Y.: Doubleday, 1955.

Sypher, F. W. *Rococo to Cubism in art and literature.* New York: Vintage, 1960.

Toulmin, S. *The philosophy of science.* London: Hutchinson University Library, 1953.

Toulmin, S. *Human understanding.* Princeton, N.J.: Princeton University Press, 1972.

Trinkaus, C. E. *In our image and likeness; humanity and divinity in Italian humanist thought.* Chicago: University of Chicago Press, 1970.

Tynianov, J., & Jakobson, R. Problems in the study of language and literature (1928). In R. de George & F. de George (Eds.), *The structuralists from Marx to Levi-Strauss.* Garden City, N.Y.: Anchor Books, 1972.

Vasari, G. *Lives of the artists.* (G. Bull, trans.). London: Penguin Books, 1965 (1550).

Veltman, K. *On Erwin Panofsky and perspective.* Atti, Milan Conference, 1979. (a).

Veltman, K. Personal communication, 1979(b).

Venturi, L. *History of art criticism* (C. Marriot, Trans.). New York: E. P. Dutton & Co., Inc., 1936.

Venturi, L. *Modern painters: Volume II, impressionists and symbolists* (F. Steegmuller, Trans.). New York: Scribner, 1950.

Venturi, L. *From Leonardo to El Greco.* New York: World, 1956.

Viator, J. (Pelerin). De artificiali perspectiva (1505). In W. M. Ivins (Ed.), *On the rationalization of sight.* New York: Da Capo, 1973.

Vignola, G. B. *La due regole della prospettiva practica.* Rome, 1611.

Vitruvius. *The ten books on architecture.* (M. H. Morgan, Trans.). Cambridge, Mass.: Harvard University Press, 1914 (25–23 B.C.).

Vygotsky, L. S. *Thought and language* (E. Hanfman & G. Vaker, Eds. and Trans.). Cambridge, Mass.: MIT Press, 1962.

Wapner, S., & Werner, H. *Perceptual development; an investigation within the framework of sensory-tonic field theory.* Worcester, Mass.: Clark University Press, 1957.

Ward, J. L. A reexamination of Van Gogh's pictorial space. *Art Bulletin,* 1976, *58,* 593–604.

Watson, W. H. *On understanding physics.* Cambridge: Cambridge University Press, 1938.

Weber M. *The protestant ethic and the spirit of capitalism* (T. Parsons, Trans.). New York: Scribner, 1958.

Weisberg, G., Cate, P. D., Needham, G., Eidelberg, M., & Johnston, W. R. *Japonisme: Japanese influence on French art, 1854–1910.* Cleveland: Cleveland Museum of Art, 1975.

Weitz, M. Genre and style. In *Perspectives in education, religion and the arts,* (Vol. 3). *Contemporary Philosophic Thought.* Albany, N.Y.: State University of New York Press, 1970.

Weitzmann, K. (Ed.). *Age of spirituality: late Antiquity and early Christian art, third to seventh century. Catalogue of the exhibition of late antique and early Christian art,* Metropolitan Museum of Art, 1977–1978. Princeton, N.J.: Princeton Univ. Press, 1979.

Weitzmann, K., Chatzidakis, M., Miatev, K., & Radojčić, S. *A treasury of icons—sixth to seventeenth centuries.* New York: Abrams, 1966.

Welliver, N. Personal communication, 1978.

Werner, H. *Comparative psychology of mental development.* New York: International Universities Press, 1948.

Werner, H. The concept of development from a comparative and organismic point of view. In D. B. Harris (Ed.), *The concept of development: An issue in the study of human behavior.* Minneapolis: University of Minnesota Press, 1957.

Werner, H., & Kaplan, B. The developmental approach to cognition; its relevance to the psychological interpretation of anthropological and ethnolinguistic data. *American Anthropologist,* 1956, *58,* 866–880.

Werner, H., & Kaplan, B. *Symbol formation: An organismic-developmental approach to the language and the expression of thought.* New York: Wiley, 1963.

Wertheimer, M. *Productive thinking.* New York: Harper, 1945.

Wheelock, A. K. *Perspective, optics and Delft artists around 1650.* New York: Garland, 1977.

White, J. *Perspective in ancient drawing and painting.* London: Society for the Promotion of Hellenic Studies, 1956.

White, J. *The birth and rebirth of pictorial space.* New York: Harper & Row, 1972 (1967).

Whyte, L. L. Introduction. In L. L. Whyte (Ed.), *Aspects of form—A symposium on form in nature and art.* London: Humphries, 1951.

Whyte, L. L. Atomism, structure and form. In G. Kepes (Ed.), *Structure in art and in science.* New York: Braziller, 1965.

Wilcox, M. M. Visual preferences of human infants for representations of the human face. *Journal of Experimental Child Psychology,* 1969, *9,* 10–20.

Wilson, J. A. *The culture of ancient Egypt.* Chicago: University of Chicago Press, 1956 (1951).

Winckelmann, J. J. *The history of ancient art.* (4 vols.) (G. H. Lodge, Trans.). Boston: J. R. Osgood & Co., 1872–1879 (1764).

Witkin, H. A. Psychological differentiation and forms of pathology. *Journal of Abnormal Psychology,* 1965, *70,* 317–336.

Wittkower, R. Brunelleschi and proportion in perspective. *Journal of the Warburg and Courtland Institutes,* 1953, *16,* 275–291.

Wolff, P. H. Cognitive considerations for a psychoanalytic theory of language acquisition. In R. R. Holt (Ed.), *Motives and thought. Psychological Issues,* 1967, *18/19,* 300–343.

Wölfflin, H. *The art of the Italian Renaissance; a handbook for students and travellers.* (W. Armstrong, Trans.). New York and London: Putnam's Sons, 1928 (1898).

Wölfflin, H. *Principles of art history: The problem of the development of style in later art.* (M. D. Hottinger, Trans.). New York: Dover, 1932 (1915).

Wölfflin, H. *Renaissance and Baroque* (K. Simon, Trans.). London: Collins, 1964 (1888).

Woodbridge, F. J. E. *Aristotle's vision of nature.* New York: Columbia University Press, 1965.

Worringer, W. *Abstraction and empathy: A contribution to the psychology of style.* (Transl., M. Bullock), London: Meridian, 1953 (1907).

Author Index

Numbers in *italics* indicate pages with bibliographic information.

Subject Index

observer in, 199–200
shading and color, 238
space, 197
Apotropic function of art, 101
Apulia, 136
Apulian Greek vases, 153
Archaic period, 12, 125, 129, 131, 138,
    142, 143, 338, 345
Architectural sculpture, 177–178
Architectural settings, 185, 186, 206
Architecture, 175
    Renaissance, 201, 202
Aristotle, 10–11, 48, 142, 190, 279
    concept of space, 276, 281, 287, 288
    De Caelo, 276
    Physics, 276
    world view, 16, 37, 190, 191–194, 195,
        282
Aristotle with a Bust of Homer (artwork),
    262
Aristotelian structure (thought), 251,
    252, 280
    rejection of, 277, 278, 279
Art, 3, 41, 363; *see also* Function of art
    creative process in, 25
    defined by cultural norm, 11, 16, 48,
        54
    dehumanization in, 346, 347
    form is essence of, 2, 21
    historical context of, 4, 362
    parallels with science, 2, 6
        Impressionism, 302–303
        post-Renaissance, 357–363
        pre-Renaissance, 190–96
        Renaissance and Baroque, 275–289
    as part of science, 225
    transformable, 355, 357
Articulation, 2, 38, 44, 45
Artist(s), 14, 15, 16, 18, 19–20, 54–55,
    188
    anonymous, 172
    identity, biography of, 139, 172, 199,
        256
    early, 26–27, 30
    interaction with prevailing style, 25–26
    potential freedom from naturalistic
        representation, 330
    role of, in construction of reality, 336
    role of, in Cubism, 326
    signed works, 139, 182, 199, 256
Asch, Solomon, 85

Aspective (pre-perspective) art, 99, 106,
    115–117, 119–120, 158, 159
Astronomy, 193–194, 279–280, 283, 285
Asymmetry, 265
    Baroque art, 266–267, 268, 270, 273
Atmospheric factors, 268
    Impressionism, 291, 292, 298
Atmospheric (aerial) perspective, 219–
    221, 238–239, 257, 265
Atomism(ists), 194, 195, 277 and n*21*
Autonomy in art, 338, 345
    struggle for, in Impressionism, 299–
        300, 318
Axis, vanishing, 153, 163, 209, 210

B
Background
    Cubism, 324
    Middle Ages art, 184
    Renaissance art, 203
    Romanesque art, 177
Bacon, Roger, 184
Balla, Giacomo, 349
Bar at the Folies Bergère, A (artwork), 265,
    303
Baroque (the), 9–10, 236, 237, 238, 241,
    252, 253, 256–275, 300, 302, 303,
    358
    bridge to Impressionism, 321
    contributions of, 290–291
    parallel development of art and sci-
        ence in, 275–289
    representational theory, 338
Baseline(s), 105, 116, 123, 132, 160
Bathers, The (artwork), 309
Battle of Greeks and Amazons, The (krater),
    132–133
Bedroom at Arles (artwork), 307, 308
Bennett, Arnold
    Clayhanger Family, The, 335
Bergson, Henri, 302
Bernard, Émile 309, 313, 316
Bernini, Gianlorenzo, 258n*20*
Beyen, H. G., 149
Binary opposition, 41–42, 192
Black Death, 11
Black-figure technique, 129, 130
Blake, William, 291
Boccioni, Umberto, 349
Bochner, Mel, 342–343

reflected in art, 4–5
revisions in, 11, 46–48
transmission of, within culture, 49–50, 51
Collage, 329
Color, 29, 31, 52, 158, 218, 305
  as autonomous value, 317–318
  Baroque art, 261–262, 264, 268, 274, 290
  Cubism, 322, 325, 327, 328, 329–330
  Fauvist Liberation of, 339
  Greco-Roman art, 134–136, 139, 147
  Impressionist and Post-impressionist art, 275, 291, 292, 295, 298, 301, 309, 312, 316–318, 358–359
  integration of shading with, 256–260
  Mannerist art, 256
  modeling of, 241
  perspective of, 238
  Renaissance/Baroque contrasted, 257
Color modulation, 316–318, 321
Color relativism (principle), 346
Complexity, 2, 7, 20, 41
Composition, 10, 36, 55
  asymmetrical, 237, 265, 273
  Baroque art, 267–268, 270, 273
  Cubist art, 327
  diagonal, 281, 290
  Lack of, in ancient art, 100
  Egyptian art, 105
  Middle Ages art, 171, 178, 185
  Modern Art, 342–343
  pre-perspective, 193
  Renaissance art, 188, 303
  Renaissance/Baroque contrasted, 257
  unified, integrated, 185, 188, 210, 225, 231, 237, 275
Conception
  shift to, from perception, 336, 340, 342, 345
Concepts
  abstract, 343
  general, 60
  simple to complex and abstract progression, 17–18
Conceptual representation (mode) 33, 34, 326–327
Conceptual theory, 6, 35–36, 59
  Cubism based on, 326–327, 332–334
  Modern Art, 338
Concrete operations (stage), 42, 45, 56,

57, 62, 63, 67–69, 71, 74, 75, 87, 88, 281, 283, 357
  Baroque art, 270–272, 274, 275
  decentration in, 85
  Impressionist art, 300
  Mannerist art, 253
  Middle Ages art, 172, 189
  modes of representation in, 241
  relinquished in Abstract Art, 345
  Renaissance art, 235–236, 238
  schemata in, 38
  shift to conceptual level, 318
  shift to formal operations, 275, 276, 281–282, 338, 362
Concrete representation (mode), 33, 34, 52, 101, 241, 326
Consciousness, 1: *see also* Self-consciousness; Self-reflective awareness
  collective, 51
  discovery of, 284
Conservation, 62–63, 67, 68, 69, 86, 237, 276
  basis and capacity for, 301
  of distance, 88, 89, 90
  in Euclidean space, 89, 90
  impersonal, interpersonal, 86
  of straight lines, distances, angles, 75
Consolidation
  mass and surface, 185, 189
  projective concepts of space, 253
Constable, John, 268, 291–292, 321
Constantinople, 169, 171
Contemporary art, 23; *see also* Modern Art
Content of art, 28, 36, 55, 285
  Baroque, 274
  classical, 173
  cultural, 357
  form liberated from, 38
  lack of, in Abstract Art, 346
  Mannerist art, 245
  Middle Ages art, 167, 172, 177 (*see also* Religious art)
  Modern Art, 341
  shifts in, 140
Continuity, 48, 70, 72, 73, 74, 75, 88, 354
Continuity principle, 92
Contour, 56, 71, 72, 73, 237–238, 240
  ancient art, 100, 101, 102, 111, 123, 124
  Post-impressionist art, 315

signifier in, 62
Separation, 70, 71, 72, 73, 74 and n8, 75, 88
Serra, Richard, 342
Seurat, Georges, 291, 303–305, 309, 312
Sextus Empiricus, 142
Sfumato, 221, 238, 239–240, 241
Shading, 52, 221
  Baroque art, 257
  Greco-Roman art, 134–136, 145–147
  Impressionism, 291
  integration of, with color, 259–260
  Mannerist art, 255, 256
  Renaissance art, 238, 239
Shadow painting *(skiagraphia)*, 134
Shadows, 29, 121, 221
  Greco-Roman art, 124, 139, 142
Shape(s), 31
Signified, 62
Signifier, 61, 62
Signorelli, Luca, 202
Simple to complex progression, 28, 30–31
  ancient art, 100
Single reference point, *see also* self and vanishing point, 153–154, 157, 208, 284, 285, 286, 288, 307, 321, 323, 333
Size, 31
  ancient art, 106
  conservation of, 89
  of objects at a distance, 145
  theories re, 153n17
  varying with distance from observer, 142
Size/distance relationship, 154–155, 200–201, 210, 216, 239
  Greco-Roman art, 157
  inverse, 155
Skenographia (scene painting), 143, 152
  defined, 153n17
Social behavior
  egocentrism and, 85–86
Social change
  ancient Egypt, 113–115
  Middle Ages, 159, 160, 164
Social context
  and cultural change, 11
Social order (organization), 3, 19, 40, 252
  impact on art, 104, 182
  Middle Ages, 182, 183–184

relation of cognitive structures to change in, 5n1
structure in, 42
Solar system, 275, 278, 279, 280, 285
Solutions (of artistic problems), 12, 18, 19, 20, 21
Space, 41, 43, 44, 56, 57, 60, 62, 70–98
  absolute, 92, 285–287, 335, 336, 347, 360–361
  ancient art, 100, 104, 117, 118, 121–123, 124
  ancient theories of, 156
  Aristotelian concept of, 276, 281, 287, 288
  Baroque art, 263–264, 265–268, 270, 272–273
  change in conceptualization of, 6–7, 52–55
  Cubism, 323, 324, 325–326, 334, 335
  in cosmology and science, 190
  development of concepts of, 21, 22, 94–97T, 98, 283, 287–288
  Egyptian art, 105, 109
  Euclidean, 56, 57, 70, 71, 72, 74, 75, 78n9, 83, 88–92, 93, 194, 195
  forms of, 1–55
  geometry of, 214, 360
  Greco-Roman art, 133–134, 138, 141–142, 157–158, 210
  homogeneous, isotropic, infinite, 1, 45, 89–90, 91, 156, 163, 188, 189, 197, 201, 206, 214, 217n19, 232, 272, 273, 275–276, 280–281, 282, 286, 287, 288, 301
  identical to matter, 285
  Impressionist and Post-impressionist, 293, 314–316, 359
  as infinite, 265–269, 270, 280–281
  integration of spectator's with picture, 265
  linear, 31, 233
  Mannerist art, 243, 244, 245, 247, 248–250, 252–253
  mathematization of, 282, 284–285
  Middle Ages art, 160–161, 164, 165, 172, 173, 175, 178, 181, 185, 189
  Modern Art, 361
  parallel development in modes of representation in art and science, 6
  perspective views of, 236
  Post-impressionism, 305–308